The Jossey-Bass Health Care Series brings together the most current information and ideas in health care fom the leaders in the field. Titles from the Jossey-Bass Health Series include these essential resources:

At Risk in America: The Health and Health Care Needs of Vulnerable Populations in the United States, Second Edition, Lu Ann Aday

Changing the U.S. Health Care System: Key Issues in Health Services Policy and Management, Second Edition, Ronald M. Andersen, Thomas H. Rice, Gerald F. Kominski, Editors

Critical Issues in Global Health, C. Everett Koop, Clarence E. Pearson, M. Roy Schwarz, Editors

Health Behavior and Health Education: Theory, Research, and Practice, Karen Glanz, Frances Marcus Lewis, Barbara K. Rimer, Editors

Health Care 2010: The Forecast, The Challenge, Institute for the Future

Health Care in the New Millennium: Vision, Values, and Leadership, Ian Morrison

Immigrant Women's Health: Problems and Solutions, Elizabeth J. Kramer, Susan L. Ivey, Yu-Wen Ying, Editors

Oxymorons: The Myth of a U.S. Health Care System, J.D. Kleinke

The Twenty-First Century Health Care Leader, Roderick W. Gilkey, Editor, and The Center for Healthcare Leadership, Emory University School of Medicine

To Improve Health and Health Care: The Robert Wood Johnson Foundation Anthology, Stephen L. Isaacs, James R. Knickman, Editors

DESIGNING AND CONDUCTING COST-EFFECTIVENESS ANALYSES IN MEDICINE AND HEALTH CARE

DESIGNING AND CONDUCTING COST-EFFECTIVENESS ANALYSES IN MEDICINE AND HEALTH CARE

Peter Muennig, M.D., M.P.H.

Contributing Editor
Kamran Khan, M.D., M.P.H.

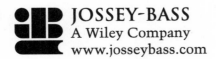

JOSSEY-BASS
A Wiley Company
www.josseybass.com

Published by

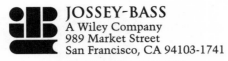

JOSSEY-BASS
A Wiley Company
989 Market Street
San Francisco, CA 94103-1741

www.josseybass.com

Jossey-Bass books and products are available through most bookstores. To contact Jossey-Bass directly, call (888) 378-2537, fax to (800) 605-2665, or visit our website at www.josseybass.com.

Substantial discounts on bulk quantities of Jossey-Bass books are available to corporations, professional associations, and other organizations. For details and discount information, contact the special sales department at Jossey-Bass.

We at Jossey-Bass strive to use the most environmentally sensitive paper stocks available to us. Our publications are printed on acid-free recycled stock whenever possible, and our paper always meets or exceeds minimum GPO and EPA requirements.

Library of Congress Cataloging-in-Publication Data
Muenning, Peter.
   Designing and conducting cost-effectiveness analyses in medicine and health care / Peter Muenning ; contributing editor, Kamran Khan.
        p. cm.
Includes bibliographical references and index.
   ISBN 0-7879-6013-6
   1. Medical care—United States—Cost effectiveness.   2. Medical care, Cost of—United States.   I. Khan, Kamran.   II. Title.
   RA410.5 .M84 2002
338.4'33621—dc21   2002016112

FIRST EDITION
HB Printing   10 9 8 7 6 5 4 3 2 1

CONTENTS

ACKNOWLEDGMENTS

I would like to thank Marthe Gold, Kim Toscano, Sonali Rana, Clyde Schecter, Marianne Fahs, and all of my students for their contributions. Special thanks go to Celina Su whose combination of economic and grammatical expertise made the book possible.

LIST OF TABLES, FIGURES, AND EXHIBITS

Tables

Figures

Exhibits

PREFACE

Though it is one of the fastest growing fields in health research, cost-effectiveness analysis has lacked an instruction manual until now. While other books address only the theoretical aspects of cost-effectiveness analysis, *Designing and Conducting Cost-Effectiveness Analyses in Medicine and Health Care* teaches students how to perform cost-effectiveness research. The art of cost-effectiveness analysis is explored by walking students through a research question in which they learn how to find and evaluate data, build a simple decision analysis model, test the model, and present the results in a research paper. Students learn how to obtain data from governmental Web sites using automated tools, and they will learn how to get the information they need quickly without having to use a statistical software package.

Designing and Conducting Cost-Effectiveness Analyses in Medicine and Health Care uses teaching techniques akin to the natural learning or immersion approach to language in which students learn by speaking rather than studying grammar. Problems are anticipated and solved in context, making the theory much easier to appreciate and learn. The book can also be read in an alternative sequence that presents cost-effectiveness theory without a practical component.

Designing and Conducting Cost-Effectiveness Analyses in Medicine and Health Care will provide students of cost-effectiveness with a basic set of economic, epidemiologic, and biostatistical tools. It is designed to be accessible to anyone with a good health vocabulary and the ability to read and critically evaluate the medical literature. Public health students, medical students, health economists, biomedical researchers, physicians, policymakers, and health managers should all find the book to be informative and fun. Because cost-effectiveness analysis is being used to evaluate medical interventions worldwide, this book includes approaches and examples that are applicable to both industrialized and developing countries. It teaches students how to evaluate interventions specific to infectious disease (a common type of analysis in developing countries) as well as chronic disease (a common type of analysis in developed countries). It also addresses issues specific to evaluating the cost-effectiveness of public health programs as well as problems specific to clinical medicine.

Designing and Conducting Cost-Effectiveness Analyses in Medicine and Health Care is written using a concise, structured format and has been tested in university cost-effectiveness courses. The first two chapters introduce the basic principles of cost-effectiveness analysis and teach students how to develop a research question and design their analysis. The third chapter reviews those methods in epidemiology and biostatistics that are needed to conduct a cost-effectiveness analysis. The remainder of the book is interactive; as concepts are introduced, students apply what they have just learned as they construct a cost-effectiveness analysis. By the end of the book, students will have completed a cost-effectiveness analysis that examines strategies for the prevention or treatment of influenza virus infections in healthy adults.

To use this book as a practical tool, students will need a computer and a connection to the Internet. Web addresses to free spreadsheet software and decision analysis software are provided. This book is also available as an e-book that will automatically link students to relevant on-line information, such as databases and other sources of information.

How to Use This Book

In addition to introducing the core concepts of cost-effectiveness analysis, *Designing and Conducting Cost-Effectiveness Analyses in Medicine and Health Care* walks students through a basic cost-effectiveness analysis that examines strategies to prevent or treat influenza virus infections. To fully benefit from this book, students should complete the exercises in each chapter; these exercises guide students through the process of obtaining electronic data, analyzing the medical literature, building a decision analysis tree, and conducting a sensitivity analysis.

Using this book for theoretical study alone. Health managers and clinicians often wish to understand cost-effectiveness analysis methods but do not wish to conduct research. While the book has been designed to allow students to understand the field of cost-effectiveness analysis using an applied approach, theory and practice have been separated for students who only wish to understand the theoretical framework of cost-effectiveness. Students wishing to learn cost-effectiveness theory or instructors using a theory-based course curricula may wish to read the book in the following order: Chapters One, Two, and Six through Nine, skipping all exercises. A theory-based approach to learning the discipline is recommended for universities on the quarter system that do not have epidemiology and biostatistics as prerequisites.

Using this book as a textbook. Instructors teaching courses that have biostatistics and epidemiology as prerequisites may skip Chapter Three without any loss in continuity; however, this chapter provides an excellent review of those concepts applicable to cost-effectiveness research. While introductory courses in cost-effectiveness analysis should skip Chapter Twelve, individuals interested in conducting cost-effectiveness research will find this chapter invaluable. Researchers wishing to conduct cost-effectiveness analysis outside of the United States may skip Chapter Four.

All of the journal articles needed for the applied analysis have been summarized in Appendix II of this book. While we cannot reproduce the articles in their entirety here, Internet links to those articles that are not subject to copyright protection are provided throughout the book. It is helpful to provide the articles summarized in Appendix II in their entirety to students.

Using Internet resources. This book provides links to data sources, journals, and other useful cost-effectiveness resources on the Internet. While the Internet has become a critical resource for cost-effectiveness research, the addresses for Web pages sometimes change. For this reason, links to specific Web pages are provided alongside links to the organizations that host these pages. When an organization changes the address of a particular page, it will occasionally be necessary to search for it from the organization's homepage. Links to the data sources mentioned in this book will be periodically updated at http://www.pceo.org/datasources.html.

A Note on Methods

In 1996, the U.S. Public Health Service's Panel on Cost-Effectiveness in Health and Medicine released methodological standards for conducting cost-effectiveness analyses. These standards were developed in response to a wide degree of variation in the ways in which such analyses were conducted. The use of disparate approaches to cost-effectiveness analysis sometimes leads to widely different study results when different research groups examine the cost-effectiveness of a single screening test or medical treatment. For example, in the introduction to its book, the Panel on Cost-Effectiveness in Health and Medicine note that the published cost-effectiveness of screening mammography for the detection of breast cancer varies from cost-savings to $80,000 (Gold and others, 1996).

To address problems with variation in the methods used from one study to the next, the Panel on Cost-Effectiveness in Health and Medicine developed a "reference case analysis." The reference case analysis renders studies more comparable, easier to understand, and more useful to a broader array of consumers of cost-effectiveness data. Though the reference case standards were designed by the United States Public Health Service, the methods are applicable to cost-effectiveness analyses conducted in any country.

Designing and Conducting Cost-Effectiveness Analyses in Medicine and Health Care adheres closely to the principles forwarded by this panel and was developed with the input of some of its members. As the Panel on Cost-Effectiveness in Health and Medicine acknowledges, a reference case analysis is not a "requirement for performing a valid cost-effectiveness analysis." The government or an insurance company may be interested in commissioning a study to answer a question that cannot be addressed within the framework of a reference case analysis. Nonetheless, because it was designed to apply to a broad array of professionals interested in the results of a cost-effectiveness analysis, the reference case analysis is comprehensive enough to provide students with all of the tools necessary to conduct any cost-effectiveness analyses. By building this book around the recommendations of the Panel on Cost-Effectiveness in Health and Medicine, we believe that this book will help students become leaders in the growing field of cost-effectiveness research.

New York, New York   Peter Muennig
November 2001

CHAPTER ONE

INTRODUCTION TO COST-EFFECTIVENESS

What Is Cost-Effectiveness Analysis?

Imagine that you are happily employed as the director of a large cancer society. Your day-to-day duties require you to conduct some research and to oversee employees who make health recommendations. One day you arise bright and early to go for a jog and, after a relaxing shower, you sit down to a cup of coffee and toast. You pick up the morning paper to find that one of your society's recommendations, that women between the ages of forty and sixty receive screening mammography for breast cancer, has made the headline news. You read that an elderly rights group is suing your society. This group argues that your recommendation unfairly discriminates against the elderly because you have implied that women over the age of sixty should not be screened for breast cancer.

You rush into the office to find that the teams that previously made the recommendation are already in a heated meeting. They have split into two factions and each group is now accusing the other of making bad decisions. But did they? You manage to calm everyone down and review the process they used to arrive at their recommendation. You learn that both groups were concerned that recommending mammograms for women over a wider age range might become very costly, thereby jeopardizing screening for women who might benefit from screening mammography the most.

One group argued that it made sense to screen older rather than younger women, because mammography works better in older women who have less dense breast tissue. Older women, they reasoned, were less likely to have a falsely positive mammogram and therefore would be less likely to suffer unnecessary procedures or surgery. Unnecessary interventions, they noted, not only place women at risk for potential complications but are also psychologically traumatic, costly, and may do more harm than good.

The other group argued that it was unwise to actively screen all elderly women with mammography, because many of these women would ultimately die from conditions other than breast cancer. Therefore, they reasoned, elderly women would be subjected to an uncomfortable and expensive screening test that would have little impact on the length of their lives.

Both factions had made arguments based on sound scientific, economic, and social research, but which group was right? You and your employees decide to conduct a more extensive analysis of the costs and benefits of breast cancer screening and plan to send out a press release to this effect. You now have the job of helping your society's policymakers decide how to resolve their internal conflict and develop more concrete conclusions. But where do you start?

You might start by having a team estimate the likelihood that older women will die of breast cancer if they are not screened and have another team estimate the number of women that are likely to have false positive mammograms at different ages. You might also wish to obtain information on the number of years of life mammography will save, the quality of life for women who have different stages of breast cancer, and the psychological impact of false positive test results. Because both teams were concerned about the costs of mammography, you may also wish to calculate the cost of screening women and the cost of all of the medical care that might be averted by detecting breast cancer at an early stage. Finally, because each team is interested in knowing whether women in both age groups might benefit from mammography, you decide that the costs and health benefits of screening each group should be compared to not screening women at all. If all of the above factors were put together in a systematic manner, you would have conducted a cost-effectiveness analysis.

Elements of Cost-Effectiveness Analysis

Screening mammography is an example of a **health intervention** (also known as a **health strategy**). A health intervention is a treatment, screening test, or a primary prevention technique (for example, vaccinating children to prevent measles). Health interventions are designed to reduce the incidence rate of disease, improve the quality of life of the people receiving them, and/or improve the life expectancy of people receiving them. Health strategies can take the form of medical screening tests, pharmaceutical treatments, surgical procedures, preventive recommendations, public health interventions, or even hospital policy changes.

One way of examining the way that a health intervention has an effect on the health of a person is to classify her according to her general state of health, or **"health state,"** and examine how the strategy changes the health state. Examples of health states include pain or the inability to walk. A health state can change naturally over time or can be improved by applying a health intervention (see Figure 1.1).

Health interventions also affect the amount of money that is spent on medical care. If the intervention prevents disease or improves the person's health state, less money will be spent on providing medical care for that person in the future. Finally, health interventions may reduce mortality associated with a disease. In Figure 1.1, a person with asthma (health state 1) is administered intravenous steroids in the emergency room (health intervention) and subsequently experiences an improvement in breathing (health state 2). That person may also be less likely to be hospitalized and may be less likely to die from the acute asthma attack.

Cost-effectiveness analysis is a research method designed to help determine which health interventions provide the most effective medical care affordable. In a cost-effectiveness analysis, a researcher gathers information from various sources on the ways in which a health intervention changes the health states of a group of people. This information is then combined with information on the ways in which the health intervention changes life expectancy and the cost of disease in society (see Figure 1.2).

FIGURE 1.1.   EXAMPLE OF THE EFFECT OF A HEALTH INTERVENTION ON THE HEALTH STATES OF A PATIENT ADMITTED TO THE EMERGENCY ROOM FOR AN ACUTE ASTHMA ATTACK.

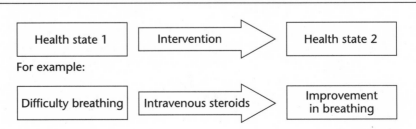

FIGURE 1.2.   DESIGN OF A TYPICAL COST-EFFECTIVENESS ANALYSIS.

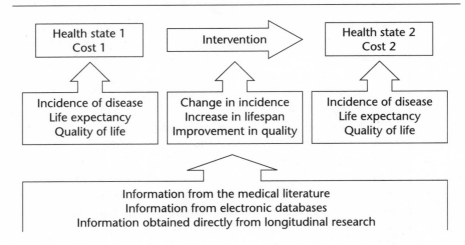

Why Conduct Cost-Effectiveness Analysis?

There are a number of ways to prevent or treat most diseases. For instance, breast cancer can be detected by self-examination, examination by a medical practitioner, screening mammography, ultrasound, or MRI. It is also possible to compare different levels of intensity of a single health intervention. For example, screening mammography might be performed every six months, every year, or every two years. Each of these **competing alternatives** is associated with a different effectiveness and a different cost. Analyses that compare two or more competing alternatives for preventing or treating a disease tell consumers how much "bang for their buck they are getting" for each strategy.

Many students of cost-effectiveness analysis in economically developed nations question the logic of choosing interventions based on both cost and effectiveness criteria rather than effectiveness alone. After all, it is argued, shouldn't we purchase the best treatments regardless of their costs? To answer this question, we must first ask what effectiveness is and then examine this concept within the framework of both industrialized and developing economies.

The importance of effectiveness. The test that detects the most cases of disease, the treatment that has the highest probability of curing or reducing the severity of a disease, or the public health intervention most likely to prevent a disease is each often thought of as the most "effective" option for managing disease. However, screening tests and treatments are sometimes associated with hidden dangers. As we saw in the example of screening mammography, a false-positive mammogram can lead to unnecessary surgery and psychological stress, and treatments can have debilitating or fatal side effects.

Public health interventions can also have negative effects. While supplementing cereal grains with the vitamin folate may greatly reduce neural tube defects in newborns, it may also lead to the under-diagnosis of vitamin B_{12} deficiency among poor or elderly populations (Haddix and others, 1996). When vitamin B_{12} deficiency is not diagnosed and treated early, it too can lead to severe neurological complications. By thoroughly examining the risks and benefits of various interventions, information on an intervention's effectiveness provides more meaningful information about various ways to treat or prevent a disease than efficacy data alone. While **efficacy** is a measure of the ability of a treatment to reduce the duration or severity of a disease, or the ability of a test to detect disease in a clinical setting, **effectiveness** is a measure of the overall risks and benefits of a health intervention in the real world.

The importance of cost-containment in industrialized nations. Given good information on the risks and benefits of a particular health intervention, should we base medical decisions on effectiveness criteria alone? In 1997, health expenditures consumed approximately 1.1 trillion dollars or 13.5 percent of the United States gross domestic product, up from about 27 billion dollars and 5.1 percent of the gross domestic product in 1960 (Kramarow and others, 1999). Even when expenditures on private health insurance are *not* counted, the United States government spends more per capita on health care than the majority of nations that provide universal health care. As McGinnis points out in the introduction to *Cost-Effectiveness in Health and Medicine,* 99 percent of these expenditures go toward the diagnosis and treatment of disease, though perhaps 85 to 90 percent of the gains in life expectancy realized in industrialized nations have come from social or public health interventions (Gold and others, 1996). The United States, which spends less of its per capita gross domestic product on social and public health interventions than any other industrialized nation, ranks twenty-fifth in the world in terms of infant mortality (Adema and others, 1996; Kramarow and others, 1999). These statistics raise serious questions about whether the United States is spending its social resources appropriately.

Depending on the country, the cost of medical care in industrialized nations is mostly borne either by insurance companies or by the government. When the price of an insurance policy increases, some people will be unable to afford health insurance. Ultimately, some of those unable to afford health insurance might then suffer or die from other illnesses as a result of the price increase. When medical costs are paid for by the government, budgets are usually fixed, so any additional expenditures will either restrict the number of people covered or the number of services provided (or both). If we know how to minimize expenditures and maximize health, more people can be covered, and more medical services can be provided.

The importance of cost-containment in developing nations. In developing nations, where government health budgets may be as low as $5 per person, the need for cost-effectiveness analysis is even more evident (McNeil, 1998). The treatment of AIDS patients with the most efficacious medications is associated with a cost exceeding $10,000 per person per year—more than the entire budget of most local health agencies in Africa (Attaran and Sachs, 2001; McNeil, 1998).

There are many examples of cost-effective strategies for reducing the incidence rate of AIDS. For example, if other sexually transmitted diseases are aggressively treated, the risk of transmitting HIV may be reduced by ridding people of genital lesions. Another relatively inexpensive and effective way of reducing the incidence of HIV is to administer anti-retroviral medications to HIV-positive mothers before a baby is delivered. This reduces the risk of transmission from mother to child. Each of these strategies has proven to be both effective and affordable in developing countries (Marseille and others, 1998).

The cost of a treatment itself can be a critical determinant of who gets treated and who does not. For example, some countries have declared AIDS a national emergency and have sought to purchase medicines that were manufactured in violation of international patent laws (Petersen, 2001). These actions, coupled with public outcry and pressure from the scientists that participated in the development of the medications, motivated pharmaceutical companies to lower the price of AIDS medicines in developing nations. This has made these drugs more affordable to some people in these countries. Whether information on the cost of an intervention is used to determine which interventions are affordable or is used to advocate for changes in the price of treatment, this information can be a major determinant of how many lives can be saved with the available medical technologies.

Using cost-effectiveness analysis to define opportunity costs. While the most effective way to detect cancer in the general population may be to conduct monthly MRI scans on everyone in society, this intervention might bankrupt most countries, leaving no money to build roads and schools, let alone to treat other medical conditions. No one would take cancer detection to this extreme simply because it is obvious that society does not have the resources to perform such an extensive intervention.

Every time society uses scarce resources in one way, it gives up the opportunity to use them in another way. In the case of an MRI machine, steel, circuits, and technical expertise are required to manufacture the equipment. Moreover, trained health professionals are required to operate the machine. All of these resources could be put to other uses in society. The value of all of these goods and services in their best alternative use is the **opportunity cost** of providing MRI scans for the general population.

Because cost-effectiveness analysis demonstrates how different approaches to treating or preventing a disease stack up in terms of both cost (resource consumption) and effectiveness (health benefits), it helps policymakers understand the opportunity cost of different interventions (Gold and others, 1996).

Scope and Aims of Cost-Effectiveness Analysis

Cost-effectiveness analyses can take many subtly different forms. Consider the case of a local health department that wishes to know the cost of screening people for tuberculosis in its clinics. It may examine the cost per case of active tuberculosis prevented when patients are screened in its clinics (relative to not providing these screening exams). This type of analysis would furnish the health department with information useful for making internal decisions, such as whether it is worthwhile to expand such programs.

On the other hand, the health department may wish to expand the analysis in order to obtain information on both the cost-effectiveness of its operations and on its broader mission of improving the longevity of the population it serves. For instance, it may wish to determine the cost of the program per year of life saved as well as the cost per case prevented.

Finally, tuberculosis is a severe disease that can require burdensome treatments, long stints in hospitals (sometimes in an isolated room) and can have an impact on people's quality of life. The health department may therefore also wish to examine the cost of tuberculosis screening relative to improvements in the quality of life of the population it serves.

While some health events, such as high-rise construction accidents, predominantly affect the quantity of life, others, such as repetitive stress injuries at work, predominantly affect the quality of life. When a measure of quality of life is added to a cost-effectiveness analysis, it becomes possible to compare health interventions that primarily affect the quality of life with those that primarily affect the quantity of life. Therefore, by incorporating an assessment of the quality of life of people with tuberculosis, the health department would also potentially be able to compare tuberculosis screening with the different programs it offers, such as those aimed at injury prevention.

Quality of life and the reference case scenario. When the Panel on Cost-Effectiveness in Health and Medicine published recommendations for standardizing cost-effectiveness analysis, it recommended that all analyses adhering to the **reference**

case scenario (a set of standardized practices for conducting a cost-effectiveness analysis, see "A Note on Methods") incorporate a quality of life measure (Gold and others, 1996). It argues that by incorporating quality into an analysis, more meaningful comparisons can be made within a single study and, potentially, across different studies.

In the tuberculosis example above, we saw that considering the quality of life improves comparisons made between two different medical conditions. Let us examine how quality considerations might improve comparisons made within a single study. A person undergoing chemotherapy and radiation therapy for breast cancer might be less able to do the things she enjoys than a person undergoing radiation therapy only. Thus, while the chemotherapy may prolong a person's life, it may also adversely affect the person's overall quality of life. If these two strategies are to be accurately compared, differences in quality of life must be compared along with changes in life expectancy. Quality is said to improve the "specificity" of an intervention because it tells you more about the impact of different interventions on a person's overall state of health than comparisons of life expectancy alone.

The methods presented in this book closely adhere to the reference case scenario, and therefore provide instruction on measuring changes in both quality and quantity of life in an analysis. After completing this book, though, you will have acquired the tools needed to perform other types of analyses because the reference case analysis is much more comprehensive than other types of analyses. We will explore the more basic types of analyses at the end of this chapter.

Cost-Effectiveness Analysis and Policy

In the above section, we learned that cost-effectiveness analyses are primarily used to compare different strategies for preventing or treating a single disease (such as breast cancer). When they are conducted according to a standard set of methods, cost-effectiveness analyses can also theoretically be used to compare medical interventions designed to evaluate many different conditions (such as repetitive stress injury and high-rise construction accidents). In this section, we will briefly explore how policy decisions are sometimes made using cost-effectiveness analyses as well as some of the controversies that have arisen as a result of such policy decisions.

Making Comparisons Across Diseases

If the cost-effectiveness of everything that is done in medicine were known, it would be possible to purchase much more health than we currently do with the social resources available. When cost-effectiveness ratios for different interventions are listed in a table, it is sometimes called a **league table.**

However tempting it might be to create a list of interventions based on their cost-effectiveness, decisions surrounding the allocation of social resources cannot be made based on numbers alone. For example, it is not possible to incorporate information on whether an intervention is fair or otherwise ethical unless it is looked at in a broader social context (Gold and others, 1996). Consider the case of people that require heart and lung transplants. Although this procedure is extremely expensive and may not result in a full and healthy life, most people would probably agree that these transplants are worthwhile because they save lives. In the extreme, if preventive interventions were generally found to be more cost-effective than treatment in a cost-effectiveness league table, it would be tempting to recommend spending the majority of a nation's social resources on preventive interventions. While this might conceivably improve national statistics such as life expectancy and infant mortality, most people would not be willing to die of a treatable condition for the sake of the larger social objective of maximizing a nation's health.

Do Cost-Effectiveness Analyses Lead to Policy Changes?

Examples of policy decisions that have been influenced by cost-effectiveness analysis include strategies for reducing parasitic infections in immigrant populations (Muennig and others, 1999), conducting cervical cancer screening among low-income elderly women (Fahs and others, 1992), and adding folate to cereal grains in the United States (Haddix and others, 1996). These studies appear to have sparked changes in the way that patients received medical care in local health departments, changes in Medicare reimbursement policies, and changes in the rules set by the United States Department of Agriculture.

Cost-effectiveness analyses can also lead to policy changes with broader implications than the authors intended. For instance, when supplementing cereal grains was found to be a cost-effective strategy for preventing neural tube defects in the United States, cost-effectiveness analysis not only helped convince the food industry that it was worth the cost, but other countries also considered similar interventions (Schaller and Olson, 1996; Wynn and Wynn, 1998).

Cost-effectiveness analysis has also proven to be a controversial tool when used without taking the broader social implications of health interventions into account. For example, in the state of Oregon, cost-effectiveness analysis was used to prioritize health interventions paid for by the state government using a league table. Those interventions deemed unaffordable were simply not paid for, creating a large statewide and national outcry for policy reform (Oregon Office for Health Policy and Research, 2001).

Principles of Cost-Effectiveness Analysis

So far, you have learned what cost-effectiveness is and how it is used. In this section, we will introduce the framework of cost-effectiveness analysis. These points will be highlighted using different scenarios illustrating the use and application of cost-effectiveness theory and practice. Throughout this book, we will build on these principles by teaching students how to design and conduct a sample cost-effectiveness analysis that evaluates strategies for the prevention or treatment of influenza virus infections in healthy adults. Students may design and conduct the sample analysis or may learn cost-effectiveness theory by simply following along (see the "How to Use This Book" section at the beginning of the book).

The Perspective of a Cost-Effectiveness Analysis

Terry Jones, the chief executive officer of a large insurance company, has received hundreds of requests for contraceptive reimbursement from the company's enrollees. He is interested in improving the company's services for the enrollees, but he is concerned that the costs might be prohibitive. On the other hand, because the company must pay for pregnancies when they occur, reimbursing patients for contraceptives might reduce the company's expenditures on hospitalization costs. Mr. Jones realizes that if the company does not reimburse for the birth control pill, most of the company's clients that wish to protect themselves from pregnancy will purchase the contraceptives on their own. However, some people will have unwanted pregnancies because it was either too inconvenient or too expensive for them to purchase the contraceptives themselves. Because pregnancy occasionally results in medical complications or even death, the company's failure to pay for contraceptives could theoretically result in litigation as well. Therefore, Mr. Jones commissions an analysis examining the cost of providing contraceptives per pregnancy prevented when the insurance company pays for contraception versus a "no pay" policy.

Jo Jo Thompson is the commissioner of a local health department in Saratoga, Illinois. Commissioner Thompson receives a report indicating that the maternal mortality rate among low-income women in Saratoga has increased over the past year. He decides to conduct an analysis to examine whether providing contraceptives to low-income women who cannot otherwise afford them is cost-effective. Commissioner Thompson wishes to know whether his health department can afford the program and whether it will be effective at reducing maternal mortality.

Finally, Tina Johanas is a United States senator interested in enacting legislation mandating that all insurance companies pay for contraceptives. Senator

Johanas' primary interest is to improve the quality of life of her constituents, but she is also concerned about the overall impact of the proposed legislation on the health care system. Therefore, she commissions a cost-effectiveness analysis examining the cost per healthy year of life gained when insurance companies pay for contraception relative to the cost of the current policy of letting insurance companies decide whether to pay for contraceptives.

In the analysis conducted from the perspective of the insurance company headed by Mr. Jones, the relevant question is whether the company pays for all of the contraceptives or none of the contraceptives. Mr. Jones decides not to include any costs incurred by patients in the analysis because such costs do not appear on his company's budget. However, he would be interested in knowing whether paying for contraceptives might reduce the number of pregnancies or the number of complications resulting from pregnancies, because such costs account for a portion of his company's expenditures.

Likewise, Commissioner Thompson is interested in costs specific to the health department, and he wishes to include only medical services and goods that the health department will pay for. These costs might include the cost of medical services paid for by the health department and the cost of the contraceptive itself. Unlike Mr. Jones, Commissioner Thompson does not wish to include the costs associated with pregnancies that occur among privately insured women, but he may wish to include costs associated with women insured by Medicaid since Medicaid payments come out of the same state budget that funds the Saratoga Health Department.

Finally, Senator Johanas is worried about the overall costs of her legislation to everyone in society. She wishes to ensure that the interests of health departments, insurance companies, and regular citizens are met. Therefore, she wishes to include all costs relevant to enacting the legislation or failing to enact the legislation.

Moreover, Senator Johanas is worried about the overall health and well-being of her constituents rather than just the number of pregnancies prevented. Because unwanted pregnancy can cause emotional as well as physical harm, she wishes to ensure that the overall quality of life of women with unwanted pregnancies is accounted for in the analysis. As an insurance company executive, Terry Jones is less concerned about abstract measures of patient well-being because his primary concern is whether the company can afford the policy change. By examining the cost per pregnancy prevented, he will capture the outcome that is most relevant to the insurance company. Finally, Commissioner Thomas decides to undertake the cost-effectiveness analysis in response to rising maternal mortality rates and is primarily concerned with whether providing contraceptives to low-income women will lower these rates.

Therefore, the party interested in the study can have an influence on which costs are included in an analysis and which outcomes are most relevant. When a particular organization includes only costs and outcomes relevant to its needs, the analysis is said to have been conducted from that party's "perspective." For example, when the study applies only to a government agency, the study is said to assume a **governmental perspective** and when the study applies to society as a whole, it is said to assume a **societal perspective.** Table 1.1 illustrates the different types of costs that might be included in a study from the perspective of an insurance company, a government agency, or society as a whole.

In Table 1.1, each of these three entities is paying for the cost of the contraceptive, medical visits, and hospitalization. Because insurance companies do not have to compensate patients for their time or pay transportation costs, environmental costs, or education costs, these costs would not be included in a study that assumes the perspective of the insurance company. However, the government would be interested in some of these costs, because it will directly or indirectly have to pay them. For example, because the local government disproportionately hires low-income women, some of the women seeking contraception might be government employees and will take time off from work to receive medical care. Some patients will also be taking public transportation that is subsidized by the city or state government. Finally, most educational institutions are public, and the intervention might therefore have an impact on school-based teen pregnancy programs or change the rate of absenteeism.

From the societal perspective, all costs must be included because "society" refers to everyone that might be affected by the intervention. Thus costs relevant

TABLE 1.1.   THE COSTS THAT WOULD BE INCLUDED IN A COST-EFFECTIVENESS ANALYSIS ON PROVIDING FREE CONTRACEPTION IF THE ANALYSIS WERE CONDUCTED FROM AN INSURER, GOVERNMENTAL, OR SOCIETAL PERSPECTIVE.

Cost	Insurance	Government	Society
Contraceptive pill	All costs	All costs	All costs
Medical visit	All costs	All costs	All costs
Hospitalization	All costs	All costs	All costs
Patient time	No costs	Some costs	All costs
Transportation	No costs	Some costs	All costs
Environment	No costs	All costs	All costs
Education system	No costs	Some costs	All costs

to the government, employers, patients, insurance companies, anyone, or anything else should be included so long as they are likely to be large enough to make a difference in the analysis. Usually, the term "society" refers to everything within the borders of a country (Drummond and others, 1997).

Since different perspectives require including or excluding different costs, the only way to standardize cost-effectiveness analyses is to require that all cost-effectiveness analyses assume the same perspective. For this reason, among others, the reference case scenario of the Panel on Cost-Effectiveness in Health and Medicine requires that the societal perspective be adopted (Gold and others, 1996).

When all costs are included, it is a simple task to exclude some of the costs not of interest to one party or another. In the insurance company's case, it might conduct a reference case analysis and then calculate cost-effectiveness ratios from the company's perspective by excluding the non-relevant costs mentioned in Table 1.1. If the company were to publish the study in the medical literature (to attract attention to its good deeds), it could simply present the reference case results along with the results of interest to the company. For example, the cost of providing free contraception relative to requiring women (or their partners) to purchase contraceptive pills might be presented as $15,000 per year of perfect health gained from the societal perspective and $77,000 per pregnancy prevented from the insurer's perspective.

The Cost-Effectiveness Ratio

Ratios put medical information into perspective. For instance, the **incidence** of a disease (the total number of new cases of a disease in a population per unit of time) tells you little about the risk of developing that disease. If a physician knows that there are 152,000 new cases of breast cancer a year in the United States, she will not be able to provide much information to a woman worried about developing that disease. The **incidence rate,** however, will provide information on the chance that any one person will develop the disease. The incidence rate is defined as the number of new cases of a disease in a population per unit of time, divided by the population at risk for the disease over the same period. If the physician has knowledge of the incidence rate of breast cancer, 1.1 cases per 1,000 women a year, she will be able to inform a patient that only about 1 in 1,000 women get the disease each year. If the physician wants to provide the patient with more specific information, she could also inform the patient of the chances of developing breast cancer in her age group, as well as how this risk compares to other diseases.

The same principles are true in a cost-effectiveness analysis. For instance, if we know the overall cost of treating a disease in a population, we might have an understanding of the economic impact of that disease but not an inkling of whether the costs justify the gains we are getting from the treatment. Likewise, if we know how many extra years of life a treatment will give us, we might be left wondering whether it is affordable relative to other available treatments.

In a cost-effectiveness analysis, the cost of an intervention, the quality of life, and the number of years of life gained are combined into a single cost-effectiveness ratio. Just as we often compare the incidence rate of one disease to that of another to get an idea of which disease occurs more frequently, by comparing the cost-effectiveness ratio of one intervention to that of an alternative strategy, we can determine how many years of healthy life each strategy will purchase.

Consider the case of oseltamivir, a new medication that can be used to treat symptomatic infection with the influenza virus (Hayden and others, 1999; Treanor and others, 2000). Doctors know that this drug is effective at shortening both the duration and severity of influenza symptoms, but is it worthwhile to give this medication to everyone who comes into the office with flu-like symptoms? We know that it is extremely rare for otherwise young and healthy adults to die from infection with influenza virus, but we also know the infection can be quite serious among the elderly or those with chronic disease (Neuzil and others, 1999; Nichol and others, 1994). Because oseltamivir reduces the duration and severity of influenza virus infection, there is a chance that the medication could save a patient's life, although the benefits would be greatest to those at high risk (the elderly and people with chronic disease). So, if doctors prescribed this medication to everyone rather than to high risk patients only, a considerable amount of money might be spent treating healthy young adults who might not get a lot of benefit from it. Although providing oseltamivir to everyone with the symptoms of influenza would probably produce health benefits, it would also likely increase health care costs considerably.

That brings us to the cost-effectiveness ratio, which indicates how much it costs to save one year of healthy life relative to other interventions aimed at treating or preventing the same disease. A year of healthy life is referred to as a **quality-adjusted life year (QALY)** in most cost-effectiveness studies. (We will return to different ways in which healthy life is measured later in this chapter.) The cost-effectiveness ratio takes the following form:

$$\frac{(\text{cost of intervention} - \text{costs averted by intervention})}{\text{QALYs gained by intervention}}$$

Equation 1.1

The cost-effectiveness ratio in Equation 1.1 is referred to as the **average cost-effectiveness ratio.** This ratio tells you how much an intervention costs relative to the number of QALYs in the cohort, but it does not provide information on how the intervention compares to other strategies for preventing or treating the disease we are evaluating. Comparisons between interventions are made using a ratio called the **incremental cost-effectiveness ratio,** which we will return to after examining the numerator and denominator values of the average cost-effectiveness ratio.

The Numerator of the Cost-Effectiveness Ratio

The **cost of the intervention** is the cost associated with actually providing a treatment or preventive test. For example, if we consider the cost of oseltamivir, we would include the price of the medication, the cost of the medical visit required to receive the treatment, and the cost of any side effects from the treatment. Most health interventions have significant nonmedical costs as well (Gold and others, 1996). For example, the time a patient spends at the doctor's should be counted in the analysis (usually at the wage the patient receives from work). Moreover, the costs of transportation and caregiving can also be significant. Sometimes, a health intervention will also be associated with relevant environmental costs or education costs, and these should be included as intervention costs when they are large enough to make a difference (Gold and others, 1996).

The **costs averted by an intervention** include future health costs that are avoided by providing that intervention. For example, patients may be less likely to develop complications related to influenza virus infection if they are treated with oseltamivir (Treanor and others, 2000). These averted complications might include future visits to the doctor or even hospitalization. Patient time costs, transportation costs, or even environmental costs can also be significantly reduced by an intervention, and these should also be included as costs averted.

The Denominator of the Cost-Effectiveness Equation

Thus, the numerator of the cost-effectiveness ratio includes *almost* all of the costs and savings associated with a particular intervention. The only costs that are not included in the numerator of the cost-effectiveness ratio are those that are captured in the denominator, such as the number of quality-adjusted life years (QALYs) gained. Why would the number of healthy years lost be considered a cost? If a productive member of society dies or becomes significantly ill, society loses out on the value of his or her contributions. Moreover, a human life has intrinsic value and is, in and of itself, a social good. (See Exhibit 1.1 for another example of how life years lost are associated with social costs.)

Of course, it is not easy to place a dollar value on something as precious and intangible as human life or on the pain and suffering caused by illness. To get

EXHIBIT 1.1. DEATH AS AN ECONOMIC PROBLEM IN SUB-SAHARAN AFRICA.

In sub-Saharan Africa, the healthy life expectancy in some countries was under thirty years of age in 2000 (World Health Organization, 2000). Tuberculosis, AIDS, and malaria have all had a profound impact on the ability of these countries to prosper economically, and these diseases at least in part explain the low economic growth rate of many countries in this continent. Some corporations hire more than one person to fill a single job posting because it is expected that one of the applicants will die prematurely. This can double, triple, or quadruple the cost of doing business in these countries. Many companies in Africa are now refusing to pay for the funeral services of their employees or to provide paid leave for death in the family of employees because the costs of doing so are prohibitive (McNeil, 1998).

around these thorny issues, cost-effectiveness analyses simply separate QALYs from any cost calculations and present them (as an additional outcome) in the denominator of the cost-effectiveness ratio. Despite the fact that deaths are also associated with the loss of wages and other goods that can be readily measured, we do not include the economic impact of death in the numerator of the cost-effectiveness ratio because we are already counting it in the denominator. If we included these costs in both the numerator and the denominator, we would be *double counting* the effect of mortality (Gold and others, 1996).

By indicating the number of QALYs separately from the numerator costs, we allow consumers of cost-effectiveness data to judge the value of healthy human life for themselves (Gold and others, 1996). A consumer of the cost-effectiveness information can then see the cost of gaining one QALY when a health intervention is applied.

How is "perfect health" measured in the denominator? The number of QALYs gained by an intervention represents the number of years of *perfect health* that would be obtained by providing that intervention. You may then ask, what is the difference between a year of life gained and a healthy year of life gained?

To answer that question, one must consider the effects of disease on both *quantity* and *quality* of life separately. Consider an example. Medications that treat migraines predominantly exert their benefit through improving quality of life, while performing the Heimlich maneuver on a choking individual mostly improves length of life. Comparing these interventions on the basis of the cost per year of life saved places the Heimlich maneuver at an unfair advantage. By adding a dimension of the quality of life lived for persons receiving each intervention, we can then level the medical playing field.

To account for quality of life, we must add some measure of pain and suffering into our calculation. It is important to consider the quality of each year of life lived for a number of reasons. First, as mentioned previously, it allows us to compare interventions that have a large impact on quality of life, but a small impact on the length of life, with those that mostly have an impact on length of life. Second, it allows us to capture the state of "well-being" of people receiving interventions that can affect their ability to participate in leisure activities, pursue relationships with others, and live a healthy quality of life. Finally, as mentioned before, if we capture the impact of a disease on a person's quality of life in the denominator of a cost-effectiveness ratio, we do not have to place a monetary value on this intangible good in the numerator of the cost-effectiveness ratio.

The use of QALYs allows researchers to combine the effects of quantity of life (for example years of life gained by an intervention) with quality of life into a single measure. But how is something as subjective as "quality" measured, and how are measures of quantity and quality of life combined? In Chapter Eight, we will learn how "quality" is measured in cost-effectiveness analysis and we will then learn how QALYs are calculated in Chapter Nine. Before moving on, though, let us look at the QALY in a very basic way.

Consider the case of a woman who dies at age sixty from complications of diabetes mellitus because the disease was not detected early and treated. If it is not treated, diabetes mellitus can lead to numerous medical complications including infections, vascular disease requiring limb amputation, blindness, heart disease, and kidney disease. In hindsight, if the woman's condition were detected earlier, her life expectancy might have been seventy years. Because she died at age sixty from a condition that could potentially have been treated, she lost ten years of life.

Let us now consider the fact that treatment for diabetes does not always prevent complications of the disease. Usually, it just delays their onset. Thus, if the woman in our example had been appropriately diagnosed and treated, her last ten years of life probably would not have been lived in perfect health. How then do we measure the quality of her last years of life lived?

To answer this question, we need to obtain information on the **health-related quality of life (HRQL)** for people with diabetes. The HRQL (sometimes abbreviated as "HRQoL") refers to the effect of a disease on the way a person enjoys life, including the way illness affects a person's ability to live free of pain, to work productively, and to interact with loved ones. The **HRQL score** is a valuation of life lived in a particular health state, and it is the basic measure of "quality" used in a cost-effectiveness analysis. In other words, the HRQL score translates a person's perception of "quality" into a number.

For example, on a scale from zero to one, individuals who consider themselves to be in "perfect health" would rate their life as a one, while someone who would just as soon be dead might rate her life as a zero. Another person with a chronic

FIGURE 1.3.   GRAPHICAL REPRESENTATION OF THE HEALTH-RELATED QUALITY OF LIFE SCORE.

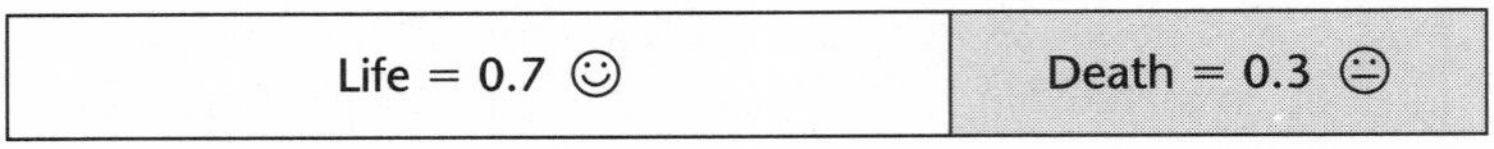

Life = 0.7 ☺	Death = 0.3 ☹

debilitating disease might rate her life as a 0.7, indicating that she values her life as only worth seven-tenths of a year of life lived in perfect health (see Figure 1.3).

The total number of QALYs in a health state is equal to the product HRQL score and the number of years lived in that health state. Therefore, one year lived with an HRQL of 0.6 is equal to $1 \cdot 0.6$ or 0.6 QALYs. Ten years lived with an HRQL of 0.6 is equal to $10 \cdot 0.6$ or 6 QALYs. In other words, while the QALY represents a year of perfect health, the HRQL score represents the *proportion* of a year that is lived in perfect health.

Suppose that, in our example of the woman with diabetes, we knew what the HRQL of the woman's life would have been each year over the last ten years of her life. Let us compare the HRQL of this woman's life over each of these ten years to the HRQL of another woman in perfect health over the same period of time (see Table 1.2).

The total number of years each woman would have lived is the same (10 years). However, when quality of life is considered, the woman with diabetes

TABLE 1.2.   HYPOTHETICAL DIFFERENCES IN HEALTH-RELATED QUALITY OF LIFE OVER A PERIOD OF TEN YEARS FOR A DIABETIC WOMAN AND A WOMAN IN PERFECT HEALTH.

Year	Diabetic woman	Healthy woman
1	0.8	1
2	0.8	1
3	0.7	1
4	0.8	1
5	0.6	1
6	0.6	1
7	0.5	1
8	0.6	1
9	0.4	1
10	0.4	1
Total score	6.2	10

would have "lived" just 6.2 QALYs while the woman in perfect health "lived" $1.0 \cdot 10$ years $= 10$ QALYs. Notice that when we tabulate QALYs on a year-to-year basis, the sum of the HRQL scores is equivalent to the number of QALYs lived over that period of time.

In Chapter Eight, we will see that the way an HRQL score is measured can bias the calculation of QALYs. Because there is no perfect way to measure a person's HRQL score, and because the HRQL can affect the way in which denominator "costs" are counted, it is important that HRQL scores are obtained and used in a consistent way. In fact, the use of something as subjective as an HRQL score affects the overall usefulness of reference case cost-effectiveness analyses (Gold and others, 1996). Still, the only way to compare different interventions across different diseases, to conduct relatively "specific" analyses, and to place a value on intangible "costs" such as the loss of health, is to include HRQL in the cost-effectiveness analysis.

Allocating Costs in the Cost-Effectiveness Ratio

So which costs are incorporated into the numerator and which costs into the denominator of the cost-effectiveness ratio? Costs associated with goods, such as medical care, diagnostic tests, or equipment, are always included in the numerator of cost-effectiveness analyses. These costs are sometimes referred to as **direct costs** because they are associated with the specific value of goods and services. Likewise, the time that a patient spends receiving an intervention (for example, the time spent in a doctor's office) and the cost of a caregiver's time are included in the numerator. These costs are sometimes referred to as **indirect costs.** While direct and indirect costs do not involve pain and suffering, the "costs" of emotional grief, pain, or suffering are captured in the HRQL score in the denominator of a cost-effectiveness analysis.

The costs associated with pain and suffering are sometimes referred to as **intangible costs** because of the difficulty in placing a specific dollar value on life or on subjective human experiences. In cost-effectiveness analysis, intangible costs related to pain and suffering (quality of life) are also often referred to as **morbidity costs,** while costs related to death are sometimes called **mortality costs.** Morbidity costs are captured in the HRQL score and mortality costs are captured as years of life lost to disease.

Tips and tricks. As a general rule, if a cost is associated with pain and suffering, it is included in the denominator of the cost-effectiveness ratio. If it is not associated with pain and suffering, it is included in the numerator of the cost-effectiveness ratio.

Some indirect costs, namely those associated with **lost productivity** and **leisure time,** are captured in the denominator because they involve a measure of pain and suffering. There are a couple of ways that an illness can affect productivity. First, illness can affect the quality and quantity of work a person performs, as well as a person's ability to enjoy his or her work. Second, the person can die from the illness. Because death and quality of life enter into the measurement of lost productivity, it is best captured in the denominator.

It is also difficult to measure the impact of illness on a person's leisure time (the time spent outside of work) since illness can affect both the quality and the quantity of leisure time a person has. To ensure that all of the accounting is done correctly, it is important to be certain that the HRQL score you use accurately captures the quality of life and incorporates the effects of illness on both people's productivity and on their leisure time (this will be discussed further in Chapter Eight).

The HRQL score, though, is only applied to those people who receive the interventions you are studying. While productivity and leisure time lost to a disease involve some aspect of pain and suffering on the part of the *patient* and should be included in the denominator, the lost productivity and leisure time of caregivers, co-workers, or others that are not afflicted with the disease (and thus do not physically suffer) are captured in the numerator.

While the costs of the time spent receiving a treatment or preventive service are generally *not* captured by the HRQL score (and are thus included in the numerator of the cost-effectiveness ratio), the time spent *recovering* from an illness should ideally be captured in the HRQL score (Gold and others, 1996). While visits to the doctor do not (theoretically) cause pain and suffering, recovering from an illness does.

Consider the case of a young man who has just had surgery for a hernia repair. Prior to surgery, he is bothered by mild to moderate abdominal pain and has a baseline HRQL score of 0.8. Following the operation, he will likely be in moderate pain for about a week and consequently will be unable to work while he is recovering. Because there is a component of pain involved, this man's quality of life will be affected, and thus recovery from illness is best captured in the HRQL score. Figure 1.4 illustrates the impact of surgery on this person's HRQL.

The terms "direct cost," "indirect cost," and "intangible cost" are sometimes used inconsistently by health economics researchers, and they sometimes have different meanings in different fields of economics, so some experts have recommended that these terms not be used (Drummond, 1997). We will refer to them here because students will frequently see these terms used in published cost-effectiveness studies.

Figure 1.5 summarizes the recommendations of the Panel on Cost-Effectiveness in Health and Medicine for the correct placement of costs in a cost-effectiveness analysis. It will be much easier to see how different costs and

FIGURE 1.4.   THE HYPOTHETICAL DAY-TO-DAY CHANGES IN HEALTH-RELATED QUALITY OF LIFE SCORE FOR A YOUNG MALE RECOVERING FROM A HERNIA REPAIR.

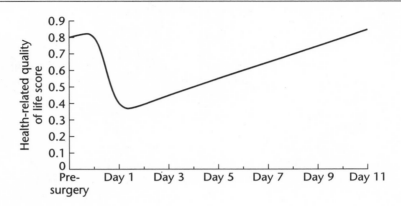

effectiveness measures are incorporated into the cost-effectiveness ratio once we begin working with real-world data in Chapter Four.

Interpreting the Cost-Effectiveness Ratio

Let us revisit the cost-effectiveness ratio (Equation 1.1). Recall that the ratio boils down to the overall cost of an intervention divided by the number of

FIGURE 1.5.   SUMMARY RECOMMENDATIONS FOR THE CORRECT PLACEMENT OF COSTS IN A COST-EFFECTIVENESS ANALYSIS.

Actual costs included in the analysis (numerator)
- Cost of health care products and services
- Cost of the time a patient spends receiving the intervention
- Cost of travel by the patient and caregivers
- Costs borne by others
- Costs not directly related to health care (for instance, environmental costs)

Theoretical costs captured in the quality-adjusted life year (denominator)
- Costs associated with mortality
- Costs associated with morbidity
- Costs associated with lost productivity and leisure time
- Cost of time spent recuperating from illness

QALYs gained:

$$\frac{(\text{cost of intervention} - \text{costs averted by intervention})}{\text{QALYs gained by intervention}}$$

Equation 1.1

Notice that if the numerator cost is high but the number of quality-adjusted life years gained by the intervention is low, the ratio becomes very large. If the cost is high but the number of QALYs is also high, the ratio will be smaller. So you can see that very expensive interventions that are also very effective may still be cost-effective relative to less expensive but less effective interventions.

Though you will not have real world information on how oseltamivir compares to supportive care or vaccination until you read through or complete the sample cost-effectiveness analysis in this book, let us look at how a hypothetical average cost-effectiveness ratio works when applied to the influenza research question.

Suppose that the average cost-effectiveness of providing supportive care is \$40/QALY, and the average cost-effectiveness of providing oseltamivir is \$50/QALY. These ratios provide us with general information about the cost and effectiveness of each intervention, but we are left wondering exactly how much more effective oseltamivir is than supportive care and how much more it costs. For example, supportive care might cost just \$4 per person but might only result in a gain of 0.1 QALYs, while providing oseltamivir might cost \$500 per person but result in a gain of 10 QALYs. It is also possible that both strategies are equally effective. If this were the case, then supportive care would simply be less expensive. Information on the differences in costs between two interventions *relative* to the difference in effectiveness is provided by the incremental cost-effectiveness ratio.

Comparing Interventions

When comparing interventions, it is important to know how much more or less costly and effective one intervention is compared to another, or compared to what is considered the current "standard of care." The standard of care refers to the status quo or existing practice that is generally accepted as the norm. Prior to the introduction of the newer medications used to treat influenza (neuraminidase inhibitors), the standard of care for treating influenza was to recommend that the person stay home, get some rest, drink plenty of fluids, and have some soup. The cost of not providing the medication can thus be called providing "supportive care." It should be noted that the supportive care option is not free of costs. In fact, persons who are not treated may be more likely to see a doctor for a complication of influenza, may be more likely to be hospitalized, or may even be more likely to die. Thus, while the supportive care option eliminates the cost of the medication and all other costs associated with distributing it, this option does not necessarily cost less than treatment.

If the patient receives oseltamivir at the onset of symptoms, the patient may still require additional medical visits and may still be hospitalized for an influenza virus infection. Our objective is to determine how much more (or less) expensive oseltamivir would be than providing supportive care and how much more (or less) effective it would be (Gold and others, 1996; Haddix and others, 1996).

To keep things simple, let us just focus on costs for the moment. Suppose that the average cost of providing medical care for influenza virus infections is \$100. If oseltamivir increases the cost of treating influenza by \$55 but reduces the cost of future hospitalization by \$5, then the total cost of providing oseltamivir would be \$100 + (\$55 − \$5) = \$150, but the incremental increase in cost would be just \$100 − \$50 = \$50. The average cost of providing oseltamivir, \$155, is meaningless unless we know the cost of providing supportive care (routine medical care alone).

Now suppose that we know that the average person who develops an influenza virus infection can expect to live 25 additional years in perfect health, while the average person who receives oseltamivir when infected with the influenza virus can expect to live 25.01 additional years in perfect health. In this scenario, providing oseltamivir to people with the flu would result in a net gain of 25.01 QALYs − 25 QALYs = 0.01 QALYs. The incremental cost-effectiveness of providing oseltamivir would be \$50/0.01 QALYs gained = \$5,000 per QALY gained. This difference in cost and effectiveness is referred to as the **incremental cost-effectiveness.** The incremental cost-effectiveness ratio is defined as:

$$\frac{(\text{total cost of intervention 1} - \text{total cost of intervention 2})}{(\text{QALYs, intervention 1} - \text{QALYs, intervention 2})}$$

Equation 1.2

When calculating the incremental cost-effectiveness ratio, the less effective intervention is always placed on the right side of the equation.

Notice that the two terms in the numerator of the incremental cost-effectiveness ratio represent the numerator terms of the average cost-effectiveness ratios (see Equation 1.1) for the two interventions being compared. Likewise, the denominator terms of the incremental cost-effectiveness ratio represent the two denominator terms of the average cost-effectiveness ratio of the two interventions being compared.

By subtracting the total cost of one intervention from the total cost of another, we are calculating the *difference* in cost between one intervention and the next. Likewise, we are calculating the difference in the total number of QALYs between these two interventions. While the average cost-effectiveness ratio indicates the cost and effectiveness of a health intervention relative to a zero cost and zero effectiveness scenario, the incremental cost-effectiveness ratio indicates the cost of one health intervention relative to another. Because we are only interested in comparisons between one intervention and the next, the incremental cost-effectiveness ratio is the only ratio that should be reported when the study is published.

Exercises 1.1–1.2

1.1. Suppose that the total cost of providing oseltamivir is $100 and the total cost of providing supportive care is $10. Suppose further that oseltamivir will result in 0.5 QALYs per person treated and providing supportive care alone results in 0.1 QALYs. What is the average cost-effectiveness of each intervention? What is the incremental cost-effectiveness of providing oseltamivir to persons with influenza relative to providing supportive care alone?

1.2. Suppose that the total cost of vaccinating an individual is $150 and that vaccination results in the gain of 0.75 QALYs per person. Using information from Exercise 1.1, calculate the average cost-effectiveness of influenza vaccination and the incremental cost-effectiveness of influenza vaccination relative to treatment.

Defining the Comparator

A cost-effectiveness analysis provides the most useful information when it indicates how much more an intervention costs when compared to current medical practice or the standard of care. By including the standard of care in our analysis, we are calculating a meaningful baseline cost and baseline effectiveness against which we can compare other interventions. For instance, by comparing treatment to supportive care, we know how much *more* treatment costs and how much *more* effective it is than supportive care. Therefore, unlike the average cost-effectiveness ratio, which presents gains relative to a zero cost and zero effectiveness baseline, the incremental cost-effectiveness ratio is dependent on how the comparator is defined.

It is often helpful to include a "no intervention" or "do nothing" comparator. A no intervention analysis will provide the consumer of the cost-effectiveness analysis with a concrete point of reference (Gold and others, 1996). If we do not treat or vaccinate people, they may still see a doctor or wind up in the hospital, and will therefore incur costs. However, they will not incur the cost of the intervention itself. Thus, the "no intervention" option is usually less expensive and less effective than other strategies in the analysis.

In our analysis, supportive care is effectively a no intervention strategy, because we are only recommending rest and hydration. If oseltamivir were widely available at the start of our analysis, some people would probably receive treatment when they visited their doctor, while others would receive supportive care only. In this case, it might be informative to know the cost-effectiveness of vaccination relative to a mixed strategy of treatment and supportive care, because this would be more representative of the current practice.

Finally, we may wish to know how the incremental cost-effectiveness of vaccination or treatment compares to other interventions that might realistically be used to treat or prevent influenza. For instance, we could consider evaluating older, less expensive medications that have been used to treat influenza. On the other hand, these medications are only active against influenza A (one of the three common types of influenza virus), they are often poorly tolerated, and they get little use by clinicians in the real world. Therefore, they are intuitively less cost-effective than either the newer medications or vaccination.

Although cost-effectiveness analyses should ideally compare all realistic alternatives to the current standard of care, this is not always possible because of limited resources. At a minimum, the most realistic alternatives to the current standard of care should be examined.

Interpreting Incremental Changes in Cost and Effectiveness

If one intervention is more effective and less expensive than another, and the intervention is ethically acceptable, there should be no question that the more cost-effective intervention is preferable. When a strategy is more effective and less expensive than others, it is said to be **dominant** (Drummond and others, 1997; Gold and others, 1996).

Usually, though, interventions that are more effective are also more costly than the standard of care option. When this occurs, the consumer of the cost-effectiveness analysis must decide whether the added effectiveness is worth the added cost (see Exhibit 1.2). For a moment, let us consider strategies in the management of influenza infection. Suppose we know that vaccination is the most effective strategy for dealing with influenza infection, but we also know that it is significantly more expensive than treatment using oseltamivir and that it therefore results in a large incremental cost-effectiveness ratio. The question then arises: If

EXHIBIT 1.2.   WHAT MAKES AN INTERVENTION COST-EFFECTIVE?

The cost-effectiveness ratio tells the reader how much it costs to purchase one year of quality life. But how do we know if something is a good buy? One study in Canada concluded that anything below US$50,000 per quality-adjusted life year is a good buy (Laupacis and others, 1992). The Federal Aviation Administration and the Nuclear Regulatory Authority, however, are willing to spend much more—sometimes more than a million dollars per year of life—to protect the health of the public.

Researchers should not state whether an intervention is cost-effective or not in medical publications because their area of expertise is research, not policymaking. Instead, it is generally preferred to simply document how the interventions studied compare with other interventions. Tengs and others (1995) produced a list outlining the cost-effectiveness of 100 different interventions so that researchers might put the results of an analysis into perspective; however, this analysis predates the reference case scenario. The most practical strategy for putting the results of an analysis into context is to compare the results of the study at hand to the results of other studies in the same country to provide some basis for comparison (Gold and others, 1996).

vaccination costs $2,000/QALY gained more than treatment with the new medication, but it is still the most effective intervention, is it worth spending the extra money?

When one intervention is more expensive than another, but is still more effective at saving lives and improving the quality of life, it sometimes becomes difficult to choose between interventions. Whether an intervention is adopted depends on its value relative to other interventions. One important factor to consider is how the public perceives the less cost-effective intervention. For example, a family might be very upset if their insurance company failed to pay $200,000 in medical bills for a life-saving organ transplant surgery but would pay for another less effective (but less expensive) intervention. On the other hand, the public may not be too upset if the government failed to recommend vaccinating all healthy adults at the start of influenza season. It is also important to consider *why* the intervention is more expensive and examine ways in which the cost might be further reduced. An example of this approach is discussed in Exhibit 1.3.

Black (1990) created a framework for conceptualizing the results of cost-effectiveness analyses called the **cost-effectiveness plane.** The cost-effectiveness plane is a graphical representation of various cost-effectiveness outcomes (see Figure 1.6). In the cost-effectiveness plane, an intervention is grouped into four quadrants based on its incremental cost-effectiveness.

Recall that when we calculate the incremental cost-effectiveness of an intervention, we first rank the interventions according to their effectiveness. We then subtract the total cost and total effectiveness of the most effective intervention

EXHIBIT 1.3.   THE CASE OF THE BETTER DRUG.

In the mid-1990s the Centers for Disease Control and Prevention (CDC) set out to determine whether patients in sexually transmitted disease clinics should be treated with doxycycline, a generic drug, or azithromycin, a brand name drug, when diagnosed with *Chlamydia trachomatis,* a sexually transmitted disease (Haddix and others, 1995). At the time of the study, azithromycin was four times as expensive as doxycycline. Apart from costs, a major difference between these two drugs is that a course of azithromycin can be taken as a single dose in front of the prescribing physician. When doxycycline is used however, it must be taken twice daily for a minimum of seven days.

   Because patients are virtually guaranteed to complete a course of azithromycin, but many will not complete a course of doxycycline, azithromycin is a more effective drug. However, from the perspective of a publicly funded clinic, the CDC found that the cost of azithromycin would have to decrease dramatically if the drug were to be used in public health clinics. By presenting this data to the manufacturer, the CDC was able to negotiate the lower rate for the drug for use in local health departments that run sexually transmitted disease clinics.

from the total cost and total effectiveness of the next most effective intervention (see Equation 1.2). Suppose that vaccination costs $50 dollars and results in a gain of 0.50 QALYs, and that supportive care costs $100 and results in a gain of 0.25 QALYs. Placing the cost of supportive care on the right side of Equation 1.2, we see that the incremental cost of vaccination would be ($50 − $100) = −$50. The cost difference in this hypothetical example is negative, so the cost lies below

FIGURE 1.6.   THE COST-EFFECTIVENESS PLANE

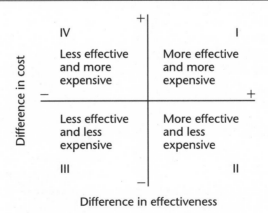

Source: Adapted from Black, 1990.
Note: The center of the graph represents the comparison intervention.

the x-axis of Figure 1.6. Likewise, vaccination is incrementally more effective and therefore lies to the right side of the y-axis.

The center of the plane represents the reference intervention. If an intervention is more effective and more costly than a reference intervention, it lays in quadrant I. If the intervention is less expensive and more effective than the reference intervention, it lies in quadrant II and dominates the reference intervention. If an intervention lies in quadrant IV, it is said to be **dominated,** because it is less effective and more costly. While interventions that lie in quadrant II and quadrant IV produce definitive results (specifically, quadrant II analyses should always be preferred and quadrant IV analyses are never preferred), interventions that fall in quadrants I or III must be evaluated within the context of the larger policy question.

Note that ratios with negative terms are not meaningful, so incremental cost-effectiveness ratios should not be presented when a ratio is cost-saving. Instead, simply report the money saved and the incremental effectiveness separately. In our hypothetical example, we would report that vaccination resulted in a savings of $50 per person and a gain of 0.25 QALYs relative to treatment, rather than report that the incremental cost-effectiveness of vaccination relative to treatment would be −$200/QALY gained.

Other Types of Analyses

Most people are familiar with the term "cost-benefit analysis," but few can concretely describe the differences between a cost-effectiveness analysis and a cost-benefit analysis. In this section, you will learn how cost-effectiveness analysis differs from the other types of economic analyses and you will learn about the related field of burden of disease analysis. Other types of economic analyses complement cost-effectiveness analysis because they provide policymakers and clinicians with different types of information.

Cost-Effectiveness Versus Cost-Utility Analysis

Although the terms are often used interchangeably (as is the case in this book), health economists sometimes distinguish cost-utility analysis from cost-effectiveness analysis. From a practical standpoint, a cost-utility analysis can be considered a specific type of cost-effectiveness analysis in which the quality of life of the study subjects is included in the denominator of the cost-effectiveness ratio. Whereas a cost-utility analysis always includes some measure of quality, such as the effect of pain or suffering on health (for example, QALYs or other quality adjusted measures), a cost-effectiveness analysis in the strictest sense compares the relationship between costs and non-quality adjusted outcomes (for example, cost per number of hospitalizations avoided, cost per number of life years gained, or cost per number of vaccine-preventable illnesses averted). When a cost-effectiveness analysis includes some measure of the health-related quality of life (HRQL), it then falls under the category of "cost-utility analysis."

There are also a number of ways in which quality measures, such as HRQL scores, are combined with quantity measures, such as the number of years of life gained by an intervention. Together, these measures of quantity and quality fall under the generic category of **health-adjusted life years (HALYs),** which include **QALYs, disability-adjusted life years (DALYs), and healthy-years equivalent (HYE),** among others. Only the QALY may be used in a reference case analysis (Gold and others, 1996).

Although analyses using any of these terms are, strictly speaking, considered cost-utility analyses, the broader term "cost-effectiveness analysis" is increasingly used instead. This may reflect a general movement toward the reference case recommendations of the Panel on Cost-Effectiveness in Health and Medicine.

When to use non-reference case cost-effectiveness analyses. Suppose a health department was interested in knowing how many vaccine-preventable diseases could be averted if a vaccine campaign were initiated. By definition, the relevant outcome in this analysis would be the cost per illness averted. A full reference case cost-effectiveness analysis would provide information regarding the effect the vaccine would have on the quality of life of everyone vaccinated and would include costs to employers and other segments of society. However, these outcomes are not relevant to the research question posed by the health department in this example. Non-reference case analyses are generally easier to complete because they require less information, and they may be more useful in circumstances where there is only one relevant outcome.

How to conduct non-reference case analyses. If a student wishes to conduct a cost-effectiveness analysis that does not incorporate quality of life measures using the societal perspective, special considerations must be made. If the outcome of interest is the number of years of life lost to disease, morbidity costs are counted in the numerator. Therefore, lost productivity and leisure time must be measured and included in the numerator. Students who wish to conduct this type of analysis can otherwise follow the procedures outlined in this textbook.

If the study is conducted from a specific perspective or includes other measures in the denominator, such as "hospitalizations averted," the costs included and the endpoints of the study must be carefully thought through. While we will not provide specific instructions on these types of analyses in this book, the general principles still apply.

The DALY is frequently used for studies in developing countries and might serve as an international standard for cost-effectiveness analyses (Murray and Lopez, 1996). It may also be used to study immigrant populations (Muennig and others, 1999). Unfortunately, as we will learn later, there are technical problems with this measure that limit its usefulness and render it incompatible with the reference case scenario (Gold and others, 1996; Muennig and Gold, 2001). Students wishing to use the DALY may follow all of the procedures outlined in this textbook and simply use the HRQL scores tabulated for DALYs by Murray and Lopez (1996). Instructions for using these scores are presented in Chapter Nine. The HYE falls to the other extreme. While it is highly regarded from a technical standpoint, it is difficult to use and might not be an appropriate measure for low-budget studies, such as those conducted in developing countries. For these reasons, the use of quality of life measures other than the QALY will only be briefly discussed in this textbook.

Cost-Benefit Analysis

An alternative to cost-effectiveness analysis that is sometimes favored by economists is the cost-benefit analysis. In this type of analysis, a dollar value is placed on both the costs *and* the effectiveness of an intervention. The final outcome is simply reported as a monetary value. Any intervention associated with cost-savings (a net benefit) should be undertaken, while any intervention associated with (excess) costs should not (unless there are other overriding concerns). Some economists argue that cost-benefit analysis is preferable to cost-effectiveness analysis because it produces a more definitive endpoint, and because the use of cost-effectiveness analysis in the health sector and the use of cost-benefit analysis in other sectors prevents reasonable comparisons of medical interventions with non-medical interventions. Others argue that it is too difficult to place a dollar value on human life, which is required in a cost-benefit analysis. By separating the number of QALYs gained from an intervention from monetary costs in analyses aimed at reducing disease or saving lives, cost-effectiveness analyses avoid the thorny issue of assigning a monetary value to human life.

Although they are sometimes used in health research, cost-benefit analyses are typically used to make decisions about projects that are not related to health care, such as constructing dams or building schools. Still, virtually all social investments have the potential to either benefit lives or adversely affect them. For example, while the construction of a dam may be beneficial in generating hydroelectric power, it may also lead to the displacement of people and communities, contribute to outbreaks of waterborne infectious diseases, or break and flood towns downstream. Because cost-benefit analyses so often affect the health and welfare of human populations, cost-benefit analyses sometimes require that a value be placed on human life regardless of whether the primary intent of the intervention was to save lives. Nonetheless, cost-effectiveness analysis has become the standard for evaluating interventions in the health care field.

Some techniques used in cost-benefit analysis differ from those used in cost-effectiveness analysis. There is a wealth of literature on the field of cost-benefit analysis, and students wishing to conduct a cost-benefit analysis should consult a textbook in that field.

Cost-Minimization Analysis

Cost-minimization analysis is useful in cases where the outcome of two interventions is similar, but the costs are different (Drummond and others, 1997). For example, patients with bacterial endocarditis (an infection of the heart) often require long-term treatment with intravenous antibiotics. Traditionally, patients with endocarditis were hospitalized while they received therapy. Today, antibiotics are sometimes administered at home, potentially reducing the costs associated with this treatment. Because both therapies are equally effective, the only relevant medical issue in evaluating each treatment is the overall cost of administering the treatment at home versus at the hospital. In this situation, a cost-minimization analysis can be used to determine the least costly treatment. Because cost-minimization analysis is easier to conduct than full cost-effectiveness analysis, it should be used whenever two or more interventions of equal effectiveness are being compared.

Burden of Disease Analysis

Burden of disease analyses do not incorporate information on the cost of a disease. Rather, they are used to determine which diseases are responsible for the most morbidity and mortality within a country, and are sometimes used by governments or nongovernmental organizations to allocate health resources.

Traditionally, the burden of a disease was measured by the number of years of life lost to that particular disease. Using that definition, diseases with high mortality rates, like malaria and tuberculosis, were thought to be the most significant health problems in the world. More recently, the World Health Organization, the World Bank, and Harvard University redefined burden of disease analyses by incorporating a measure of quality of life, the disability-adjusted life year (DALY), into their definition. Once quality of life was included, depression, which previously ranked near the bottom of the list, moved up to become one of the world's most significant health problems (Murray and Lopez, 1996).

The DALY is not without its problems. First, as in cost-effectiveness analysis, when measuring quality of life we are left using subjective and imperfect tools in lieu of more objective and definitive measures like death rates. Because people of different nationalities and cultures have different perceptions of human suffering and quality of life, the limitations in generating the health-related quality of life scores are exaggerated when conducting cross-national comparisons. To get around this limitation and to simplify the collection of HRQL scores, quality of life is measured using the input of experts, rather than people residing in a specific culture (Murray and Lopez, 1996). For technical reasons that will be discussed in Chapter Eight, this renders the DALY incompatible with the reference case scenario of a cost-effectiveness analysis (Gold and others, 1996). Therefore, despite a large number of studies incorporating DALYs, this outcome measure is not comparable to the QALY.

CHAPTER TWO

DEVELOPING A RESEARCH PROJECT

In this chapter, you will learn how to develop a cost-effectiveness research project. We will use our sample cost-effectiveness analysis on strategies to prevent or treat influenza virus infections in healthy adults to illustrate how a research question is developed and how to design a cost-effectiveness analysis.

The Ten Steps to a Perfect Research Project

Cost-effectiveness analyses are conducted using a series of intuitive methodological steps, most of which may be generalized to any scientific research project. These steps are presented in Figure 2.1.

Let us briefly review each of these steps.

1. *Develop a research question.* A research question is a well-defined statement about your hypothesis on a particular subject or topic. To test this hypothesis, you must clearly indicate which interventions you will be comparing, which subjects you plan to include, and how your analysis will be conducted.

2. *Design your analysis.* In designing a cost-effectiveness analysis, a researcher must thoroughly review the background information on the disease and health interventions under study and then chart out the different twists and turns a disease might take when different health interventions are applied.

FIGURE 2.1.   THE TEN STEPS TO A PERFECT RESEARCH PROJECT.

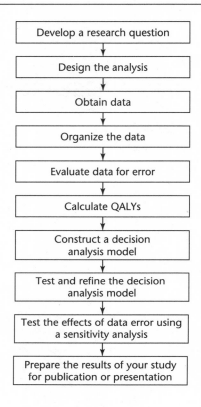

3. *Obtain data relevant to your cost-effectiveness analysis.* Data relevant to your analysis may come from published studies in the medical literature, from electronic databases, or from other sources, such as medical experts.

4. *Organize your data.* Lack of a good organizational system can dramatically increase the time required to conduct a cost-effectiveness analysis. Data are typically organized using spreadsheet programs and notes describing the sources from which the data were obtained.

5. *Evaluate your data for error.* In cost-effectiveness analysis, it is at least as important to understand the shortcomings of the data you include in the analysis as it is to find the most error-free data available.

6. *Calculate QALYs.* Cost-effectiveness analysis should use QALYs as at least one of the outcome measures so that the analysis can be compared with other cost-effectiveness studies.

7. *Construct a decision analysis model.* A decision analysis model melds together all of the data you have collected.

8. *Test and refine the decision analysis model.* Usually decision analysis models will have omissions, oversights, or incorrect formulas entered into them. These must be detected and fixed before the model can be used.

9. *Conduct a sensitivity analysis.* No data are entirely free of error. A sensitivity analysis will evaluate how the errors in your data sources might affect the cost or effectiveness of each of the medical interventions you are studying.

10. *Prepare the study results for publication or presentation.* Once you have finished your study, you will need to present it in a way that anyone can understand. Adopting standard publication formats helps you achieve this goal (and get published).

This book is organized following the ten general steps outlined above. For teaching purposes, we will discuss evaluating data sources for error prior to discussing how the data elements are obtained and organized, so that you will have a better understanding of the limitations of each source we discuss. We will also calculate QALYs after constructing the decision analysis model, so that beginning students are not overburdened with cost and effectiveness data at the same time. Once each of these ten steps is completed, you will find a Project Map indicating how far along you are in the analysis.

Developing a Research Question

The first step in any research project is developing a research question. The data you will collect, the way you will think about analyzing it, and the way in which you will present it will vary according to the question you are trying to answer. A well-thought-out research question will help eliminate false starts and put the study into perspective.

Project Map

1. Develop a research question.
2. Design your analysis.
3. Understand the sources of error in data.
4. Obtain data.
5. Organize data.
6. Construct a decision analysis model.
7. Calculate quality-adjusted life years.
8. Test and refine the decision analysis model.

9. Conduct a sensitivity analysis.
10. Prepare the study results for publication or presentation.

The question should be as comprehensive as possible, but concise. A comprehensive question will compare all realistic alternatives and will include an evaluation of the costs and benefits of not performing the intervention (for example, "usual care," "presumptive treatment," "supportive care," "no program," and so on).

It is important to be careful of the language you use to describe the reference arm of your study, as a poorly worded description of this arm can lead to false assumptions about the intervention on the part of the people who will read your study. Poor wording can also lead you down the wrong path when it comes time to collect data and build a model. "Usual care" or "current practice" implies that interventions are being compared to a mixture of medical interventions that reflect the current practice standards (Gold and others, 1996).

The research question should state what you are comparing, how you are conducting the comparison, to whom you are targeting the intervention, and how frequently the evaluation is being performed. When broken down into these basic components, the research question naturally presents itself to both the reader and to the researcher. (See Table 2.1 for examples of how these principles apply to different research questions.)

In Table 2.1 we see how three research questions might be developed. If we wished to question the practice of obtaining a blood pressure on everyone who walks into a medical clinic, we must ask what the logical alternative to this practice might be. Clearly, we would not want to do away with blood pressure cuffs altogether. One possible alternative would be to screen only those people who are most likely to have high blood pressure, such as people over the age of forty-five.

TABLE 2.1.   EXAMPLES OF VARIOUS RESEARCH QUESTIONS IN COST-EFFECTIVENESS ANALYSIS.

Comparison	What?	How?	Who?	How Often?
Screen all asymptomatic persons versus screen only patients over 45 years of age	Hypertension	Cost-effectiveness	Visitors to clinics	Each visit
Screening mammography versus breast self-exam versus current practice	Breast cancer	Cost-effectiveness	Females age < 50	Every 2 years
Screen with RPR versus screen with VRDL versus no screening	Syphilis	Cost-effectiveness	Immigrants aged 17 and over	On entry to U.S.

Another alternative strategy might be to evaluate blood pressure screening at different frequencies, such as once a year rather than at each visit.

In this book, the art of cost-effectiveness will be taught using a simple cost-effectiveness analysis that was carefully designed specifically for teaching purposes. This study will examine whether it is more cost-effective to treat persons who develop symptoms of influenza during the flu season with oseltamivir, or to vaccinate all healthy adults at the start of each influenza season. We will compare both of these options to "supportive care," or giving people what their moms gave them when they were young: soup, crackers, something for the cough, and something for the fever.

Because the cost-effectiveness of vaccination has been firmly established among older adults and persons with certain chronic conditions, it makes sense to limit the study to younger, healthier populations. In addition, because oseltamivir has not been tested in children, it also makes sense to limit the study to persons over the age of fifteen.

We must be careful in defining what we mean by "healthy," however. The influenza vaccine is currently recommended for people with chronic lung disease, diabetes, and heart disease, among other conditions ("Prevention," 1999). Though it may be worthwhile to evaluate the cost-effectiveness of influenza vaccination or treatment in this group, an analysis of adults without these conditions would be more useful. If any strategy is found to be cost-effective when applied to people without these conditions, it will almost certainly be cost-effective when applied to people with these conditions.

Our research question might take the form: "Is treatment, vaccination, or supportive care the most cost-effective way to manage influenza-like illness among healthy adults?" (See Table 2.2.) Influenza-like illness is a cluster of diseases that produce symptoms similar to those people have when infected with the influenza virus. These symptoms may be induced by the influenza virus itself, or by a number of other respiratory tract viruses or bacteria. The World Health Organization (WHO) defines influenza-like illness as the presence of fever ($>100°F$) plus a sore throat or cough (Kendal and others, 1982).

TABLE 2.2.   RESEARCH QUESTION FOR THE SAMPLE COST-EFFECTIVENESS ANALYSIS.

Comparison	What?	Study (How?)	Population (Who?)	How Often?
Vaccination versus treatment versus supportive care	Influenza-like illness	Cost-effectiveness	Persons residing in the United States age 15–65	Each influenza season

There are two reasons for evaluating influenza-like illness rather than influenza itself. First, when we evaluate the cost-effectiveness of the treatment arm, we wish to reproduce real life situations as closely as possible. Physicians will often treat patients based on their symptoms, rather than on the results of laboratory tests. Therefore, it makes more sense to use a symptom-based definition. Second, most of the studies in the medical literature examine influenza-like illness rather than influenza virus infection (in part because it is so difficult to differentiate influenza from some of these other respiratory pathogens).

We should keep in mind, however, that this definition is a technical definition. Many illnesses that physicians would not diagnose as influenza fall under the heading of "influenza-like illness." For example, an otherwise healthy patient that presents to the physician a fever, cough, sore throat, and sinus pain might be diagnosed with sinusitis rather than influenza-like illness. Still, for the purposes of scientific research, it makes sense to limit the definition of the disease we are studying to something that is tangible and measurable.

Another reason for using influenza-like illness is that the definition captures some illnesses that arise from a prior infection with the influenza virus. These **secondary illnesses** (illnesses that arise as a result of a previous illness or a co-existing medical condition) include sinusitis and bacterial pneumonia. Bacterial pneumonia, for example, is often associated with a fever, cough, and chest pain. The presence of fever and cough is sufficient to classify this disease as an influenza-like illness, though like sinusitis, few physicians would mistake it for influenza.

To fully evaluate the research question, and to gain perspective on the types of costs and benefits we will need to collect for our analysis, we should ask:

1. *Have we included all of the important interventions?* When considering treatment options, we could include the older anti-influenza medications in our analysis, we could compare different doses of oseltamivir, or we could include the inhaled cousin of oseltamivir, zanamivir (Monto and others, 1999).

In an ideal situation, all logical comparisons would be included in a cost-effectiveness analysis. The ideal is not always possible though, given the limited resources available to most researchers. Therefore, those interventions that *are* included should make sense from a policy standpoint. For example, the older antiviral medications are less effective, are sometimes associated with severe side effects, and are rarely used for the treatment of influenza today, so we can safely exclude them from our research question. Zanamivir is more difficult to use and is about as effective as oseltamivir. If the resources were available, we might also consider evaluating zanamivir, because it would be important for doctors and policymakers to know how this drug compares to oseltamivir (to simplify the analysis, we will not include it in this book). Finally, higher doses of oseltamivir offer little in terms of improved effectiveness but double the cost of treatment while increasing the chances of side effects. Therefore, the most logical interventions to include in the analysis are vaccination and treatment with the standard dose of oseltamivir.

The reference case scenario recommends that the standard of care be included as a comparator (Gold and others, 1996). It also suggests that the next best alternative to the intervention under study and a no intervention strategy be included.

2. *How will we decide how the disease is usually diagnosed or treated?* In the case of oseltamivir, it may be necessary to examine the cost-effectiveness of testing patients before treating them with oseltamivir versus treating patients **presumptively** (presuming the patient has the illness and treating him or her without further testing for the illness). Alternatively, we might study the costs and benefits of treating patients based on the results of a laboratory test for the influenza virus, or a combination of the presumptive treatment and laboratory testing approaches.

If the treatment were more expensive than the test, had side effects, or might cause the influenza virus to become resistant to treatment, it would be prudent to include a test and treat option in the analysis, because the question of whether to test before treating is itself a relevant policy question. However, de Andrade and others (2000) found that presumptive treatment is more economical than testing, so there is a rational basis for excluding testing from our analysis. To keep things simple, we will exclude laboratory testing from the analysis presented in this book, though we will discuss laboratory testing in detail in Chapter Twelve. Thus, our research question will compare supportive care, presumptive treatment with oseltamivir, and influenza vaccination for persons with influenza-like illness. Unless we include a mixture of influenza virus testing and presumptive treatment in our analysis, we will not be testing real-world treatment patterns and should be careful to outline this fact in our research question.

3. *Is the clinical setting relevant?* Oftentimes, it is important to consider the place where a patient will receive the intervention(s) you are studying. For example, policymakers may be interested in knowing whether patients should be vaccinated in the workplace, or whether a patient should make a special trip to the doctor each season to ensure the receipt of an influenza vaccination. If patients are to go to their doctor specifically for a vaccination, the cost of vaccination will be higher than if patients are vaccinated at their workplace, because patients will incur transportation costs and additional medical costs if vaccination is the sole reason for their medical visit. Therefore, the strategy of vaccinating in the workplace is intuitively more cost-effective than making a special trip to the doctor for the vaccination. Our research question should therefore focus on workplace vaccinations or vaccinations in situations where no special effort is required on the part of

the patient or the physician (for example, during a medical visit for some other reason, vaccinations in prisons, and other similar situations).

4. *Are we comparing two different interventions or different levels of a single intervention?* Consider two questions: 1) Is it more cost-effective to treat influenza-like illness with a low dose of oseltamivir or a higher dose of oseltamivir? 2) Is it more cost-effective to treat influenza-like illness or to prevent it with vaccination? In the first example, we are concerned primarily with how much more the higher dose of oseltamivir will cost than the lower dose, as well as how much more effective it is than the lower dose. An analysis that compares different levels of an intervention can be simple relative to comparing two entirely different interventions because the data requirements for such an analysis are minimal. This type of analysis is called a **marginal** analysis because the costs and effects of the more aggressive program are analyzed above and over (on the margin of) the less aggressive program (Haddix and others, 1996). In the second example, it is necessary to dig up information on both the vaccine and the treatment. This is called an **incremental** analysis. Our research question examines two entirely different approaches to preventing complications of influenza-like illness, rather than two different levels of a preventive intervention. Therefore, we will conduct an incremental analysis.

Marginal analyses can take many forms. For instance, preventive interventions, such as screening mammography, must often be repeated throughout the patient's lifetime. But how frequently should this occur? If screening tests are performed frequently, the cost of screening will increase, but the chances of catching the disease early will also increase. Therefore, screening interventions should contain an analysis examining the cost of screening at different frequencies (Gold and others, 1996).

5. *What type of study is appropriate?* This book focuses only on cost-effectiveness analyses with a strong emphasis on cost-utility analysis (because this is the subtype of cost-effectiveness analysis recommended by the Panel on Cost-Effectiveness in Health and Medicine). Nevertheless, the reader should be aware that there are other ways of evaluating health interventions, such as through a cost-benefit analysis, and should consider all options when formulating a research question (Drummond and others, 1997; Gold and others, 1996; Haddix and others, 1996). Generally, if the primary reason to do the intervention is to save lives or reduce disease, a reference case cost-effectiveness analysis should be performed. On the other hand, if the intervention is going to be compared with non-health related investments, a cost-benefit analysis may be more useful. For example, in a study of the economic benefits of air bags, a cost-benefit analysis may be preferred because the consumers of the information (car companies and federal regulators) will prefer the familiar and more definitive cost-benefit ratio. (Recall that a

cost-benefit ratio indicates whether the intervention should be done, rather than how much it will cost to save a year of quality-adjusted life). However, economic analyses tend to complement one another so the existence of a cost-effectiveness analysis does not preclude a cost-benefit analysis.

6. *Who will we conduct the study for?* In some cases, a researcher will be asked to conduct a study for an insurance company or the government. In other instances, the study will be designed for publication in the medical literature. The audience of the study determines which costs and outcomes are to be included. For example, when conducting a cost-effectiveness analysis, an insurance company may only be concerned with how much money it will have to spend and how much it might save on a treatment or preventive intervention. It is unlikely that the insurance company will be very interested in whether a patient has to spend money on gas or take a taxi to get to the hospital for a preventive intervention. Moreover, its representatives probably will not be too concerned about lost productivity costs or other indirect costs that the patient's employer has to absorb. On the other hand, they will certainly be interested in how much the intervention costs and how much it will save, because they will have to pay for the difference. The audience of the study determines the perspective of the analysis (Drummond and others, 1997; Gold and others, 1996; Haddix and others, 1996).

7. *To whom does the study apply?* In most cost-effectiveness analyses, data from many different studies are analyzed as if each study were part of one larger study. Therefore, the analyses do not usually have a defined cohort. This allows researchers to define the characteristics of the population they wish to study; cost-effectiveness analyses usually analyze study outcomes for a **hypothetical cohort.** For example, if we were examining the cost-effectiveness of various interventions to prevent sexually transmitted HIV infection among children and adolescents in South Africa, we might, in our hypothetical cohort, include all sexually active persons between the ages of ten and eighteen residing in South Africa. We would then collect and analyze information from different sources that pertains only to our hypothetical cohort.

Ensuring that the data you collect match the characteristics of the hypothetical cohort you are studying is not an easy task. Most diseases are more severe for persons of lower socioeconomic status. If we collect data from a study of health maintenance organization (HMO) enrollees, the data will underestimate the severity of disease in the general population because HMO enrollees tend to be affluent and, by definition, have insurance. It is therefore important to ensure that the demographics of the subjects in the studies you choose to include in your analysis are similar to the demographics of the cohort you wish to evaluate in your cost-effectiveness analysis (Drummond and others, 1997; Gold and others, 1996).

8. *How far into the future do we need to capture outcomes?* In the case of influenza, a person is ill for a short period of time and then recovers. The **time frame** of an analysis is the period over which the immediate costs and benefits of an intervention occur. Influenza is a seasonal disease, and costs are only incurred over influenza season. However, it is much simpler to calculate the costs of this disease over the period of a year because most of the data sources we will use do not provide month-to-month information.

The **analytic horizon** is the period over which all costs and outcomes are considered (Haddix and others, 1996). For example, though vaccination is mostly only effective for one year, it will save future years of life. Thirty-year-old people who die today from influenza might have otherwise lived to be seventy-five, so we must count each year of future life lost in the denominator of our cost-effectiveness ratio. Typically, a study will have an analytic horizon equal to the life expectancy of the cohort you include in your study.

9. *Where will we draw the boundaries of our analysis?* In the case of influenza-like illness, the disease may be transmitted person-to-person. When people are vaccinated, the chance of person-to-person transmission of the disease is greatly reduced. Consider the case of a man with an influenza-like illness. He might infect two other people who might then infect four more. Eventually, a large portion of a community of unvaccinated people may become infected.

This one person would cause a wave of costs, morbidity, and possibly mortality that will crash at some point. Ideally, we should account for all of the money spent treating all of the people that this person made ill and capture all the sickness he caused. In reality, this would be a very difficult task, so the researcher must draw a boundary around which costs and consequences are captured, and this boundary should be defined at the outset of the analysis (Drummond and others, 1997; Gold and others, 1996; Haddix and others, 1996).

10. *Are there enough data to answer our question?* Some cost-effectiveness analysis questions are not possible to answer because the data are not available. Cost-effectiveness analyses may use data from electronic databases, from the medical literature, from ongoing studies, or even from expert opinion. When one key data element is missing, it is possible to conduct a **threshold analysis.** If we did not know how many people become infected with influenza each season, a threshold analysis would tell us the incidence rate at which vaccination would be the more cost-effective option, as well as the incidence rate at which treatment would be the more cost-effective option (Gold and others, 1996).

Developing a research question for the sample analysis. Let us now review the research question for our sample cost-effectiveness analysis. As the research question is described, try to identify each of the elements discussed in the preceding section.

We will conduct a cost-effectiveness analysis evaluating strategies to prevent or treat influenza-like illness among healthy persons aged fifteen to sixty-five residing in the United States. For the purposes of our analysis, a healthy adult is defined as a person who does not have chronic lung disease, heart disease, diabetes, or other chronic conditions that place him or her at greater risk for complications of influenza infection. We decided to evaluate only healthy adults because currently there is uncertainty as to whether the optimal strategy to manage influenza infection in this population is to 1) provide vaccination at the beginning of the influenza season, 2) provide treatment with oseltamivir only if illness develops, or 3) provide supportive care only if illness develops. We will evaluate each of these strategies from the societal perspective using an incremental cost-effectiveness analysis that adheres to the reference case guidelines.

Subjects in our hypothetical cohort receiving supportive care who become ill with an influenza-like illness may visit their doctor or become hospitalized, but they will not receive antiviral therapy or laboratory testing for the influenza virus. Instead, they will be sent home with instructions to care for themselves, or if hospitalized, they will receive standard hospital care. None of the subjects in this arm of the analysis will have been vaccinated at the start of the influenza season.

Subjects in the oseltamivir arm of the study who become ill with an influenza-like illness will receive oseltamivir presumptively (without laboratory testing) if they visit a physician for their illness. This may or may not reduce their chances of experiencing severe symptoms associated with influenza virus infections.

Subjects in the vaccination arm of the analysis will receive the influenza vaccine at the start of the influenza season. The vaccine will be administered either at the subjects' place of employment, as part of a medical visit unrelated to vaccination, or in another institutional setting. If the vaccine fails, these subjects may require hospitalization or other medical care.

The time frame of the analysis will be a single influenza season and the analytical horizon will be life, because influenza-like illnesses may be associated with fatalities in a healthy adult population. The study is targeted to clinicians who may benefit from guidance on how to optimally manage influenza-like illness in the clinical setting.

Now that we have developed a concrete research question, we may begin to think of how we might design the analysis.

Designing Your Analysis

To study the effect of an intervention on a disease, you will need to learn just about all there is to know about the disease. For instance, in our research question we will need to know how people get influenza, what the normal course of an infection is, and all of the potential complications of influenza. We will also need information on each of the interventions we are evaluating to prevent or treat it.

There are three steps to gathering information about a disease and the interventions to prevent or treat it. The first step is through simple learning. This requires reading medical textbooks and review articles to get a thorough understanding of what you are about to tackle. The second step is to process the information you have learned by charting out the course of the disease when different interventions are applied. This will give you a better idea of the specific data elements you will need to collect.

Project Map

1. Develop a research question.
2. **Design your analysis.**
3. Understand the sources of error in data.
4. Obtain data.
5. Organize data.
6. Construct a decision analysis model.
7. Calculate quality-adjusted life years.
8. Test and refine the decision analysis model.
9. Conduct a sensitivity analysis.
10. Prepare the study results for publication or presentation.

The third step to gathering information about the disease and interventions is to collect the pieces of information you will need to actually conduct your analysis, such as incidence rates, mortality data, and costs. These data are obtained from the medical literature, electronic datasets, or other sources. Once you have charted out the course of the disease when different interventions are applied and have made a list of all of the data elements you will need, you will be ready to begin collecting data.

In the following sections, we will tackle each of these three steps in order.

Step 1: Learn About the Disease

To learn about the natural progression of a disease and the effect different interventions might have on a disease, it is necessary to read medical textbooks, summary articles, and clinical practice guidelines. Clinical practice guidelines describe the optimal way to manage a disease and are especially helpful because they usually contain flowcharts and other useful tools for visualizing the progression of a disease. (One good place to obtain clinical practice guidelines is through the Agency for Health Research and Quality (http://www.ahrq.gov/clinic/cpgsix.htm).) Clinical practice guidelines can also sometimes be obtained by medical societies such as the American Cancer Society. Since we cannot expect you to learn all about influenza virus infections just to get through the sample cost-effectiveness analysis, we will summarize the basics of the disease here.

Symptoms of influenza virus infection. Influenza is usually an acute self-limited illness that lasts around five to seven days. It usually causes a fever, fatigue, headache, runny nose, cough, and sore throat. Often, the symptoms appear so quickly that people can recall the moment they knew that they first felt ill. Typically, people with influenza are so tired that they cannot get out of bed, eat very little, and sometimes need someone to take care of them (Keech and others, 1998). Of course, this often means missing work, though many people will go to work if possible so that they do not use up the vacation days they might better use when feeling well.

Differences between influenza and influenza-like illness. It is often difficult to tell the difference between infection with the influenza virus and other viral or bacterial infections of the respiratory system. Many viruses and bacteria can produce a sore throat, runny nose, cough, and fatigue. It would be expensive and time-consuming for a doctor to test every patient that comes into his or her office for influenza or the other diseases that produce these symptoms. Most studies of the influenza virus therefore examine "influenza-like illness" instead. As we have seen from the studies by Bridges and others (2000), Nichol and others (1995), and Treanor and others (2000) listed in Appendix Two, the way that influenza-like illness is defined varies from study to study. Though this complicates the development of a cost-effectiveness analysis on strategies to prevent or treat influenza virus infections, it makes for a good teaching tool, because most of the data will need to be critically examined or adjusted before they are used. We will use the formal definition for influenza-like illness used by the World Health Organization (WHO). It defines influenza-like illness as "feverishness or a measured temperature of at least 37.7°C (100°F) plus cough or sore throat" (Kendal and others, 1982).

While most diseases are diagnosed using a basic set of clinical criteria (fever plus cough), these diagnoses are usually supported by laboratory testing. For most medical conditions, clinicians provide a concrete name to a particular constellation of symptoms and laboratory data. For example, a patient who experienced crushing chest pain and who had laboratory evidence of heart muscle destruction is said to have had a myocardial infarction (heart attack). Influenza-like illness, on the other hand, is a constellation of *diseases* that produce similar symptoms.

Most patients that visit their doctor with a fever and a cough or sore throat are given a specific diagnosis. This might include streptococcal infections of the throat, bronchitis, or influenza. Few clinicians would mistake a throat infection for influenza. However, throat infections may be counted among the cases of influenza-like illness simply because they can produce "feverishness" along with a sore throat. A practical advantage of using this definition is that most of the research in the medical literature has been conducted on influenza-like illness rather than influenza virus infections. By using this definition, we will have more data available to us. Another advantage of using this definition is that some of these seemingly unrelated infections that happen to produce a fever, cough, and sore throat may have been caused by a recent infection with influenza. Bacterial pneumonia and other secondary infections sometimes arise from a recent infection with the influenza virus.

Complications, transmission, and treatment. Severe manifestations of influenza virus infection are rare in healthy adults and include primary influenza pneumonia, secondary illness, and aggravation of existing medical conditions (LaForce and others, 1994; Neuzil and others, 1999; Nichol and others, 1995; Sullivan and others, 1983). In rare instances, influenza can progress into primary influenza pneumonia. This is a serious illness that causes bleeding and inflammation in the lungs. More frequently, people recovering from influenza develop a secondary bacterial pneumonia, sinusitis, or otitis media (ear infection). Of these secondary illnesses, bacterial pneumonia can be fatal. Influenza virus infections can also aggravate other medical conditions, such as heart disease or lung disease.

Influenza viruses fall into three categories: influenza A, B, and C. Only influenza A and B are susceptible to neuraminidase inhibitors, such as oseltamivir. Each season, different strains of influenza virus circulate through the population. Though the influenza vaccine is targeted toward three circulating strains of influenza A or B, the match between the virus and the vaccine is not always perfect. About once in every ten influenza seasons, the vaccine is poorly matched to the circulating strains of influenza virus. When this occurs, the vaccine is only effective in a small proportion of people.

Influenza A and B are responsible for the majority of influenza outbreaks; however, influenza A is responsible for all of the severe outbreaks. Virtually every influenza season there are outbreaks of the illness. Once every ten to fifteen years there is a global **pandemic** (worldwide epidemic). During the 1957 pandemic, there were approximately 70,000 **excess deaths** due to influenza or pneumonia in the United States. The term "excess deaths" refers to the number of deaths that occur beyond the average number of deaths outside of the influenza season. During the average influenza season, there are approximately 114,000 hospitalizations and 20,000 excess deaths attributed to influenza virus infection ("Prevention," 1998).

When many people are immunized, a phenomenon called **herd immunity** generally occurs. When a large proportion of the population is immune to a virus, there are fewer people that can transmit the disease, so unvaccinated people will be at a lower risk for the disease. Unfortunately, the percentage of people that must be vaccinated for herd immunity to occur is not known. In fact, the influenza virus has been known to spread in communities with high rates of vaccination and barely touch communities in which virtually no one has been vaccinated (Barker and Mullooly, 1980).

You have already learned about the randomized controlled trials of the influenza vaccine and oseltamivir in healthy adults. Each of these studies is summarized in Appendix II. To follow the examples presented in this chapter, it will be necessary to refer to the summaries of these studies.

Step 2: Chart Out the Course of the Disease

To get a good idea of which data elements you will need in your cost-effectiveness analysis, you should sketch out the natural progression of the disease that you are studying. For example, we know that people with influenza-like illness might miss work, need someone to take care of them, might need to see a doctor, and, if the infection is serious, might end up in the hospital or even die. After recovering from the disease, the person might then develop a secondary illness that, in turn, might require a medical visit, result in hospitalization, or result in death. If each of these events is charted out, you will have a much better idea of which data elements you will need to collect for your analysis. The course of different events that can occur in a cost-effectiveness analysis is sometimes called an **event pathway.**

Beginning students find that it is easiest to draw a flowchart indicating the different courses the disease might take. (See Figure 2.2 for a partial flowchart of the course of influenza-like illness.) A separate flowchart should be made for each health intervention under study, because each intervention will presumably modify the course of events in an illness. Oftentimes, clinical practice guidelines will chart out the natural course of disease for you.

FIGURE 2.2.   PARTIAL FLOWCHART INDICATING THE CLINICAL COURSE OF INFLUENZA-LIKE ILLNESS.

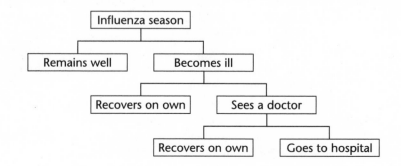

Almost all of the "events" in an event pathway are associated with a cost. In Figure 2.2, for example, ill people might see a doctor or might recover on their own. If they see a doctor, they will incur the cost of driving to the doctor, the cost of the doctor's visit, and so on. Each of the events is also associated with a probability. For example, the chance that a person will become ill during influenza season is equal to the incidence rate of influenza-like illness during that season. To conduct our cost-effectiveness analysis, we will need to know the probability of each event and the cost of each event.

Create an event pathway for each intervention. The probabilities and costs you obtain will generally be different for each intervention under study. For instance, if a man is treated with oseltamivir, chances are that he will be less likely to be hospitalized than if he received supportive care.

It is also possible that the course of the flowchart will change when an intervention is applied. For instance, oseltamivir is only effective if it is given within forty-eight hours after the onset of the illness. The illness may assume a different course if the medication is administered on time rather than if it is administered after forty-eight hours. Therefore, the flowchart outlining the course of illness among treated people may contain additional boxes representing events that would not occur in an untreated population.

Once you have sketched out each of the possible events that might occur when a person receives supportive care, is treated, or is vaccinated, you can begin to generate a list of the elements you will need for your cost-effectiveness analysis. Even with a flowchart, students conducting a cost-effectiveness analysis for the first time are bound to miss some of the twists and turns that can occur over the course of disease. For this reason, we will discuss the parameters that are usually needed in designing a cost-effectiveness analysis in the next section. In Chapter Seven, you will learn how to create an event pathway using a decision analysis model.

Step 3: List the Data Elements That You Will Need

Imagine that you were evaluating 100 subjects at the beginning of influenza season and that the flowchart in Figure 2.2 is a giant funnel. If you poured the subjects into the top of the flowchart, they would trickle through it over the course of the influenza season, some going one way and others going the other way. Each fork in your flowchart represents a chance event. The first fork in the flowchart thus represents the chances of becoming ill.

The chance that someone will become ill is equal to the incidence rate of influenza-like illness. Thus, if the incidence rate of influenza-like illness were forty-nine cases per 100 persons, forty-nine would end up in the "Becomes ill" box and fifty-one would land gently in the "Remains well" box. There is a chance that some ill people will need to see the doctor, will be hospitalized, and so on. The chance of each of these events must be collected.

While each fork in Figure 2.2 can be thought of as a probability, each box can be thought of as a cost. For example, people that end up in the "Becomes ill" box will probably take some medicine for the fever and sore throat and will incur costs for medications. If they decide to visit a doctor, they will incur the cost of a medical visit. Thus, listing the probabilities and costs is a relatively simple task once the disease has been fully charted out. Over the next few chapters, you will learn how to obtain and analyze the costs and probabilities used in a cost-effectiveness analysis. In Chapters Five and Six, you will learn how to work with the different costs and probabilities typically used in cost-effectiveness analysis.

CHAPTER THREE

WORKING WITH DATA

Overview

One of the things that makes cost-effectiveness analysis fun is that you get to criticize everyone else's hard work. One of the most often used sources of information in cost-effectiveness analysis is the medical literature, and you must be good at tearing it apart to be certain that you are obtaining the highest quality data possible. Data for cost-effectiveness analyses are also obtained from electronic data sources, expert opinions, the authors of published studies, or in some cases, from ongoing randomized controlled trials. While it is not as fun to criticize electronic data as it is to criticize the medical literature, the same basic sources of error are present in both.

In this chapter, you will receive the tools needed to evaluate sources of error and to work with data. To understand data commonly used in cost-effectiveness analysis, you will need to know how to work with rates, how to work with distributions, how to weight means, and how to critically evaluate the medical literature. In Chapter Five, you will apply what you learn in this chapter as you begin to obtain data for the cost-effectiveness study on strategies for preventing or treating influenza-like illness.

Project Map

1. Develop a research question.
2. Design your analysis.
3. **Understand the sources of error in data.**
4. Obtain data.
5. Organize data.
6. Construct a decision analysis model.
7. Calculate quality-adjusted life years.
8. Test and refine the decision analysis model.
9. Conduct a sensitivity analysis.
10. Prepare the study results for publication or presentation.

Review of Rates

To understand the medical literature and to use data in electronic datasets, you should have a basic understanding of rates and know how to calculate them. Rates fall into three broad categories: crude rates, specific rates, and adjusted rates. We will discuss each of these rates in this section.

A **crude rate** is defined as:

$$\frac{\text{number of events occurring in a given year}}{\text{susceptible population at the midpoint of the year}} \cdot 10^n$$

Equation 3.1

The "number of events" in the numerator of Equation 3.1 refers to the number of diseases, hospitalizations, deaths, and so on that occur in a population of people. The "susceptible population" in the denominator is the population in which an event might conceivably have occurred. For example, if we knew the number of cases of uterine cancer in the United States during 1999, the population at risk would be all females in the United States at the midpoint of 1999. The midpoint population is usually used because it is the best estimate of the average population over the period in which people could have experienced one of the events in the numerator. Occasionally, rates are defined over a shorter or longer period.

The exponential function 10^n is usually tacked onto the end of a rate to make the rate easier for consumers to understand. While it is not easy to grasp the meaning of the mortality rate for stroke, 0.00013, it is easy to grasp the mortality rate of stroke per 100,000 persons, 13 per 100,000 persons. Very common events are usually described per 100 persons (10^2), while very uncommon events, such as death, are usually described per 100,000 persons (10^5).

Crude rates apply to everyone in the population that could have experienced an event and therefore do not account for differences in the characteristics of different groups of people, such as the elderly or the poor. Older people are generally at much greater risk of disease and death than young people, and poor people are generally at much greater risk of disease and death than wealthy people. In cost-effectiveness analysis, it is important to examine differences between different subgroups in a population, so it is necessary to use **specific rates,** or rates specific to a particular group.

Age-specific rates refer to the number of events occurring in a particular age group. For instance, the rate of influenza among twenty- to twenty-five-year-olds is defined as:

$$\frac{\text{total cases of influenza among 20--25-year-old persons}}{\text{midpoint U.S. population, persons aged 20--25}} \cdot 10^n$$

Equation 3.2

One of the sad facts of life is that as people get older, the risk of illness and death increases. If we do not carefully account for differences in the rate of disease for each age group, our estimate of the rate of disease may lead to errors in our analysis.

Consider the case of a hypothetical cost-effectiveness analysis (CEA) cohort and a cohort obtained from a study in the literature, each with 164,000 subjects (see Table 3.1). Suppose that we wish to apply the mortality rates from the study to our cost-effectiveness cohort, but our cohort contains more elderly persons, and the study cohort contains more children and adolescents. Multiplying the age-specific mortality rates from the study in Column 1 by the number of subjects in Column 2 yields the predicted number of deaths (Column 3) among persons of different ages in our hypothetical cohort. In Row 9, we see that the total number of subjects in the cost-effectiveness cohort and the study cohort is identical, but the total number of deaths in the cost-effectiveness cohort is higher than the study cohort because there is a larger number of elderly persons subjected to a higher mortality rate. The crude mortality rate in each cohort is calculated by dividing the total number of deaths by the total number of subjects. For example, the crude mortality rate in the cost-effectiveness cohort is calculated by dividing the value in Column 3 Row 9 by the value in Column 2 Row 9. In Row 10, we see that the crude mortality rate is also higher in the cost-effectiveness cohort (2.86 deaths per 1,000 subjects) than it is in the study cohort (1.89 deaths per 1,000 subjects). If we were to use the crude mortality rate in that cost-effectiveness analysis, we would greatly underestimate the overall number of deaths in the cohort.

TABLE 3.1. HYPOTHETICAL EXAMPLE OF TWO POPULATIONS WITH EQUAL NUMBERS OF SUBJECTS AND IDENTICAL AGE-SPECIFIC MORTALITY RATES BUT DIFFERENT POPULATION DISTRIBUTIONS BY AGE.

Row		1	2	3	4	5
			CEA Cohort		*Study Cohort*	
	Age	Rate	Number Subjects	Deaths	Number Subjects	Deaths
1	0 to 10	0.00010	10,000	1.00	25,300	2.53
2	10 to 20	0.00015	15,000	2.25	37,060	5.56
3	20 to 30	0.00023	20,000	4.50	30,250	6.81
4	30 to 40	0.00045	40,000	18.00	24,200	10.89
5	40 to 50	0.00090	25,000	22.50	18,150	16.34
6	50 to 60	0.00270	30,000	81.00	12,100	32.67
7	60 to 70	0.00810	15,000	121.50	10,890	88.21
8	70+	0.02430	9,000	218.70	6,050	147.02
9	Total		164,000	469.45	164,000	310.01
10	Crude rate · 10^3			2.86		1.89

Adjusted rates (or standardized rates) are rates that account for differences in the characteristics of people in two or more populations. While specific rates apply to subgroups *within* a population, adjusted or standardized rates account for differences in the characteristics of subgroups *between* two or more populations. In cost-effectiveness analysis, rates are mostly used to estimate the risk of disease or death. Although adjusted rates can tell us how one population compares to another population, they cannot be used to calculate risk. Because standardized rates are not often employed in cost-effectiveness analysis, we will not discuss how they are adjusted in this book. Students wishing to explore the calculation of adjusted rates should consult an epidemiology textbook.

Prevalence Versus Incidence

Prevalence refers to the total number of cases of a disease in society (prevalence is also referred to as **prevalent cases**). The **prevalence ratio** is the total number of prevalent cases divided by the number of people at risk for the disease. The prevalence ratio is often erroneously described as **prevalence rate.** Because it refers to the proportion or percent of people with a disease, rather than the number of cases that *develop* over a period of time, it is a ratio rather than a rate.

Recall from Chapter One that the incidence refers to the number of *new* cases over a period of time, usually one year. The incidence rate refers to the number of new cases divided by the population at risk of the disease over a defined period of time. Therefore, the incidence rate of diabetes in the year 2000 would only include persons who were newly diagnosed with the condition in the year 2000.

The Relationship Between Risks and Rates

Rates, such as incidence rates and mortality rates, are usually good estimators of the risk of disease. The risk of disease is defined as:

$$\frac{\text{number of events over period}}{\text{susceptible population at the beginning of period}}$$

Equation 3.3

As you can see, the formula for rates, Equation 3.1, is very similar to the formula for risk, Equation 3.3. Notice that the denominator of Equation 3.1 incorporates the midpoint population for the year in which the events occurred as an estimator of the population in which the events can occur, while Equation 3.3 includes all subjects over the same period (Jeckel and others, 1996).

Suppose that we followed a group of 1,000 people over a year to see how many would develop influenza-like illness. If 410 subjects develop an influenza-like illness, the risk is 410/1,000 = 0.41. Rates, on the other hand, are typically calculated using information from the general population. In the general population, people are constantly moving, dying, and being born, so we usually estimate the denominator value using the midpoint of the period over which the events were tabulated. Because a rate does not usually provide information on how many people there were at the beginning of the period, it is an imperfect estimator of risk. Imagine that there was a horrible influenza epidemic in February that wiped out 15 percent of the population. If we were to use the midpoint population of that year, we would be underestimating the population in which the events (cases of influenza) actually occurred in, because these people were already dead by the time the census workers got around to counting them. This would result in an overestimation of the risk of influenza, because the denominator would be smaller than it would have been if the true population of persons at risk for influenza had been known.

Technically speaking, any calculation of the risk of influenza, or any other disease that occurs early or late in the year, should be adjusted to better reflect the risk of disease before it is used in a cost-effectiveness analysis. However, for most diseases, the difference between a risk and a rate will not be large. There are four things to consider when deciding whether a rate is a good estimator of risk.

First, the period over which the events occur in the rate should be short (one year or less). If the period is long, the population in the denominator is likely to change. Second, if the event is a death, the proportion of the population affected by the event in the rate should be small (less than 3 to 5 percent). If many people die from the event, the population that is susceptible to the event (the denominator) will shrink, resulting in a rate that is larger than the risk. Third, we must consider whether the event occurs once or many times over the period. This problem commonly occurs when examining hospitalization data and will be discussed in detail in Chapter Five.

Finally, we must be certain that the susceptible population in the denominator of the rate is truly the population at risk of the event. For example, if we knew the total number of influenza cases and were to apply Equation 3.1, it would be tempting to divide the total number of cases in each age group by the total population in each age group. However, some people in the general population will have received the influenza vaccine and will not be susceptible to infection. If we were epidemiologists rather than cost-effectiveness researchers, we might be more interested in the rate of influenza in the general population rather than the rate of influenza among unvaccinated people, because we would be more concerned with the severity of the epidemic than some abstract notion of risk. However, in cost-effectiveness analysis, we are more interested in knowing the chances of contracting influenza virus infections among unvaccinated and vaccinated people, and we should be careful to include only unvaccinated subjects in the denominator. In Chapter Five, we will learn how to calculate the risk of influenza and influenza-like illness using the percentage of people who have received the vaccine and the efficacy of the vaccine by age group.

Tips and tricks. Always be careful to remove the constant (10^n) multiplier when using rates to estimate the risk of disease. This may seem obvious, but some published rates appear in decimal form despite the 10^n multiplier. For example, the crude mortality rate per 100,000 persons for tuberculosis was 0.2 in 1997. To obtain the actual mortality rate, this number must be divided by 100,000, yielding a rate of 0.000002.

Risk over a Long Period of Time

Occasionally, it is necessary to calculate rates over a period of time longer than a year. For example, to study the number of deaths among foreign- and native-born black and white residents in New York City, Fang and others (1996) combined four years of mortality data (1988 to 1992) for each group and divided these deaths by the midpoint population of this four-year period (1990). It was necessary to combine data from four years to obtain reliable estimates of the total number of deaths among foreign-born black and white residents of New York City.

When events are summed over many years, the rate of a disease will differ from the risk of disease. As people move into the area under study or move out of the area under study, the denominator changes relative to the numerator. Unfortunately, there is no steadfast way to estimate the risk of a disease over a long period of time. If prospective studies are available, they can sometimes be used to estimate the risk of disease, but only if they address subjects that are demographically similar to the cohort you wish to study. (See "Review of Medical Study Designs" below.)

Understanding Error

For every measurement, rate, probability, and cost value used in a cost-effectiveness analysis, there exists a true mean value that is applicable to the hypothetical cohort. For example, there is an average risk of developing influenza-like illness in any given year. Unfortunately, only an omniscient being would know what this value is. Being fallible, humans must rely on imperfect scientific methods to estimate the true value of each input into a cost-effectiveness model. The extent to which the measured value of an input is representative of its real value is referred to as the **accuracy** of that measurement. If the value of the input is similar each time that it is measured, it is said to be **reproducible** or **reliable.**

Once you have obtained the articles from the medical literature that you need to conduct your cost-effectiveness analysis, you must determine whether the information you extract from these articles is likely to be accurate. To evaluate the data for accuracy, you will need to have a basic understanding of the common types of error, of statistical distributions (such as the normal distribution), and you will need to understand the different ways in which studies are conducted.

The more you read and systematically analyze the methods sections of original research articles, the more comfortable you will become with judging the quality of these articles. Though the basic elements of biostatistics and epidemiology presented in this section will be sufficient to understand the basics of error estimation, students who have never had exposure to these disciplines or who have never had to critically read the medical literature may require further study before they are ready to conduct a publishable cost-effectiveness analysis.

Common Types of Error

The most common types of error found in the medical literature are **random error** and **bias.** The extent to which a value is subject to random error is dependent on the size of the sample from which it was derived. Random error is sometimes referred to as **sampling error** and can be reduced by increasing the size of a statistical sample. We will see examples of how this works in the section "Frequency Distributions and Random Error."

Bias, or **non-random error,** occurs when error affects the data in a systematic way. For example, surveillance data are obtained by asking physicians to fill out a card and send it to a local health department when the physician sees a patient with a communicable disease of public health importance. Because only some physicians actually take the time to fill out the reporting card, reportable diseases are almost always undercounted. This type of error is called non-random because the error in the number of cases reported always occurs in one direction. Because non-random error is systematic, it is sometimes referred to as **systematic bias** or **differential error.**

To understand the difference between random error and non-random error, consider the case of two different people shooting arrows at a target. A highly trained but cross-eyed sharpshooter's target might look like Figure 3.1, while a clear-sighted amateur's target might look like Figure 3.2.

In the first case, the sharpshooter's problem was systematic error or bias. In the second case, the amateur's arrows did not miss the target in a systematic way. Rather, the arrows were randomly distributed around the target. Most medical data will either contain random or non-random error simply because it is very

FIGURE 3.1.   NON-RANDOM ERROR.

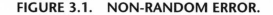

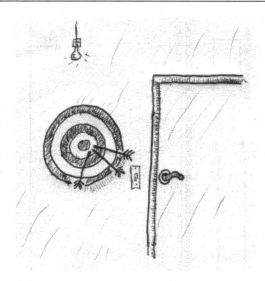

FIGURE 3.2.   RANDOM ERROR

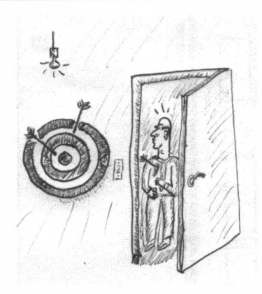

expensive to eliminate both types of error. For example, the National Health Interview Survey (NHIS) (Adams and others, 1996) is a health survey of about 100,000 people living in the United States. Because it is administered to a large number of people, it is relatively free of random error when it is used to tabulate the incidence or prevalence of common diseases. The NHIS asks subjects to recall whether they were ill over the preceding year and to record which diseases they had. Because people have trouble remembering whether they were sick, they are likely to forget the number of illnesses they had. (If this seems difficult to grasp, try to remember how many times you had a cold over the last year.) Thus, for some diseases, the NHIS will hit below the bull's eye (produce an undercount of the number of diseases respondents had), and it will do so consistently.

The NHIS has a sister survey, the National Health and Nutrition Examination Survey (NHANES), that is relatively free of bias; however, the sample size is small (Centers for Disease Control and Prevention, 2001). In this survey, the government parks a huge white van outside the door of unsuspecting citizens and invites them into the van to have their health checked. Once inside, they are poked, prodded, and tested for a number of diseases. By actually testing subjects, the study greatly reduces bias (non-random error), but the testing is very expensive, so only a small sample of subjects can be tested.

Managing Error in Cost-Effectiveness Analysis

Virtually every source of data you will use in cost-effectiveness research will be subject to random or non-random error. Cost-effectiveness researchers must therefore learn how to manage error and demonstrate how error affected the accuracy and reliability of the cost-effectiveness ratios they present to the people that read the analysis.

While random error is usually easy to measure, non-random error cannot always be perfectly quantified. Sometimes, though, it is possible to estimate the extent to which an input is subject to non-random error and adjust the input accordingly. This process is akin to nudging the sharpshooter depicted in Figure 3.1 a little to the left.

For example, the amount a hospital charges its clients is known to consistently be an overestimate of the actual cost of providing medical services (Chrischilles and Scholz, 1999). Because of this, health economists have studied and attempted to estimate the magnitude of difference between the dollar amount a hospital charges for a medical service and the actual cost of that medical service to society. Using this information, it is possible to reduce the systematic bias inherent in hospital charge data. You will learn how to adjust for systematic bias in charge data in Chapter Six. In the following section, "Frequency Distributions and Random Error," you will learn how to estimate the extent to which your data are subject to random error.

Still, understanding the error in your analysis is only three-quarters of the battle. You will also need to examine the impact this error might have on your cost-effectiveness ratios and, by using a sensitivity analysis, should present the effect of this error to the consumers of your study results. A sensitivity analysis is a way of testing the effect of error inherent to each input on the overall cost and effectiveness of each of the interventions under study. Suppose that you found that the cost of a treatment is between $5 and $10, and you choose to use $7.50 as the most likely value in the analysis. A sensitivity analysis will examine the effect of each extreme cost in the analysis, as well as values in between, on the overall cost of each strategy. (You will learn about this in Chapter Ten.)

Exercises 3.1–3.3

3.1. The National Health Interview Survey (NHIS) is subject to recall bias, because subjects are asked to remember the diseases and the number of medical visits they had over the past year. Would you expect the NHIS to undercount some diseases more than others? Which ones?

3.2. How might the methodology used to collect survey data affect the extent to which the data are subject to bias?

3.3. How might the type of bias you encounter affect the sensitivity analysis you perform on your study?

Frequency Distributions and Random Error

When we think of the rate of a disease, the cost of a medication, or the number of deaths that occur in a given year, we generally imagine these values as fixed because they are often presented like facts. In reality, however, these figures are often only approximations of the actual or true values. For example, after the 1999 West Nile virus outbreak in New York City, the newspapers reported that seven people died after developing the illness. In reality, the number of deaths reported was likely lower than the actual number of deaths, because some cases likely escaped the attention of health experts or were misdiagnosed by physicians. For the same reasons, when conducting a cost-effectiveness analysis it is important to recognize that the exact value for each input is generally not known, and that each input must be thought of as having a range of possible values. For example, if we were to evaluate the efficacy of public health interventions aimed to reduce the spread of the West Nile virus (such as spraying with pesticides to kill mosquitoes that transmit the virus), experts might assume that the actual number of deaths was somewhere between five and fifteen. All inputs used in a cost-effectiveness analysis may be thought of as **variables,** because the true value of the inputs you use in a cost-effectiveness analysis is not known. Variables do not have a fixed numerical value and are therefore represented by a range of possible values.

For example, suppose we obtain cholesterol test values from 100 people that vary between 115 and 290 mg/dl, the range is 290–115 = 175 mg/dl. Most of the subjects will have a cholesterol value somewhere close to the mean of these values, but a few will have values around 130, and a few others will have values around 270. If we were to list the number of people that had a cholesterol level between 115 and 135 mg/dl, 135 to 155 mg/dl, and so on, we would have a **frequency distribution** of these cholesterol levels (see Table 3.2).

If we were to show Table 3.2 graphically, it would take the form presented in Figure 3.3. The frequency of events can also be described as a probability. For example, the 30 values between 155 mg/dl and 175 mg/dl, out of the 100 subjects in the sample, can be expressed as 30/100 = 0.3. When frequency distributions are expressed as probabilities, they are known as **probability distributions.** Figure 3.4 shows the data in Table 3.2 as a probability distribution rather than a frequency distribution. Most frequency distributions or probability distributions

TABLE 3.2. FREQUENCY DISTRIBUTION OF HYPOTHETICAL CHOLESTEROL VALUES OBTAINED FROM 100 SUBJECTS.

Cholesterol Level (mg/dl)	Number of Subjects
115 to 135	3
135 to 155	15
155 to 175	30
175 to 195	25
195 to 215	12
215 to 235	7
235 to 255	5
255 to 275	2
275+	1
Total	100

in medicine form a roughly bell-shaped curve known as a **normal distribution** (also known as a **Gaussian distribution** to those of you who like to pay tribute to the people who bring us scientific discoveries). When perfectly bell-shaped, the peak of the bell (the part that you would hang by a string if it were actually a bell) represents the mean of the sample.

When the sample size is small, curves tend to look more like abstract representations of a bell rather than a perfectly drawn bell. (**Skewness** refers to a shift

FIGURE 3.3. GRAPHICAL REPRESENTATION OF THE 100 CHOLESTEROL VALUES IN TABLE 3.2.

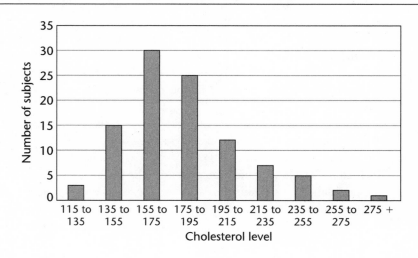

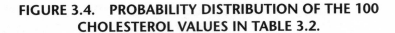

**FIGURE 3.4. PROBABILITY DISTRIBUTION OF THE 100
CHOLESTEROL VALUES IN TABLE 3.2.**

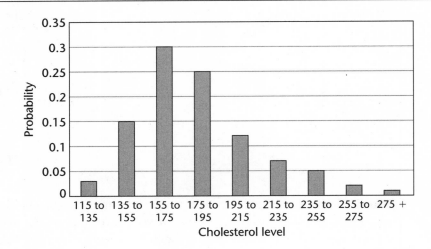

in the peak of a curve to the left or right). Though skewness is usually due to factors other than random error, Figure 3.3 will serve us well in understanding how the shape of a distribution changes with sample size and how statistical tests work.

If we were to increase the sample size however, the chances are that more people with high cholesterol levels would be randomly selected, thereby rounding out the curve; as the sample size taken from a normally distributed population increases, the distribution of values looks more and more like an actual bell. If we had a sample size of 1,000 subjects rather than 100 subjects, the probability distribution in Figure 3.4 would probably appear more like Figure 3.5. We can see that the mean value of the sample of 100 subjects (Figure 3.4) is slightly different than the mean of the sample of 1,000 subjects (Figure 3.5). Thus, as the sample size increases in an unbiased sample of values, the accuracy of the mean value is generally improved.

Statistical tests are tools for measuring the effects of sampling error on the differences between two sample means. Suppose for a moment that we obtained the cholesterol level of another 100 people (the dashed line in Figure 3.6). By chance, the mean of the new population appears to be higher than the mean of our original population. A statistical test (in this case, we might choose a student's t-test), would tell us whether the differences between these two population sample means were likely due to chance or were probably not due to chance. If we were to

FIGURE 3.5. HYPOTHETICAL PROBABILITY DISTRIBUTION OF 1,000 CHOLESTEROL TEST RESULTS.

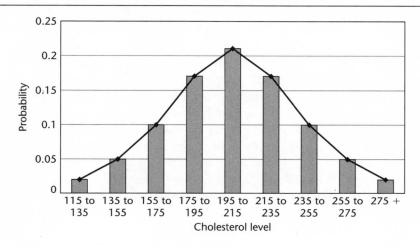

FIGURE 3.6. COMPARISON OF ORIGINAL SAMPLE OF 100 CHOLESTEROL LEVELS (SOLID LINE) WITH NEW SAMPLE OF 100 CHOLESTEROL LEVELS (DASHED LINE).

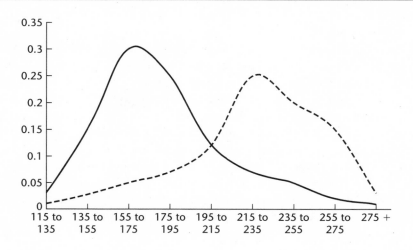

increase the sample size of each population in Figure 3.6, we would expect the two populations to increasingly appear as if they were a single population, taking on the appearance of Figure 3.5. Therefore, a smaller difference between sample means is needed for statistical significance as the sample size increases.

Studies in the medical literature often compare two or more sample means. For example, a sample of people who are treated with a cholesterol-lowering drug might be compared with a sample of people who are not. If the drug works, the mean cholesterol level in the treated population should be lower than the mean cholesterol level in the untreated population. However, if the sample size is small, differences between the two population means must be fairly large for a statistically significant difference to be detected. In other words, if the sample size is too small, it is less likely that a real difference between two population means will be detected. The ability of a statistical test to detect a difference between two population means is referred to as statistical **power.** When a real difference between two populations exists, but no difference is detected by statistical testing, it is referred to as a **type II error.** When a difference between two populations is detected by statistical testing, but no difference between the means actually exists, it is referred to as a **type I error.**

The possible values of true population means are often presented in the medical literature as measured sample means with **95 percent confidence intervals.** The 95 percent confidence intervals refer to *the range of possible values of the mean* over which we can be 95 percent certain the true value of the parent population mean is represented. Thus, if the mean cholesterol value in the above example were 178.5 mg/dl, and the 95 percent confidence values were 120 mg/dl and 260 mg/dl, we would know that there is only a 5 percent probability that the mean value of cholesterol levels in the real world is less than 120 or greater than 260.

We would also know that the chance of seeing a value of 255 mg/dl would be relatively small and the chance of seeing a value of 180 mg/dl would be relatively large. Notice in Figure 3.5, for example, that only about 0.05 percent of the subjects have a value in the 255 mg/dl to 275 mg/dl range, but over 20 percent of all subjects have a cholesterol level in the 175 mg/dl to 195 mg/dl range.

Usually, researchers are willing to accept a 5 percent probability that the difference between two samples is due to chance alone. When this threshold is set lower, the chance of making a type II error increases and the chance of a type I error decreases. Conversely, when this threshold is set higher, the chance of a type II error decreases and the chance of a type I error increases.

For each variable used in a cost-effectiveness analysis, there is a value that most likely represents the actual cost, probability, or effectiveness measure that we would expect to see in the real world. This number is sometimes called the **baseline value,** because it will be used to determine the principle cost-effectiveness ratio you will publish in your study. There will also be high and low values for this variable that are plausible (for example, the highest and lowest observed price of a drug on the free market). Because the chance that you will actually observe extreme values in the real world is very small, each variable included in a cost-effectiveness analysis can be weighted according to the chance that it might be observed. For instance, referring to Figure 3.5, we see that there is a 22 percent chance of observing the mean cholesterol value and a 5 percent chance of seeing a value in the 135 to 155 range. We will discuss how different values can be weighted and tested in a sensitivity analysis in Chapter Ten.

In cost-effectiveness analysis, researchers will often know that the baseline value is pretty likely and that the high and low values are pretty unlikely, but they will not have any information on the distribution of these values. In these instances, the **triangular distribution** is typically used (see Figure 3.7). Let us return to the example of drug costs. Suppose you call ten pharmacies across the country to obtain the cost of oseltamivir. The ten values you obtain might average $53 for a full course of the medication. While the discount drug chains you called were able to sell this medication for less than the mean value, the expensive drug boutique on Rodeo Drive sold it for more. The chance that the actual mean value of this medication is as high as the one you found on Rodeo

FIGURE 3.7.   EXAMPLE OF A TRIANGULAR DISTRIBUTION.

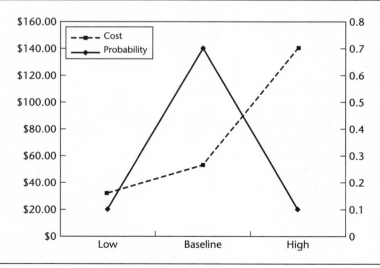

Note: The solid line represents the probabilistic weight assigned to each cost value (dashed line).

Drive is very small, and the chance that the mean value is as low as the cheapest drugstore blowout in Joplin, Missouri is very small. Though you do not have a true statistical sample and do not know the distribution of the values, you want to have a way of telling your decision analysis model that these extreme high and low values are very unlikely. Because you are not certain exactly *how* unlikely they are, you can simply distribute the probabilities in a triangular shape around the baseline value of $53.

When a triangular distribution is used, values that are more likely representative of the true mean (the baseline values) are assigned a heavier weight than values that represent less likely estimates of the true mean value. In Figure 3.7, the mean cost (about $53 on the left y-axis) is assigned a high probability of occurring (about 0.7 on the right y-axis), based on a subjective assessment of the chance that this is the most likely value for the cost of oseltamivir. Likewise, the extreme low value and extreme high value are subjectively assigned a low probability of occurring. We shall return to this discussion in Chapter Ten.

Calculating Weighted Means

Weighted means are commonly encountered in cost-effectiveness analysis. Imagine that you had three groups of people that were randomly selected from the United States population to have their blood cholesterol levels measured. Suppose further that you wanted to know the mean cholesterol level of all of the subjects together. If you knew the number of people in each group and the mean cholesterol value of each of these groups, you could estimate the overall mean cholesterol level of all of the subjects combined by calculating a weighted mean. A weighted mean is the average value of a set of numbers that are each weighted by some factor, such as the number of subjects in a group.

In cost-effectiveness analysis, it is often necessary to calculate weighted means for the data that you will ultimately use in your cost-effectiveness analysis. If data from many small cross-sectional surveys are available, a weighted mean can improve the accuracy of a parameter estimate. It is also useful for adjusting data retrieved from data extraction tools or from printed tabulations of data. A weighted mean is calculated using the formula:

$$\frac{\begin{array}{c}(\text{events in population 1} \cdot \text{number of persons in population 1} \\ + \text{ events in population 2} \cdot \text{number of persons in population 2})\end{array}}{(\text{number of persons in population 1} + \text{number of persons in population 2})}$$

Equation 3.4

Evaluating Study Limitations

In this section, you will learn how to identify limitations of studies and will be presented with some tips for avoiding research efforts that contain mistakes. However, identifying mistakes on the part of researchers is tricky (and sometimes impossible) given the limited amount of information published in the methods section of a research paper.

Review of Medical Study Designs

Medical studies are usually conducted to evaluate risks or rates. For example, they might indicate the risks associated with smoking or the risk of morbidity or mortality among people treated with a new medication relative to untreated people. Alternatively, they might indicate the probability that a screening test will correctly identify people who have a disease. Because cost-effectiveness analyses are constructed using the probabilities of different events, virtually all cost-effectiveness analyses will require information from medical studies.

Medical studies are usually described according to how they follow subjects over time. While cross-sectional studies give us a slice of information at one point in time, retrospective studies examine factors that occurred in the past (*retro-* = "backward" and *-spective* = "looking"), and prospective studies are designed to examine events that will occur in the future. Each of these different study designs has different limitations, and it is important to understand them.

Cross-sectional studies. In a cross-sectional study, data are obtained at one point in time. Cross-sectional studies are useful for obtaining the prevalence of disease or enumerating the number of people at risk for a particular disease (for example, identifying the number of smokers in different age groups). In Chapter Five, we will examine the Behavior Risk Factor Surveillance System (BRFSS), a cross-sectional survey, to determine the percentage of adults who are vaccinated against the influenza virus (http://apps.nccd.cdc.gov/brfss/index.asp).

Retrospective studies. Retrospective trials are generally designed to identify risk factors for disease. In a retrospective study, people with a disease are paired up with a control group of people who are similar in most ways but do not have the disease. Each group is then examined for a past exposure to some risk factor for the disease (see Figure 3.8). For example, a group of new mothers whose children had cleft palate might be asked about a potential contributing cause, such as having taken a medication while pregnant. A group of mothers whose children were free of birth defects and who gave birth in the same hospital might then be interviewed to determine whether they too had taken that particular medication during pregnancy.

FIGURE 3.8.   RETROSPECTIVE STUDY DESIGN.

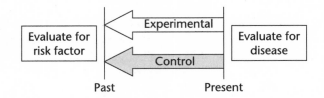

Retrospective studies are especially susceptible to bias. In a retrospective study, recall bias occurs when the group without the disease fails to remember whether they were exposed to the risk factor. In the case of the new mothers, those mothers whose children had a birth defect may be much more motivated to try to remember whether they had taken medications during pregnancy than those who did not. If the control group reports having taken fewer medications simply because people in this group did not remember having taken the medication, the medication may be falsely implicated as a cause of the birth defect.

Another common type of bias specific to retrospective studies is **confounding.** This occurs when the control group does not match the experimental group with respect to another risk factor for the disease. For example, one study examining the relationship between coffee drinking and heart disease found a strong association. However, because coffee drinkers are also significantly more likely to smoke than people who do not drink coffee, the control group contained fewer smokers than the experimental group (Thelle and others, 1983; Urgert and others, 1996). (Do not worry, coffee was subsequently found to be relatively safe.)

Prospective studies. Like retrospective trials, prospective trials are generally designed to identify risk factors for disease. Prospective trials offer a number of advantages over retrospective trials. First, they reduce bias by examining a group of people with a putative risk factor and a group of people without the potential risk factor before they develop disease, then follow them over time to see whether the people with the risk factor are more likely to develop the disease (see Figure 3.9). Second, they allow for the calculation of incidence rates and **risk ratios.** A risk ratio indicates how much more likely people with the risk factor are to develop disease than those who do not have the risk factor.

The risk ratio is calculated as the incidence rate of disease among people with the risk factor over the incidence rate of disease in people without the risk factor, or:

$$\text{risk ratio} = \text{incidence}_{\text{risk factor}}/\text{incidence}_{\text{no risk factor}}$$

Equation 3.5

FIGURE 3.9.   PROSPECTIVE STUDY DESIGN.

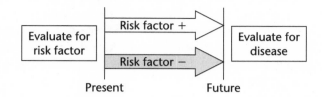

which is often written as:

$$\text{risk}_{\text{risk factor}}/\text{risk}_{\text{no risk factor}}$$

Equation 3.6

The risk ratio is also referred to as **relative risk.** (Both are conveniently abbreviated "RR.")

Tips and tricks. Technically speaking, Equation 3.5 refers to a rate ratio rather than a risk ratio. This term is sometimes used when it is important to distinguish between a ratio of rates rather than a ratio of risks. In practice, these terms are often used interchangeably. (See "Review of Rates" earlier in this chapter.)

The risk ratio produces a number that is easy for most people to understand. For example, the relative risk of developing lung cancer among smokers is about 9.0, indicating that smokers are at nine times the risk of developing lung cancer as non-smokers (Doll and Hill, 1956). Retrospective trials allow for the calculation of odds ratios rather than risk ratios, a measure that only reflects risk when applied to relatively rare conditions. The use of relative measures of risk will be thoroughly described under the "Efficacy and Measures of Risk" section in Chapter Five.

Prospective studies are expensive to conduct and are therefore often generally applied only to major research questions relating to common diseases. Older prospective trials were often only targeted toward white male cohorts, and the results may not always be generalizable to other populations (this limitation will be discussed in more detail in the "Evaluating the Medical Literature" section).

Another problem with prospective studies is that subjects who are willing to participate in a study may differ from those not willing to participate. People who are willing to take part in a randomized controlled trial without reimbursement may be healthier, more ideological, or more affluent than people who do not. This can distort the overall severity or impact of a disease. Imagine a study that examines the overall impact of smoking on health outcomes. If mostly healthy subjects enroll in the study, people with diabetes might be excluded from both the experimental and control groups. Because a diabetic who smokes is at much greater risk of heart disease than the cumulative risk of both of these conditions separately, smoking may appear to be less harmful than it really is.

The tendency for volunteer study subjects to be healthier than the general population is called the **healthy volunteer effect.** If we were to evaluate a non-smoking intervention in a cost-effectiveness analysis using data obtained from a cohort of mostly healthy smokers, the benefits of smoking cessation would be artificially reduced. Likewise, people who drop out of studies differ from people who stick with a study to the end. For example, in a famous prospective study of risk factors for heart disease conducted in Framingham, Massachusetts, subjects who dropped out of the investigation were later found to have a much greater risk of heart attack and death than the subjects who stayed in the study (Dawber and others, 1951). Prospective studies are commonly referred to as **longitudinal studies,** because patients are followed over time.

Randomized controlled trials. The randomized controlled trial is probably the most often used source of information in the field of cost-effectiveness analysis. A randomized controlled trial is a type of prospective study designed to determine whether those who receive a particular intervention have better health outcomes than those who do not. In this design, subjects are randomly assigned to either an intervention group or a placebo group (see Figure 3.10). They are then followed over time to see if there are differences in the rate or severity of disease between the two groups. The only difference between a randomized controlled trial and other prospective studies is that some subjects in other prospective studies have something (such as a smoking problem) that may increase their risk of disease, and some subjects in a randomized controlled trial are given something (such as smoking cessation advice) that may reduce their risk of disease.

In a randomized controlled trial, it is possible to control for the placebo effect (see Exhibit 3.1). Unfortunately, in the field of cost-effectiveness analysis we are interested in how interventions work in the real world. In the real world,

FIGURE 3.10.   RANDOMIZED CONTROLLED TRIAL STUDY DESIGN.

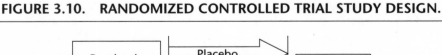
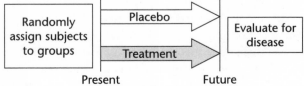

EXHIBIT 3.1.   PLACEBO CONTROLLED STUDIES.

The placebo effect is a powerful biopsychological phenomenon. People administered dummy pills or sham surgery will often experience improved health outcomes relative to those that do not. For example, when coronary artery bypass surgery was first evaluated, subjects with angina (chest pain) randomized to the placebo group were given nothing more than a superficial cut on the skin of their chest. (Today, this practice would probably not be deemed ethical.) Subjects in the experimental group underwent open-heart surgery. While 70 percent of the patients who received the surgery reported long-term improvement, all of the patients in the placebo group reported long-term improvement (Fisher, 2000).

people who take a medication benefit from both the treatment effect and the placebo effect. When a medical intervention is compared with a placebo, and the placebo has an impact on the illness under study, the cost-effectiveness of an intervention will be underestimated. Consider the case of clinical evaluations for minoxidil solution, a topical treatment for male pattern baldness. Balding men do not usually spontaneously grow hair. However, this is exactly what happened with men in the placebo group of the randomized controlled trial evaluating the clinical efficacy of this drug. If we were to measure the effectiveness of the drug relative to the placebo, the drug would appear to be less effective than if it were measured relative to each subject's hair pattern when the study was started.

Other subconscious cues, such as the body language of a researcher, can also have an impact upon treatment outcomes in a randomized controlled trial. For this reason, the researchers that actually interact with patients are often made unaware of whether the patient has received the intervention or not. When neither the patients nor the researchers that interact with the patients know who received the placebo and who received the treatment, the study is said to be **double blinded.**

To keep both the patients and the researchers unaware of who is in the experimental group and who is in the placebo group, patients must be randomly assigned to either group. The status of each patient is hidden until the end of the study, at which point the study is "uncovered" and the effects of the intervention are examined. It is therefore important to examine the characteristics of the patients that were **randomly allocated** to the placebo group or the control group (these characteristics are almost always presented in the first table in the article describing the study). Sometimes chance works against researchers, and subjects receiving the placebo have a lower average income or smoke more often than subjects in the intervention group. When the subjects in the placebo group happen to have more risk factors for disease than the subjects in the experimental group, or imperfections in the randomization process occur, the intervention may appear to be more or less effective than it would have been under perfect conditions. For these reasons, it is important to make sure that the experimental and control groups used in the study are demographically similar.

Meta-analysis. A meta-analysis is a systematic analysis of many studies published in the medical literature. In this design, data are obtained from different prospective or randomized controlled trials and then combined into a single study. For example, if one study evaluated a treatment for heart disease in Chicago and another study evaluated the same treatment using a similar study design in San Francisco, the subjects in the experimental group from each study would be combined into a single group. Likewise, the subjects from the control groups would be combined into a single group. The effect of the treatment on the combined experimental group relative to the combined control group would then be analyzed.

As with any other study, the quality of meta-analysis studies is variable. One recent meta-analysis in a major peer-reviewed journal found that mammography was not effective at reducing mortality rates for breast cancer (Gotzshe and Olsen, 2000). However, the authors chose to exclude all of the studies demonstrating the clinical effectiveness of this technique because they felt that these studies had problems with the random allocation of subjects. Most experts agree, however, that mammography is effective because the mortality rate for breast cancer has declined more rapidly than improvements in treatments would suggest.

When many studies exist pertaining to a particular parameter of interest in a cost-effectiveness analysis, cost-effectiveness researchers will sometimes conduct their own meta-analysis on these studies. For example, if it were necessary to generate an estimate of the incidence rate of influenza infection for the United States, but only regional estimates were available, a meta-analysis of all of these studies might provide a better estimate of the rate of influenza nationwide. Meta-analytic techniques are too advanced for an introductory textbook, and we encourage students to read further before attempting to conduct a meta-analysis on their own.

Primary cost-effectiveness studies. In rare instances, a longitudinal study will be primarily directed at collecting cost and effectiveness data. In this study design, a group of subjects are administered a standard of care intervention and one or more health interventions with the primary goal of determining the cost-effectiveness of a particular strategy. In other words, subjects are allowed to behave as they might in a real-world setting and costs are measured as they are incurred.

For instance, if the study were evaluating a new antibiotic, patients may see the physician as they normally do. The time spent during the medical encounter is measured, the cost of the antibiotics is recorded, and no unusual measures are taken to ensure that they have taken all of their medications. If patients have side effects to the medication, the researchers determine whether the side effects led to additional medical visits or other costs. Finally, the time patients spend receiving caregiving, driving, and other costs are recorded.

The advantage of a primary cost-effectiveness analysis is that most sources of error can be carefully controlled, costs can be obtained directly from the study, and cost-effectiveness analyses can simulate real-world conditions better than standard longitudinal analyses. Unfortunately, try as the researchers may, this approach still yields results obtained under experimental conditions, rather than real-world conditions. For instance, patients might be followed in university hospitals where medical care differs from that in other clinical settings. In a traditional cost-effectiveness analysis (an analysis that uses secondary sources of data), it is often possible to examine longitudinal studies from many different parts of the country and in different clinical settings, improving the validity of the analysis.

Exercise 3.4

3.4. Would recall bias generally make observed risks more apparent or less apparent in retrospective studies? How might this problem be managed in a cost-effectiveness analysis?

Evaluating the Medical Literature

When evaluating the medical literature, there are two questions that should immediately come to the cost-effectiveness researcher's mind. The first is, "Was this study carefully designed and executed?" The second is, "Are the results of this study generalizable to my study population?" If these two questions are consistently asked, cost-effectiveness researchers should be able to get a better idea of whether the data that they wish to extract from the study will be useful. Let us look at these two questions in more detail.

Are the results generalizable to your study population? A study with **external validity** will produce results that are generalizable to groups other than those under study. One criticism of medical research conducted in the twentieth century is that the majority of studies examined only the health effects of white men, raising questions as to whether the study results were valid for other groups in the United States. It may be the case that one type of antihypertensive medication is better for African-American males while another is better for white women, but these differences in treatment response are usually not known because those cohorts were not represented in the studies. Sometimes, the results of studies are undergeneralized as well. Until recently, women with crushing chest pain were sometimes sent home from the emergency room simply because heart disease was thought of as a "male problem."

Studies applied to specific subgroups of a population can be especially problematic for cost-effectiveness researchers. For example, a cost-effectiveness analysis examining screening mammography versus no screening among African-American females would require tricky assumptions on the part of researchers, because most studies of the effectiveness of screening and the effectiveness of various treatments were conducted on white women.

The following subsets of questions should help you determine whether the results of a published study are generalizable to your study population:

- Was the study population localized to a particular geographic region? Results of studies conducted in a specific geographic region of the country may not apply to all persons nationwide. For example, the rate of influenza-like illness in a study conducted in New York City (where winters are cold and people are packed into subways) may not apply to persons living in Los Angeles (where the weather is nice and people spend most of their time alone in cars). It would be best to obtain a national estimate of influenza-like illness or estimates from other parts of the country for comparison.
- Are the characteristics of the subjects in the study similar to the characteristics of the population you are studying? Often, researchers will conduct studies in specific settings such as a Veterans Affairs hospital or in a health maintenance organization (HMO). In the former case, the patients may be likely to be older and have many coexisting illnesses. In the latter case, the subjects may be more likely to be employed and middle or upper middle class than the general population.
- What were the inclusion and exclusion criteria? Sometimes, studies examining a treatment for a disease will exclude people with preexisting medical conditions. For example, studies on the efficacy of the influenza vaccine almost always exclude subjects that have diseases that put them at high risk of hospitalization or death from influenza virus infections. Subjects with chronic diseases are excluded from vaccine efficacy studies, because subjects in the placebo group have a moderate risk of death if they actually contract influenza. Since we are only interested in the efficacy of the vaccine in healthy adults, this research will be useful to us. However, if we were interested in the efficacy of the vaccine in *all* adults, the results of these studies would be of little use, because an important subset of our hypothetical cohort would have been excluded ("Prevention," 1999).

- Does the definition of illness differ in any meaningful way from the definition you are using, or does it differ from the definition used in other studies you are including in your analysis? We will discuss this problem in detail in Chapter Five.

Are the study results valid at all? Studies may contain design problems that limit the accuracy of the results or introduce bias. These problems compromise the study's **internal validity.** For example, a study that has a small number of subjects might exaggerate or underestimate the efficacy of a treatment or screening test you wish to evaluate.

Likewise, a study that contains systematic bias might produce results that underestimate or overestimate the difference between an experimental and control group. Consider a randomized controlled trial that is evaluating the efficacy of a cholesterol-lowering drug in reducing mortality. Suppose that, by chance, the group receiving the treatment is slightly younger than the group that is not receiving the treatment. The efficacy of the treatment might be overestimated because younger people are less likely to die over the duration of the study than older people. There are a number of common pitfalls in study design that can introduce non-random error, which are outlined by the following questions:

- Did the subjects who failed to complete the study differ from subjects who successfully completed the study? Oftentimes, subjects who drop out of a study or subjects who fail to complete surveys are sicker than the general population or at higher risk of disease. If a large number of subjects failed to complete a prospective study, the risk ratio for the factor under study is likely to be larger in the real world than in the study. A survey with a large number of non-completers may undercount the total number of cases of a disease. As a very general rule of thumb, at least 80 percent of the subjects should complete the study. However, if 100 percent of the subjects in the group without the risk factor under study completed a prospective study and 80 percent of the subjects with the risk factor completed the study, we can expect the results to be skewed.
- If the study was retrospective, what were some of the potential sources of bias? Retrospective studies are subject to many different types of bias, such as recall bias. (Some of these will be discussed further in Chapter Five.) The direction of the bias (the way in which the bias may affect study results) should be taken into consideration when including data from these studies in your cost-effectiveness analysis.
- If the study is a randomized controlled trial, how did the treatment and placebo groups differ in demographic composition and risk factors for disease? In an economic analysis of influenza vaccination (Bridges and others, 2000), a

significantly higher number of subjects exposed to secondhand smoke at home were randomly assigned to receive the influenza vaccine than subjects who were randomly assigned to receive the placebo injection (see Appendix II) in the 1997–1998 influenza season. In that season, the influenza vaccine was poorly matched to the circulating strains of influenza virus, and the subjects who received the vaccine had higher rates of influenza-like illness and more medical visits than subjects in the placebo group.

• Did the study examine the efficacy of a screening test in reducing morbidity or mortality? Studies on the efficacy of screening tests are subject to unique sources of error, **lead-time bias** and **length bias,** which will be discussed in detail in Chapter Five (see "Efficacy and Measures of Risk").

Other ways of identifying error in the medical literature. It has become standard practice for authors to discuss the limitations of their studies in the discussion section of their research articles. Here, you will often find a good deal of qualified language surrounding the major problems with the analysis. In some cases, authors provide in-depth discussions of the problems they encountered with their research. If an editorial accompanies the article, it may identify additional problems with the research. A final forum for identifying problems with a study is to read the letters to the editor in the months following the study. Outside readers who identify problems with a research article will often write to the journal to point them out. Medline searches will help identify the volume and issue in which the letters were published.

CHAPTER FOUR

FINDING THE DATA YOU NEED

Overview

Cost-effectiveness studies often synthesize information from a number of different sources. Usually, researchers require information on the incidence or prevalence of a disease, risk ratios, and costs, among many other inputs. These inputs can be obtained from the medical literature, from electronic datasets, from unpublished sources (such as ongoing longitudinal studies), or from experts on the disease you are studying. In this chapter, we will examine different sources of publicly available electronic data, briefly discuss the ways in which alternative data sources can be used, and forward a system for organizing the data you collect.

Project Map

1. Develop a research question.
2. Design your analysis.
3. Understand the sources of error in data.
4. **Obtain data.**
5. Organize data.
6. Construct a decision analysis model.
7. Calculate quality-adjusted life years.
8. Test and refine the decision analysis model.

9. Conduct a sensitivity analysis.
10. Prepare the study results for publication or presentation.

Finding Information in the Medical Literature

It is generally easy to find the medical literature that you will need for your cost-effectiveness analysis. PubMed is a popular and comprehensive search engine for scientific research that is run by the government and can be accessed on the Internet at http://www.ncbi.nlm.nih.gov/entrez/query.fcgi. This Web page has a helpful tutorial that will assist you in finding the literature in which you are interested.

As you learned in the last chapter, the studies you use should be evaluated for sampling error and non-random error along with other problems with the study design. Electronic datasets are subject to the same types of error. Unlike studies in the medical literature, though, it is relatively easy to identify error in an electronic dataset, because most datasets are accompanied by detailed descriptions of the limitations of the data they contain.

Using Electronic Datasets

Health datasets provide a wealth of information that is useful for conducting cost-effectiveness analyses. Using these datasets, you can obtain much of the information on medical costs, disease prevalence rates, hospital discharge rates, or just about any type of cross-sectional health-related data in which you are interested. Other datasets provide information related to transportation, crime, and education, all of which are useful for estimating the non-medical costs of medical interventions or diseases.

Though the words "electronic" and "dataset" instill a sense of fear in most people, obtaining data from electronic databases is not as difficult as it sounds. In fact, there are a number of tools designed specifically to make the information that electronic datasets contain more accessible to nontechnical types. These tools take the form of computer programs or Web pages that guide would-be researchers through the step-by-step process of obtaining the information they need. These programs or Web pages are sometimes referred to as **data extraction tools.**

It is also possible to obtain cost-effectiveness data using printed tabulations of these datasets. These are large documents containing lists of useful data, such as hospitalization rates or mortality rates, as well as the most commonly used **cross-tabulations.** A cross-tabulation lists the outcome of interest (such as a hospitalization rate) by some other characteristic (such as gender). Appendix III, for example, is a cross tabulation listing the United States population by age-interval and the year the census was taken. To find out how many five- to nine-year-olds there were in 1997, simply follow the row values for five- to nine-year-olds to the column labeled 1997. (There were 19,749,000.) Virtually all major health datasets are either associated with a data extraction tool or are available as a printed tabulation (see Table 4.1).

For students who are more experienced in using statistical analysis programs, it is also possible to download an entire dataset and then obtain the information you need using a statistical software package. The advantage of working with an entire dataset is that you will have more control over the ways in which different pieces of information are combined, making it possible to conduct more sophisticated analyses. The disadvantage is that most datasets require familiarity with a statistical package and sometimes require that the user format all of the data by hand. Unformatted datasets contain seemingly random lists of numbers or words that the researcher must put into some semblance of order. Because this is a beginner's textbook, we will focus on obtaining data from sources that do not require the use of a statistical software package. As you build the sample cost-effectiveness analysis evaluating strategies to prevent or treat influenza-like illness, you will use printed data tabulations or data extraction tools rather than unformatted electronic data.

In this section, we will explore ways to identify the sources of data you will need and provide Internet links to most of the major sources of data useful for cost-effectiveness analysis in the United States. We will also examine the different data extraction tools that are available in the United States. While it is not possible to list all of the data sources commonly used for international cost-effectiveness research here, most governments collect health data and make that data publicly available. Analyses conducted in developing countries will most often have to rely upon the medical literature or ongoing prospective trials; however, the World Health Organization (WHO) maintains useful data repositories (http://www.who.int). In the following sections, we will discuss how you can obtain printed data tabulations, how to obtain data from ongoing studies, and how to estimate an input using expert opinion.

Finding the Electronic Data That You Need

Though electronic datasets are rich sources of information, you will have to familiarize yourself with the contents and limitations of each of the datasets commonly used in cost-effectiveness analysis. Once pointed in the right direction, though, it will be relatively easy for you to find the information that you are looking for.

TABLE 4.1.   MAJOR U.S. HEALTH DATASETS AVAILABLE TO THE PUBLIC.

Dataset	Description
Healthcare Cost and Utilization Project-3 (HCUP-3) ⬚ www.ahrq.gov	This dataset contains information on hospital discharges from 22 states. Data may be obtained for specific states or weighted for national averages. Contains information on the number of discharges by disease, and hospital charges.
National Hospital Discharge Survey (NHDS) www.cdc.gov/nchs ⬚	A smaller sample of hospitals than the HCUP-3. This dataset is available in electronic and published form.
Medical Provider Analysis and Review www.hcfa.gov/stats/medpar/medpar.htm	This dataset contains charges to Medicare, reimbursable charges, and actual payments made by Medicare. It is useful for formulating cost-to-charge ratios or for determining hospital charges by diagnosis-related groups (DRGs).
Medical Expenditure Panel Survey (MEPS) www.meps.ahrq.gov ⬚ ⬚	Contains survey data from clinicians, nursing homes, and the general population regarding health care use, expenditures, insurance status, and many other useful variables. Useful for generating ambulatory care costs.
National Ambulatory Medical Care Survey (NAMCS) ⬚ www.cdc.gov/nchs	This is a national survey of physicians that includes over 36,000 patient records for ambulatory care services. Does not include hospital outpatient or emergency room data.
National Hospital Ambulatory Medical Care Survey (NHAMCS) ⬚ www.cdc.gov/nchs	This dataset supplements the NAMCS with hospital and emergency room data.
National Nursing Home Survey (NNHS) www.cdc.gov/nchs	This dataset provides information about 8,000 randomly selected nursing home patients.
National Home and Hospice Care Survey (NHHCS) www.nchs.gov	This is a national sample of 1,500 home and hospice care agencies.
Surveillance, Epidemiology, and End Results System (SEER) ⬚ www-seer.ims.nci.nih.gov	This dataset contains information on most major cancers. Variables specific to race, gender, and country of birth are linked to census data.
National Health and Nutrition Examination Survey (NHANES). ⬚ www.cdc.gov/nchs	This nationally representative dataset contains data from physical examinations and clinical and laboratory tests. Prevalence data are available for specific diseases and health conditions.
National Health Interview Survey (NHIS) ⬚ ⬚ www.cdc.gov/nchs	A nationally representative survey of the health status, mobility limitations, and disease for non-institutionalized persons. Also contains the total number of medical visits for each subject.

(Continued)

TABLE 4.1. (*Continued*)

Dataset	Description
Multiple Cause of Death Datafile www.cdc.gov/nchs 🖹	This dataset contains information on all deaths by ICD-9 code and includes the decedent's place of birth, education level, location of the death, as well as the underlying cause of death and other conditions the decedent had.
Combined Health Information Database http://chid.nih.gov 🔧	Contains a number of datasets related to chronic disease.
Bureau of Labor Statistics www.bls.gov	Government agency that tracks wages for many professions. This is useful in estimating time costs for patients who undergo an intervention.

🔧 Indicates that a data extraction tool is available.

🖹 Indicates that printed tabulation is available.

Every health dataset was designed to meet a particular research need. Therefore, datasets tend to have themes, much the same way that a novel will have a central protagonist and plot. Like novels, some datasets essentially replicate the themes of other datasets with varying degrees of success. They differ from novels, though, in that researchers must often examine data from all of the similar datasets to get the full story about the information they are looking for.

For example, the National Hospital Discharge Survey (NHDS) is a dataset containing hospital discharges for approximately 300,000 patients from about 500 hospitals (474 hospitals in 1997). These data were obtained from both electronic hospital tapes and transcripts of actual hospital records (Owings and Lawrence, 1999). The Healthcare Cost and Utilization Project-3 (HCUP-3) only contains data obtained from hospital billing systems, but it is composed of a weighted sample of approximately half of all the hospital discharges in the United States (Healthcare Cost and Utilization Project, 2001). Both datasets contain information on the total number of discharges by diagnosis, information on the patients' demographics, and discharge status (for example, whether the patient was discharged to home, died in the hospital, or was discharged to a nursing home). Because the NHDS was (in part) built using actual hospital transcripts, it contains less non-random error than the HCUP-3 dataset. The HCUP-3, on the other hand, is derived from a very large sample and is relatively free of sampling error.

Table 4.1 provides a description of the most commonly used datasets in cost-effectiveness analysis, Internet links to the agency that collected the data, and information on the availability of data extraction tools or printed summaries of the data. To find the data you are looking for, read through the descriptions of each dataset in the table and then visit the Web site of the agency that collected the data. When looking for a particular input, such as the prevalence of a disease, refer to Table 4.2, which lists the sources of information that researchers typically turn to when in need of commonly used parameters in cost-effectiveness analyses.

One unique source of cost data listed in Table 4.2, the Health Care Financing Administration (HCFA), provides data on the costs associated with ambulatory surgical centers, laboratory fee schedules, physician fees, and home health care costs, among other useful costs, and it contains nationwide data as well as data specific to different regions of the country. To obtain a complete list of the datasets produced by HCFA, visit http://hcfa.gov/stats/pcat0401.pdf. Another HCFA site (www.hcfa.gov/stats/carrpuf.htm) provides the researcher with a complete package of spreadsheets, manuals, and coding books relating to physician payments (Macintosh users must click on the ".zip" files rather than the ".exe"

TABLE 4.2.   DATASETS USEFUL FOR FINDING FREQUENTLY NEEDED COST-EFFECTIVENESS PARAMETERS

Variable	Possible Sources
Prevalence rate	NHIS, medical literature, NHANES.
Incidence rate	Medical literature, NHIS (acute diseases only), NHANES, SEER.
Mortality rate	Medical literature, Multiple Cause of Death Dataset, Mortality follow back, SEER, WONDER.
Risk ratio	Medical literature.
Population data	U.S. Bureau of the Census, WONDER.
Disease severity/distribution	NHIS, NHANES, SEER.
Medical utilization (number of hospitalizations, outpatient visits, and so on)	HCFA, HCUP-3, Medicaid, NMES, SEER-Medicare, NAMCS.
Cost of medical care	HCFA, medical literature, HCUP-3, Medicaid, NMES, SEER-Medicare, BLS.*
Cost of transportation, labor, environmental impact, and so on	U.S. Bureau of the Census, BLS,* medical literature, Internet search engines, University of Michigan.

*BLS = Bureau of Labor Statistics.

Note: See text and Table 4.1 for descriptions of these datasets.

files). Note that HCFA plans to change its name to the "Centers for Medicare and Medicaid Services."

Periodically updated versions of Table 4.1 and Table 4.2 are maintained on-line at New School University's Program in Cost-Effectiveness and Outcomes at http://www.pceo.org/datasources.html.

Which Dataset Should You Use?

Students often wonder whether it is best to begin a search for a piece of information in the medical literature or whether it is better to start with electronic data. The answer is simple. You should always obtain as much information as possible about any parameter you are looking for and should look to both sources. Before the advent of data extraction tools, researchers sometimes chose to forgo the task of digging through complicated datasets to find information they were able to easily obtain from the medical literature. Today, it is so easy to obtain electronic information that there is no excuse for failing to take a peek at parameters that can quickly be obtained from datasets.

Students also wonder whether data from the medical literature is superior to data from electronic sources or vice versa. When information is available from both published studies and from electronic datasets, it is important to weigh the limitations of each source. The medical literature is often the best source of information for data that is difficult to capture in a dataset, such as the incidence rate of a disease or risk ratios. On the other hand, electronic datasets are often populated with nationally representative information, greatly improving their external validity.

Generally speaking, electronic datasets are more useful for obtaining descriptive data (such as costs), rates (such as medical utilization rates), and the prevalence of a disease. In some cases, electronic data are far superior to published data. For example, while it would be highly unlikely that you would find a nationally representative sample of cholesterol test results for African-American women in the medical literature, you would be able to find such information from the National Health and Nutrition Examination Survey (NHANES).

While almost all of the datasets listed in Tables 4.1 and Table 4.2 are offered in their entirety for free as downloads from the Internet, high-speed Internet access is needed to obtain them. They can also be purchased on CD-ROM through the National Technical Information Service (NTIS), which is a clearinghouse for federal data (http://www.ntis.gov). For most research projects, though, researchers will be able to use the plethora of free data extraction tools or printed data tabulations available for downloading from various government agencies.

Using Data Extraction Tools

Most data extraction tools retrieve information about a particular disease using International Classification for Disease (ICD) codes. In the ICD system, diseases are assigned a five-digit number. The first three digits are used to identify the disease, and the last two are used to identify subtypes of the disease. For example, influenza with pneumonia is classified as 48700, and influenza with respiratory manifestations is classified as 48710. Most data extraction tools provide a mechanism for looking up the ICD code for the disease you are interested in (for those that do not offer lookup tools, the codes can be obtained from http://www.eicd.com; http://www.wonder.cdc.gov; or through the NCHS at http://www.cdc.gov/nchs/datawh.htm). The NCHS has ICD-9 codebooks dating back to 1996 and provides tables that may be used to cross-reference codes from one year to the next. After the ICD code has been entered into the data extraction tool, you will be taken through a series of simple steps that will help you obtain the information you are looking for.

While ICD codes provide the most specific information, there are many other ways in which diseases are classified. One of the most useful classification schemes is the Clinical Classifications for Health Policy Research (CCHPR) system. In this system, diseases are grouped together in ways that are meaningful for health policy research. For instance, influenza virus infections for ICD codes 48700–48799 are grouped together. The codes themselves are called Clinical Classification Software (CCS) codes. For more information on the CCHPR system, including examples of the different ways codes are combined, visit http://www.ahrq.gov/data/hcup/ccs.htm.

Finally, Diagnosis Related Groups (DRGs) are groupings of diseases that are similar in cost. For example, DRGs clump infectious and inflammatory conditions of the respiratory system together. These conditions are further broken down according to whether the patient experienced complications with the disease or did not experience complications. In Chapter Six, we will see how each of these different systems can be used to calculate costs for medical services.

Software that takes you step by step through a problem is often referred to as a "wizard." As you proceed through each extraction tool's wizard, you will be asked information about the demographics of the group you are studying, such as age, race, and income. Unfortunately, these categories often cannot be modified, so you are stuck with the age groups predefined by the tool. Once you have finished, the tool will present you with tables containing the information you need.

Examples of data extraction tools include SEER*Stat (go to http://www.seer.ims.nci.nih.gov/ to obtain a free CD-ROM disk by mail), which contains cancer statistics, and HCUPnet (www.ahrq.gov), which allows researchers to obtain data on the number of hospitalizations, in-hospital deaths, and hospital charges nationwide.

The most comprehensive data extraction tool is maintained by the Bureau of the Census. This tool, called the Federal Electronic Research and Review Extraction Tool (FERRET, http://ferret.bls.census.gov), contains both census and health-related datasets. One of the nice features of the FERRET tool is that it allows you to either download any part of a dataset you are interested in or to generate cross-tabulations of data. For a partial listing of available datasets from FERRET, see Table 4.3.

Another comprehensive data extraction tool, WONDER, is maintained by the Centers for Disease Control and Prevention (www.wonder.cdc.gov). To use this system, you must register to receive a password, but registration is free. (For a listing of available datasets, see Table 4.4.)

Tips and tricks. WONDER now contains links to most major datasets used in health research. These datasets, which were compiled for Healthy People 2010, can be accessed at http://wonder.cdc.gov/DATA2010. (Free registration is required.)

Data from local health departments, including surveillance data and mortality data should be available online in the near future. Currently data are available for the New York area at http://www.infoshare.org (there is a user fee for this service, however).

Every data extraction tool has quirks and limitations, but they are generally very easy to use. Students who have never turned on a computer before have produced publication quality analyses using these tools.

TABLE 4.3.   SELECTED DATASETS AVAILABLE VIA FERRET.

- The Current Population Survey (CPS). A monthly sample of the United States population.
- Mortality—Underlying Cause-of-Death dataset.
- The National Health and Nutrition Examination Survey (NHANES). See description in Table 4.1.
- The National Health Interview Survey (NHIS). See description in Table 4.1.
- The National Hospital Ambulatory Medical Care Survey (NHAMCS). See description in Table 4.1.
- The National Ambulatory Medical Care Survey (NAMCS). See description in Table 4.1.

TABLE 4.4.   SELECTED DATASETS AVAILABLE VIA WONDER.

- AIDS dataset. Contains AIDS surveillance data.
- Census. Contains population estimates by age groupings and race.
- ICD9 Finder (lookup ICD9 codes). Allows users to look up the ICD-9 code for a particular disease.
- Linked Birth/Infant Death datafile. Used for examining infant mortality.
- Birth datafile. Contains information reported from birth certificates.
- National Institute for Occupational Safety and Health (NIOSH). Contains mortality data for work-related injuries.
- Cancer Surveillance, Epidemiology, and End Results (SEER) datafile. See Table 4.1 for description.
- Sexually Transmitted Disease datafile. Contains surveillance data for sexually transmitted diseases.
- Tuberculosis datafile. Contains surveillance data for tuberculosis.

Exercises 4.1–4.4

4.1. Obtain the total number of discharges, in-hospital charges, and the average length of stay (ALOS) from the HCUP-3 dataset for influenza-virus infections (ICD-9 code 487) by age group.

4.2. Calculate the hospitalization rate using the data you obtained from Exercise 4.1. You may use Appendix III or the U.S. Bureau of the Census Internet site (http://www.census.gov/population/www/estimates/nation2.html) to obtain population data.

4.3. Calculate a weighted mean charge and weighted mean length of stay using the data you retrieved in Exercise 4.1.

4.4. Calculate the rate of hospitalization and the weighted mean hospitalization charge for influenza virus using the Clinical Classification Software (CCS) coding system (CCS code 123).

4.5. Why might the hospital charges we obtained differ when the CCS system and the ICD systems are used?

4.6. In the sample cost-effectiveness analysis, we are interested in hospitalizations among healthy adults. What are some ways in which we might examine hospitalizations and hospital charges for persons that do not suffer from chronic illnesses?

Using Printed Tabulations of Electronic Data

A very simple way to obtain information is via the use of printed tabulations of data. Like most data extraction tools, data printouts force the researcher to work with the age, race, and gender groupings the publishers see fit to use. If you use a printed data tabulation, the information must be retyped into your spreadsheet program, but when the data needs are minimal, they are much easier to use than unformatted electronic data. The National Center for Health Statistics (NCHS) offers printed information from the National Health Interview Survey (NHIS) and mortality data, as well as other types of data, for free on its Web site (http://www.cdc.gov/nchs). To search for a printout of tabulated data, click on the search button on the Web Page and type in the name of the dataset. The major sources of tabulated data are listed in Table 4.1 (marked with a document symbol 📄) and Table 4.5.

A catalog of publications from the National Center for Health Statistics is also available that contains a complete listing of all of its tabular and non-tabular data (http://www.cdc.gov/nchs/data/catpub98.pdf).

Exercise 4.7

4.7. Calculate the incidence rate of influenza using data from the National Health Interview Survey. The data are available from the National Center for Health Statistics (www.cdc.gov/nchs or http://www.cdc.gov/nchs/data/ 10_200_1. pdf). Assume that influenza season begins in October and ends in March.

TABLE 4.5.   SELECTED SOURCES OF PRINTED DATA TABULATIONS.

Hourly wage by profession: http://stats.bls.gov/oes
Contains information on the hourly wages of people in different professions.

Hourly wage by race and gender:
http://www.census.gov/hhes/www/income.html
Contains annual earnings for everyone in the United States, earnings by state, gender, and race.

Health of the United States: http://www.cdc.gov/nchs/data/hus99ncb.pdf
Synthesizes data from multiple sources to produce overall health statistics for the United States.

National Health Interview Survey:
http://www.cdc.gov/nchs/data/series/SR_10/SR_10_200.pdf
Contains information on acute and chronic diseases, perceived health status, and activity limitations by race and gender.

National Hospital Discharge Survey:
http://www.cdc.gov/nchs/data/sr13_144.pdf
Contains information on hospital discharges by diagnosis.

Mortality data: http://www.cdc.gov/nchs/data/nvs47_19.pdf
Tabulated data for 72 selected causes of death.

Linked birth/death data: http://www.cdc.gov/nchs/data/nvs48_12.pdf
Useful for calculating infant mortality rates by cause of death.

International health data: http://www.cdc.gov/nchs/data/ihdrg99.pdf
Contains summary statistics by country, including birth rates and death rates.

Understanding Error in Electronic Data

Electronic health datasets produced by the United States government are usually accompanied by a printed discussion of the limitations of electronic data sources. This discussion often includes formulas for evaluating the error that they contain. Occasionally, researchers will need to use smaller datasets that do not include a detailed description of the data limitations. In these instances, it will be necessary to contact one of the authors to discuss the various limitations of the data, including potential sources of non-random error.

While the primary limitation of studies in the medical literature is random error, electronic data are more frequently limited by non-random error. For example, hospitalization data and mortality data are primarily affected by **misclassification bias.** Misclassification bias arises when the physician who fills out the death certificate writes down the wrong cause of death. Imagine that a patient developed heart disease as a result of diabetes mellitus. Sometimes, the doctor filling out the death certificate is unsure whether to list the diabetes or the heart disease as the cause of death. Therefore, the enumeration of the number of deaths attributed to these medical conditions may be incorrect.

The HCUP-3 dataset is a weighted sample of half of all of the hospitalizations in the United States. Mortality data from the NCHS are not obtained from a sample at all—they contain every recorded death in the United States. Therefore, these datasets are not subject to random error.

The manuals that accompany hospitalization and mortality datasets provide instructions for adjusting these data for underreporting, for performing statistical tests, and so on. Though mortality data are not subject to sampling error and can be adjusted for underreporting, they cannot usually be adjusted for misclassification bias. Using the Multiple Cause of Death Datafile, which lists all conditions that the patient might have died from, can minimize misclassification bias. Using discharge data from the National Hospital Discharge Survey (NHDS) can minimize misclassification bias in hospital datasets, since specially trained health workers obtained a subset of these data directly from medical records. For rare conditions and for data on hospital charges, the Healthcare Cost and Utilization Project-3 (HCUP-3) dataset must be used, because it is a much larger and much more comprehensive database.

Using Data from Unpublished Research Projects

For some cost-effectiveness studies, it will be possible to obtain unpublished data directly from the authors of studies published in the medical literature. Oftentimes, a research project will only publish selected results of studies, leaving out precisely the information you are looking for. Tracking down the authors of a study is usually a simple task. Authors may be contacted via the medical journal or the institution with which they are affiliated. Contact information for authors is published on the first page of articles in most medical journals, including institutional affiliations. One of the fastest and easiest ways to find an author is to visit the personnel directory on an institution's Web page.

When you are in need of information on a medication, most pharmaceutical companies will readily provide data they have collected on the drugs they manufacture. When information is obtained directly from a pharmaceutical company, you should mention the source in any publications you produce, because these companies may be motivated to portray their medications in a favorable light and could conceivably produce biased data.

Using Data from Piggybacked Studies

Suppose that a pharmaceutical company wishes to know the cost-effectiveness of a drug that it is currently studying for efficacy. If the company simultaneously collects information on the efficacy of the drug and the cost-effectiveness of the drug, it will be able to kill two birds with one stone. Adding an economic evaluation to an ongoing randomized controlled trial is called **piggybacking** (Gold and others, 1996; Haddix and others, 1996). When the primary objective of the study is to collect cost and effectiveness data, the study is called a primary cost-effectiveness analysis. In these study designs, data on the cost and efficacy of the health intervention under study are collected over the course of the analysis.

Because any single study cannot capture all of the costs or changes in mortality rates that result from a health intervention, it is usually necessary to supplement the data that the researchers are collecting with information from other studies or from electronic datasets. For example, Bridges and others (2000, see Appendix II) examined the efficacy of the influenza vaccine in preventing influenza-like illness while simultaneously collecting information on the number of medical visits, hospitalizations, and medications consumed in the vaccine and placebo arms of their study. They then used the MEDSTAT MarketScan Databases (Medstat, 2001) to estimate the cost of each medical visit and each hospitalization that occurred. Using this information, they conducted a cost-benefit analysis of influenza vaccination.

Unfortunately, their sample size was too small to detect differences in hospitalization rates and mortality rates between the placebo group and the vaccine group, and they did not supplement these data with outside sources of information. Therefore, the results of their economic analysis were skewed in favor of not vaccinating.

In addition to problems associated with collecting comprehensive data, the piggyback study design usually cannot directly compare the intervention under study with other potentially useful health interventions for preventing or treating a disease. For example, if a pharmaceutical company wishes to compare the product it is evaluating to other products currently on the market, it would be necessary to add more study arms to the randomized controlled trial, which can be very expensive.

Because piggyback studies or primary cost-effectiveness analyses usually require supplementary data, students who are learning cost-effectiveness analysis to add an economic component to a randomized controlled trial will still need to have good data retrieval skills.

Using Expert Opinion

Sometimes, information on a parameter is not available through published, electronic, or unpublished sources. When this occurs, the value of this parameter can be estimated using the opinion of experts. While it would be unusual for a group of experts to correctly guess the true value of a cost-effectiveness input (for example, the number of people a single syphilis patient will infect on average), they will very likely be able to guess the highest and lowest possible values for that parameter. When cost-effectiveness data are collected using the opinion of experts, the reference case analysis requires that a formal process be used called the **Delphi method.**

In the Delphi method, a group of experts is brought together. Each expert secretly provides his or her best guess of the value of the input of interest to a facilitator. The facilitator then communicates the results of each expert's anonymous guess to the group and the experts revise their estimates until consensus is reached (or at least until most people can agree on a realistic range of possible values). There are many different variations on this technique, which will not be discussed here.

Organizing Your Data

The bane of any researcher's existence is organizing data. Nevertheless, it is nearly impossible to conduct a research project without a good organizational system. Of course, a good filing system will be necessary to keep track of all of the different medical articles. But it is just as important to keep track of the parameters you will use when it comes time to put all of the information you have collected into a decision analysis model.

There are two major goals to organizing data. The first is to create a summary of each dataset and each study from the medical literature that you will be using. This will allow you to quickly review the benefits or the pitfalls of each data element before it is used. The second is to have a source of key data elements you will be using to construct your decision analysis model.

Project Map

1. Develop a research question.
2. Design your analysis.
3. Understand the sources of error in data.
4. Obtain data.
5. **Organize data.**
6. Construct a decision analysis model.
7. Calculate quality-adjusted life years.
8. Test and refine the decision analysis model.
9. Conduct a sensitivity analysis.
10. Prepare the study results for publication or presentation.

No matter how carefully you read a study or a summary of a dataset, you will forget many of its key elements. Having each dataset and study summarized concisely allows you to refer to it quickly. When the Centers for Disease Control and Prevention (CDC) set out to summarize the medical literature on community preventive services, they hired a small army of public health students and junior researchers. These students summarized the data from each of the thousands of studies they reviewed so that they could quickly put all of the information together in a way that made sense, and so that the authors could easily refer to the materials if they had questions (your author was one of those lackeys in his youth). You would do well to heed their example, albeit on a much smaller scale.

Summarizing Journal Articles

When obtaining parameters across studies, it is important to note how the study design, the participants, the intervention, and the outcomes differ from one another. All studies will differ from one another in important ways and these differences must be tracked. For example, if we are to include data from Nichol and others (1995) ("The Effectiveness of Vaccination Against Influenza in Healthy, Working Adults," see Appendix II), and Treanor and others (2000) ("Efficacy and

Safety of the Oral Neuraminidase Inhibitor Oseltamivir in Treating Acute Influenza," see Appendix II), we should note the following factors:

- Treanor and others (2000) defined the influenza season as January to March, included healthy adults aged eighteen to sixty-five, excluded persons with serious chronic disease, and defined influenza-like illness as fever *and* one or more respiratory symptoms *and* one or more constitutional symptoms. Respiratory symptoms included cough, sore throat, or nasal symptoms. Constitutional symptoms included headache, malaise, muscle aches, sweats, chills, or fatigue. The study design was a multi-center blinded randomized controlled trial. The subjects were volunteers and were mostly middle class and white.
- Nichol and others (1995) defined the influenza season as December through March, included only subjects in the Minneapolis-St. Paul area, included healthy eighteen- to sixty-five-year-old subjects, excluded persons with serious chronic disease, and defined influenza-like illness as a sore throat associated with either a fever or cough that lasted twenty-four hours or over. The study design was a blinded randomized controlled trial, and the subjects were recruited from the surrounding community.

We see that the major ways in which these two studies differ greatly are in the location of the study, the time frame of the study, and the definition used for influenza-like illness. If we obtained an incidence rate estimate from Treanor and others (2000), it would have greater external validity because it was a **multi-center trial.** In a multi-center trial, subjects are drawn from clinics or hospitals in different geographic locations. Moreover, some data from Treanor and others (2000) will not be directly comparable to data from Nichol and others (1995) because the latter group of researchers used a broader definition of influenza-like illness. A broader definition will identify more people with influenza-like illness and thus make the incidence rate of the disease appear higher than the rate reported in Treanor and others (2000). It will also result in lower rates of complications and medical visits, because any subject that meets a looser definition of illness will be less likely to actually be infected with the influenza virus. If we lose sight of these important study design differences, we will likely run into data quality problems. Table 4.6 lists one example of a journal summary table.

Summary sheets for electronic datasets are much easier to compile because most of the problems and benefits of the data are summarized in the manual describing the data (see Table 4.7).

Major parameters of interest obtained from a dataset or journal can be safely maintained on a separate type of sheet we will call a "data sheet."

TABLE 4.6. EXAMPLE OF A JOURNAL SUMMARY SHEET.

Author:	Name of the authors.
Title:	Title of the study.
Reference #:	Number used in reference section of paper (this need not be entered until you have begun to write the paper).
Methods study design:	Randomized controlled trial, retrospective, prospective, and so on.
Location:	Geographic location of study.
# of subjects:	Number of subjects in each arm of the study.
Inclusion criteria:	Were there any demographic or medical criteria the subjects had to meet to be included in the study?
Exclusion criteria:	Where there any medical conditions or other restrictions that precluded a subject from enrolling in the study?
Subject demographics:	Income, race, education level, and age of the subjects.
Equal allocation?	If the study was a randomized controlled trial, were both groups similar?
Results of interest:	Tables and any other data that might be useful.
Other notes:	Study design limitations and differences between the study cohort and your hypothetical cohort.

TABLE 4.7. EXAMPLE OF A SUMMARY SHEET FOR AN ELECTRONIC DATASET.

Name:	Name of the dataset.
Source:	Institution that collected the data including contact information.
Reference #:	Number used in reference section of paper.
Methods study design:	Self-report survey, medical records review, billing data, or other method.
Population:	Does the data pertain to the entire U.S. population or some subset?
# of subjects:	Total number of subjects included in the dataset.
Sources of error:	What is the standard error of each data element? Is the data subject to some other type of bias, such as misclassification bias?
Subject demographics:	Income, race, education level, and age of the subjects.
Other notes:	Limitations of the data, formulas for correcting error and calculating rates, and notes on how the data are formatted. Advanced students using statistical analysis programs may wish to keep notes on variables.

Summarizing Data

Data sheets list all of the information you will include in your cost-effectiveness analysis. There are three elements that must be tracked for every variable you use: 1) the most likely value of the parameter, 2) the lowest likely value of the parameter, and 3) the highest likely value of the parameter. Oftentimes, estimates you obtain will be associated with a range of values (due to error) and will be accompanied by information on the distribution of these values (for an explanation of distributions, see Chapter Three). It is important to keep track of the information on the distribution of values because you will need this information when you conduct a sensitivity analysis. Finally, it will be necessary to calculate some of the parameters you will use in your analysis, and you will need to keep track of how these items were calculated. For example, you may have obtained information on the total number of hospitalizations and the total number of people at risk of hospitalization, but you will still need to know the hospitalization rate.

Because there are so many things to keep track of, and because you will need a dynamic medium for tracking this information, it is best to use a spreadsheet program as a data sheet. (See Table 7.1 in Chapter Seven for instructions on downloading free spreadsheet software.) So, if we are keeping track of all of the variables we will be using on a data sheet, why bother keeping summary sheets of the medical literature? First, you will never be able to obtain all of the information you need from a study on the first try. Typically, you will have to dig up an article you are interested in ten or more times throughout the course of a cost-effectiveness analysis. Second, you will think of things that need to be cross-referenced and will need to make qualitative comparisons between studies

TABLE 4.8.   EXAMPLE OF A DATA SUMMARY SHEET.

Variable or Source	Base Value	High	Low	Distribution	Notes
Incidence rate (per capita)					
Bridges and others	0.23	0.24	0.215	Normal	Region = Michigan
Nichol and others	0.69	0.55	0.73	Normal	Definition = Upper respiratory illness
NHIS	0.591	0.42	0.78	Triangular	Assumed triangular distribution
Duration of illness (hours)					
Treanor and others	92	104	72	Normal	Hours of illness

frequently. Summary sheets will allow you to quickly refer to the most import elements of the studies you will use in your analysis. This will all become evident as we proceed through the sample cost-effectiveness analysis.

Table 4.8 outlines what a data summary sheet might look like. Notice that each variable heads each list and that all of the possible values are listed below it by the source from which it was obtained. The distribution of each variable is provided by source, and notes specific to each source are listed along with the data. Notice too, that the units of each source are presented next to the heading (for example, "Duration of illness" is denoted in hours).

Now that you have an idea of how to evaluate, obtain, and organize data that are commonly used in cost-effectiveness analysis, you can begin to develop these skills as you apply them to the sample cost-effectiveness analysis. Over the next two chapters, you will learn how to work with the probabilities and costs commonly used in cost-effectiveness analyses by drawing on the literature review and data retrieval skills you learned in this and the previous chapter. In Chapter Seven, you will combine all of this information using a decision analysis model that evaluates the cost of each of the strategies to prevent or treat influenza-like illness.

CHAPTER FIVE

WORKING WITH PROBABILITIES

Overview

If cost-effectiveness analysis were a building, probabilities would be its scaffolding. Probabilities indicate how likely subjects are to become ill, how likely subjects are to see a doctor, and so on. Therefore, they provide a framework for deciding how much an intervention will cost and how effective it will be. In our partial flowchart outlining the course of influenza-like illness (see Figure 2.2), each branch point represents a chance event. For example, at the first branch point, there is a chance that subjects will either develop an influenza-like illness or remain well. These probabilities can be estimated using rates or other types of ratios. For instance, the incidence of influenza-like illness indicates the probability of developing an influenza-like illness, and the ratio of the number of people visiting the doctor over the total number of ill people indicates the chance that a subject will visit a doctor when he or she develops an influenza-like illness (see Table 5.1).

In this chapter, we will explore how data from the medical literature or electronic datasets are used to estimate the probabilities that are needed to construct a cost-effectiveness analysis. We will also demonstrate how to work with probabilities in our sample cost-effectiveness analysis, discussing the advantages and disadvantages of various methods and approaches. Should you choose to

TABLE 5.1. COMMON PROBABILITIES USED IN COST-EFFECTIVENESS ANALYSIS.

Probability	Definition	Use in Cost-Effectiveness Analysis
Incidence rate	Probability that a subject will develop a disease.	To determine the percentage of subjects that will become ill and to calculate QALYs.
Prevalence ratio	Probability that a subject will have a disease.	To determine the number of subjects screened who will have a disease or to determine the number of subjects with the disease at the start of the intervention.
Secondary transmission of infectious disease	Probability that an infected subject will spread the infection to another person.	Analyses that evaluate infectious disease.
Duration of illness	Time spent with a disease.	To calculate QALYs, to set the analytic horizon of the study, and to design decision analysis models.
Distribution of illness	Probability that a subject will have a disease given the age, income, or race of the subject.	Analyses examining interventions designed to treat or prevent chronic disease, interventions targeted toward demographically defined groups, and to adjust data.
Side effects	Probability that a subject will develop side effects to a treatment or procedure.	Interventions using medical treatments or invasive surgical procedures.
Medical utilization	Probability that a subject will visit a doctor, be hospitalized, or receive long-term care.	To determine the costs associated with medical care.
Efficacy	Probability that a treatment or preventive intervention will reduce or detect disease in a clinical setting.	To determine the effectiveness of a treatment or preventive exam, to allocate costs.
Secondary illness	Probability that a person will develop a disease as a result of having the disease under study.	Interventions designed to prevent or treat diseases that place subjects at risk of other diseases (for instance, hypertension or diabetes).
Sensitivity and specificity	Probability that a subject will test positive or negative for a disease given the presence or absence of disease.	Interventions evaluating screening tests or diseases detected by screening tests.
HRQL score	Quality of life with disease.	To calculate QALYs.
Mortality rate	Probability of death.	To calculate QALYs.

complete the exercises in this chapter, be sure to save the information you obtain. These probabilities will be put to use in Chapter Seven when we begin to construct our decision analysis model. If you decide not to complete the exercises, but wish to practice building a decision analysis model, you may simply look up the values in Table 7.3 in that chapter.

As you proceed through this chapter, keep in mind the hypothetical cohort in the sample cost-effectiveness analysis. Recall from Chapter Two that we will need information for: 1) the supportive care arm of the analysis, 2) the treatment arm of the analysis, and 3) the vaccination arm of the analysis. Subjects receiving supportive care are neither vaccinated at the beginning of the influenza season nor treated when they develop an influenza-like illness, but otherwise receive any necessary medical care. Subjects in all three arms are between the ages of fifteen and sixty-five and may have any illness but heart disease, diabetes mellitus, or chronic lung disease. Finally, influenza-like illness is defined as feverishness or a measured temperature of at least 37.7°C (100°F) plus cough or sore throat (Kendal and others, 1982). All of the data that we obtain should apply to the characteristics of this cohort.

Incidence and Prevalence

Virtually every cost-effectiveness analysis will require information on either the incidence of a disease or the prevalence of a disease. These parameters are used to determine the chance that a subject in a hypothetical cohort will have or will develop a disease, and they are also used to calculate QALYs. Recall from Chapter Three that incidence of a disease refers to the number of *new* cases of disease over a defined period, and that the incidence rate refers to the number of new cases over a defined period divided by the midpoint population in that period. Recall, too, that prevalence refers to the number of *existing* cases over a period, while the prevalence ratio refers to the number of existing cases divided by the midpoint population of that period. Thus, incidence data are used to determine the chance that a subject will develop a disease, while prevalence data are used to determine the chance that a subject will have a disease at the outset of the analysis.

Incidence rates are usually obtained from the medical literature or from ongoing prospective trials, though some incidence rates may be obtained from electronic datasets. Prevalence rates can be obtained from the medical literature or from electronic datasets. Care must be taken to differentiate incidence rates (the rate of new diagnoses) from prevalence ratios (the ratio of existing cases to the number of persons at risk for these cases). Most electronic datasets contain only prevalence information, since they are derived from cross-sectional surveys of the population (see Chapter Three for a description of cross-sectional surveys). However, because some acute infectious diseases have a rapid onset and resolution, it is sometimes possible to obtain the incidence rate for these diseases from electronic datasets. Some electronic datasets also contain data from prospective trials or from a series of cross-sectional studies using the same subjects, so these data can sometimes be used to obtain incidence rates for chronic diseases.

Generally, population surveys such as the National Health and Nutrition Examination Survey (NHANES) or the National Health Interview Survey (NHIS) are used to calculate either incidence or prevalence rates (Adams and others, 1999). In contrast, because ambulatory care utilization or hospitalization data only capture a subset of all subjects with a disease, medical utilization datasets cannot be used to calculate incidence or prevalence rates. Instead, these datasets are used to estimate the number of medical visits in a given year. This will be discussed in the "Medical Care Utilization" section below.

There are a number of important sources of error to consider when evaluating incidence rates. Foremost, studies that include incidence rates often come from prospective investigations that were conducted in a specific geographic location. Thus, incidence rates obtained from a study in one region of the country are usually not generalizable to other regions of the country or world. (That is, they are not externally valid.) To overcome this problem, it is usually necessary to calculate the average incidence rate across studies conducted in many different parts of the country to which your study applies.

Finally, the incidence rate of some diseases is also subject to **seasonal variation** (a change in the incidence rate of disease between winter, spring, summer, and fall). This is especially true of infectious diseases such as influenza, most of which are more common in the winter than they are in the summer in nonequatorial countries. The incidence rate of a disease can also vary from year to year.

Incidence Rate of Influenza-Like Illness

Our goal in this section is to estimate the incidence rate of influenza-like illness. The incidence rate of influenza-like illness may be estimated using published data reports and prospective trials. Self-report data obtained from the National Health Interview Survey (NHIS) indicate that the incidence rate of "influenza virus" infections in persons between ages eighteen and sixty-five is about forty-five cases per 100 people (see Figure 5.1). Self-reported rates of "influenza virus" infection are likely to approximate self-reported rates of influenza-like illness, because most people will have been either self-diagnosed or diagnosed presumptively. (Recall

FIGURE 5.1.   THE INCIDENCE OF SELF-REPORTED INFLUENZA VIRUS INFECTIONS AND OTHER CONDITIONS, 1982 THROUGH 1996.

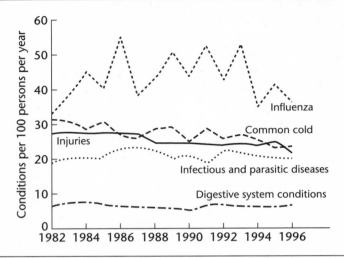

Source: Current estimates from the National Health Interview Survey, 1996. National Center for Health Statistics. Vital Health Stat 10(2000). 1999. Figure 2.

that a presumptive diagnosis is made by a clinician based on symptoms or findings on a physical exam without the assistance of laboratory data.)

However, because data from the NHIS are subject to recall bias, results from this survey may underreport the true incidence rate of disease. Moreover, these data were obtained from the general population, some of whom received the influenza vaccine at the start of the influenza season. Because some people were vaccinated, we would expect the reported incidence of influenza-like illness to underestimate the rate of influenza-like illness in an unvaccinated population. On the other hand, people are likely to think they have "the flu" whenever they are ill, so these data are also subject to misclassification bias. The nice thing about these data is that they are nationally representative and available over many seasons.

Analyzing the medical literature. The medical literature contains estimates of the incidence of influenza-like illness from specific geographic sites. However, because the rates of influenza-like illness vary from region to region and from year to year, incidence data from the medical literature, like incidence data obtained from the NHIS, are limited in that they can only provide us with an idea of what the average annual incidence rate of influenza-like illness is nationwide. Unfortunately, we are stuck between using survey data, which has good external validity but poor internal validity (national survey data), and prospective data, which has good internal validity but poor external validity (the medical literature).

Another problem with the medical literature is that some studies use a different definition of influenza-like illness than others. If the definition is very strict, fewer people will meet the definition of influenza-like illness and the incidence rate will appear to be lower than it will in studies that use a looser definition. In this section, we will provide a detailed analysis of the medical literature to illustrate some of the dilemmas faced by cost-effectiveness researchers and will put some of the material you learned in Chapter Three in context. Let's examine the studies reporting the incidence rate of influenza-like illness in more detail (all of these studies are summarized in Appendix II).

Bridges and others (2000) conducted a randomized controlled trial of the influenza vaccine among a population of workers at the Ford Motor plant in Dearborn, Michigan. They examined differences in the rate of influenza-like illness and upper respiratory illness over two years, 1997–1998 and 1998–1999. They intentionally used a definition of upper respiratory illness that was identical to the definition used by Nichol and others (1995) so that comparisons could be made between the two studies. The average seasonal rate of influenza-like illness in the group receiving a placebo (a sterile saline injection) was 22 cases of influenza-like illness per 100 subjects (0.22 cases per subject) over the two-year study period. (This was calculated by adding the number of ill subjects over each influenza season together and then dividing this sum by the total number of subjects over both seasons.) The average seasonal rate of upper respiratory illness over this two-year period was 34 cases per 100 subjects (0.34 cases per subject). In the first year of the study, the influenza vaccine was poorly matched to the strains of virus circulating in the community and the group receiving the vaccine had a *higher* rate of influenza-like illness and upper respiratory illness than either of the placebo groups (0.28 cases per subject for influenza-like illness and 0.45 cases per subject for upper respiratory illness). When the group that received the ineffective influenza vaccine is included, the overall incidence of influenza-like illness in this study becomes 24.4 cases per 100 persons (0.244 cases per subject).

In vaccine trials, we generally choose to examine the incidence rate of illness in the placebo group alone, so that we know what the base incidence of illness is among unvaccinated persons. Because the influenza vaccine reduces the risk of developing influenza virus infection and the secondary complications of influenza infection, vaccinated groups generally have a lower rate of influenza-like illness than unvaccinated groups. There are two things to consider, however, when studying the incidence rate of disease in placebo groups. First, as pointed out in Chapter Three, placebos are good at treating (and possibly good at preventing) disease. If a placebo cream can help a balding man grow hair, it is conceivable that a placebo injection could prevent influenza-like illness (see Exhibit 3.1). Second, people that enroll in randomized controlled trials are usually healthier than the general population (see "Prospective Studies" in Chapter Three). If subjects receiving placebo injections were less likely to contract an influenza-like illness than the average healthy adult, the incidence rate of influenza-like illness reported in a study might be lower than we would expect in the general population.

Campbell and Rumly (1995) found that the incidence rate of influenza-like illness among unvaccinated textile workers in North Carolina during the 1992–1993 season was 49 percent. Monto and others (1995) used **passive surveillance** reports of influenza-like illness from a number of physicians in Michigan. Passive surveillance systems rely on physicians to report a disease to a local health department and typically undercount the total number of cases (because the physicians forget to fill out the reporting form). These authors minimized underreporting by using a select group of physicians who agreed to report all cases of influenza-like illness they saw. These researchers found that the rate of influenza-like illness in Michigan was approximately 40 percent during the 1989–1990 season and approximately 50 percent during the 1990–1991 season.

Adjusting for different disease definitions. This section demonstrates how creative researchers can adjust data when faced with limited information on a parameter estimate. Though creativity is not encouraged in the sciences, it is sometimes needed when the cost-effectiveness analyst is faced with a drought of information. Here, we will see how we might adjust the data from Nichol and others (1995), who examined the costs and benefits of influenza vaccination in preventing upper respiratory illness rather than influenza-like illness. We will do so by capitalizing on the fact that Bridges and others (2000) collected incidence data for both influenza-like illness and upper respiratory illness.

Nichol and others (1995) found that the incidence rate of upper respiratory illness was about 69 per 100 persons in Minneapolis-St. Paul, Minnesota in 1997. To adjust the data from Nichol and others (1995), we multiply their incidence rate of upper respiratory illness by the ratio of the incidence rate of influenza-like illness to the incidence rate of upper respiratory illness in the placebo group of the Bridges and others (2000) study. Thus, the incidence rate of influenza-like illness (ILI) for the Nichol and others (1995) study is mathematically estimated as follows:

$$\text{incidence rate } \cancel{\text{URI}} \text{ (Nichol and others, 1995)} \cdot \frac{\text{incidence rate ILI (Bridges and others, 2000)}}{\text{incidence rate } \cancel{\text{URI}} \text{ (Bridges and others, 2000)}}$$

Equation 5.1

Here, we see that the upper respiratory illness (URI) terms cancel out, leaving us with an estimated rate of influenza-like illness.

Correcting for the differences in the definition of illness used in these studies produces an incidence rate that is around $0.22/0.34 = 0.65$, or 65 percent that of the upper respiratory illness definition. If you recalculate these rates using the numbers of subjects provided by the authors, you should obtain a ratio of 0.67. These numbers differ due to rounding error. Thus, multiplying the rate of upper respiratory illness from Nichol and others (1995), 0.69, by this correction factor, 0.67, yields an estimated incidence rate of 0.46. In doing this, we are assuming that the ratio of influenza-like illness to upper respiratory illness was the same in both studies, which is not very likely. However, it is still useful to get a general idea of what the incidence rate of influenza-like illness might have been in the Nichol and others (1995) study, because so few data are available.

Obtaining an estimated rate of influenza-like illness. Our summary sheet for influenza-like illness incidence rates might look like Table 5.2.

We see that the median value for the incidence rate of influenza-like illness, 0.45, is very close to the rates published in other studies. Mean values are usually used as baseline values when the data do not contain either very high or

TABLE 5.2. ESTIMATES OF THE INCIDENCE RATE OF INFLUENZA-LIKE ILLNESS FROM VARIOUS SOURCES IN THE MEDICAL LITERATURE.

Source	Base	High	Low	Distribution	Notes
Bridges and others (2000)	0.24	0.28	0.22	Normal	Region = Michigan. Years = 1998 + 1999.
Nichol and others (1995)	0.69	–	–	–	Definition less stringent. Region = Minnesota. Year = 1994–1995.
Nichol and others (1995)	0.46	–	–	–	Corrected using data from Bridges and others.
Monto and others (1995)	0.45	50	40	–	Surveillance data. Year = 1989–1990 and 1990–1991. Base value = mean of high and low.
NHIS (Adams and others, 1999)	0.45	60	40	–	Self-report data. Base value = mean of high and low.
Campell and Rumly (1995)	0.49	–	–	–	Region = North Carolina. Year = 1991–1992.
Mean Score	0.42	–	–	–	Includes only the calculated value from Nichol and others.
Median Score	0.45	–	–	–	

very low values; otherwise, the median value is generally preferable. In this case, the incidence rate of influenza-like illness obtained by Bridges and others (2000) is much lower than the other values we found. We see that the mean value, 0.42, is lower than the value reported in all but one study, making the mean value a less likely estimator of the true incidence rate of influenza-like illness.

The median value of a set of numbers is used when some numbers in the set are unusually high or low. Very high or very low values can skew the mean value of a set of numbers. For instance, economists typically use the median income in a country because multibillionaires tend to artificially increase the mean in wealthy nations. Likewise, extremely poor people tend to skew the mean downward in developing nations. However, a relatively large set of numbers must be available for a median value to be useful.

The lower rate in the Bridges and others (2000) study could have been spurious or could be attributable to the demographic characteristics of the cohort. We will discuss the differences in the demographics of the cohort in the "Distribution of Illness" section below.

Secondary Transmission of Infectious Disease

When contagious diseases are included in a cost-effectiveness analysis, it is important to try to estimate the chance that one person will infect another and propagate the disease. **Secondary transmission** of infectious disease occurs when a person who is infected with a disease transmits the disease to another person. A mathematical model is usually needed to estimate how many people will be infected, on average, from a single person with a communicable disease. However, the estimated risk of secondary transmission is sometimes published in the medical literature.

The reference case scenario of the Panel on Cost-effectiveness in Health and Medicine recommends that real life situations be modeled as closely as possible. In real life, secondary transmission of infectious disease should usually be modeled because preventive interventions are rarely applied to all subjects in a hypothetical cohort. Some people will receive medical interventions and some will not. Let us use syphilis as an example. Those who do not receive treatment might reinfect some of those that did. Likewise, if some people remain infectious despite having received treatment, they may reinfect other persons who were successfully treated and now need to be retreated. Hypothetical cohorts can be quite promiscuous.

There are some uncommon instances in which it is not necessary to develop a mathematical model for secondary transmission. First, if a sufficient number of subjects can be treated or vaccinated to produce herd immunity (see Chapter Two), there may be too few secondary cases to bother counting. Second, if the intervention is clearly cost-saving relative to all other interventions, *and* modeling secondary transmission will only deepen those savings, it is not necessary to include such modeling.

Recall that herd immunity occurs when so many subjects are vaccinated that too few susceptible subjects remain to spread the disease from person to person. The number of people that must be vaccinated for herd immunity to occur depends on the disease and the efficacy of the vaccine (or treatment) under study.

If an intervention is less expensive *and* more effective than the other health interventions under study, it is possible to avoid incorporating costs that are very difficult to capture, provided that adding these costs would make the intervention even more cost-saving. Any intervention that saves money and lives should always be implemented (provided that it is ethically acceptable to the population that will receive it).

Secondary Transmission of Influenza

Because the task of incorporating secondary transmission in a model can be daunting, it is best to find out if this task can be skipped altogether. The level at which herd immunity protects people from the influenza virus is not known. Influenza has been known to spread through nursing homes in which virtually everyone was vaccinated and to skip over large populations of unvaccinated people. Our last hope is that influenza vaccination or treatment will be cost-saving relative to supportive care. It is best to complete the study without incorporating secondary transmission to see if we can be saved from this difficult task.

Duration of Illness

The **duration of illness** is defined as the time from the clinical onset of a disease until the time of resolution of the illness or death. The duration of illness is one of the most important elements of a cost-effectiveness analysis and is used to calculate quality-adjusted life years and to estimate the future costs of disease (Gold and others, 1996; Murray and Lopez, 1996). For infectious diseases, estimates of the duration of illness may be obtained from the medical literature, from ongoing randomized controlled trials, or using expert opinion. For a disease that is lifelong, such as diabetes mellitus, the average duration of illness is equal to the life expectancy with the disease minus the mean age of onset. We will see how life expectancy is calculated in Chapter Twelve. The mean age of onset can either be calculated using electronic data or obtained from the medical literature. Estimating the duration of illness of diseases that may be lifelong if untreated, but may also be cured, usually requires the opinion of experts.

Duration of Influenza-Like Illness

Treanor and others (2000) examined the duration of illness in people with laboratory-confirmed influenza virus infection, people with influenza-like illness, and people treated with various doses of oseltamivir. In their study, influenza-like illness was defined as fever, respiratory symptoms, and constitutional symptoms (for example, fatigue and malaise).

Exercises 5.1–5.2

5.1. Obtain the duration of influenza-like illness in hours from the Treanor and others (2000, see Appendix II).
5.2. How will the differences between the definition of influenza-like illness used by Treanor and others (2000) and the definition used in our analysis bias our estimate?

Efficacy and Measures of Risk

Whether the health intervention under study is a medication, a vaccine, a screening test, or a public health intervention, it is necessary to know how good the intervention is at preventing morbidity, improving quality of life, and/or preventing mortality.

The extent to which an intervention reduces the risk of morbidity, mortality, hospitalization, and so on is termed the **efficacy** of the intervention. Recall from Chapter One that efficacy tells us how good an intervention *can be* under experimental conditions and effectiveness tells us how good an intervention *is* in the real world. When evaluating the efficacy of a medical intervention, it is important to consider factors that distinguish efficacy from effectiveness (Gold and others, 1996). For example, under study conditions, patients are usually closely monitored to see whether they are taking their medications, are shamed into adhering to their smoking cessation program, and so on. The researchers also make sure that physicians are correctly administering a screening test, correctly administering a primary prevention program, or correctly diagnosing a disease. As we proceed through our sample cost-effectiveness analysis, you will learn techniques for estimating real-world effectiveness using efficacy data.

Suppose that we wanted to determine the efficacy of the influenza vaccine in preventing influenza virus infections. The efficacy of the influenza vaccine would be:

$$\text{vaccine efficacy} = 1 - \frac{\text{incidence rate of disease, vaccinated}}{\text{incidence rate of disease, unvaccinated}}$$

Equation 5.2

For example, if the incidence rate of influenza were 10 cases per 100 persons in the general population, but 2 cases per 100 persons among those who received the vaccine, the vaccine efficacy would be $1 - (0.02/0.10) = 1 - 0.20 = 0.80$ or 80 percent.

Oftentimes, you will see the efficacy equation presented as:

$$\text{vaccine efficacy} = \frac{\text{incidence rate in unvaccinated} - \text{incidence rate in vaccinated}}{\text{incidence rate in unvaccinated}}$$

Equation 5.3

which is mathematically equivalent to Equation 5.2.

Tips and tricks. Some epidemiology textbooks use the term attack rate rather than incidence rate when presenting Equations 5.2 and 5.3. The attack rate is equal to the number of ill persons divided by the number of persons exposed to the disease. Since it is not ethical to intentionally expose healthy subjects to a disease, studies typically examine incidence rates during the peak season and use this as a proxy for the attack rate.

The basic formula remains the same no matter what outcome you are looking at or what preventive intervention you are evaluating. For instance, if you are interested in knowing the efficacy of treatment at reducing mortality, the efficacy of the treatment would be:

$$\text{treatment efficacy} = 1 - \frac{\text{risk of death, treated}}{\text{risk of death, untreated}}$$

Equation 5.4

The time frame during which an intervention is evaluated should be clearly indicated to place the result in context. For example, if you calculated the efficacy of a chemotherapy regimen at reducing the number of deaths, and you followed patients for five years after the therapy was administered, you would call your result a "five-year treatment efficacy." The results you obtain will be dependent upon the time frame of the intervention under study.

There are a number of different methods for determining risk in cost-effectiveness analysis. These include risk ratios, odds ratios, and the attributable risk.

Risk ratios. The most common measure of risk is the risk ratio. Recall from the section on prospective studies in Chapter Three that the risk ratio is defined as the incidence rate of disease among people with a particular characteristic (or risk factor) divided by the incidence rate of the disease among people without the characteristic. The risk ratio is often used to define the risk of an outcome, such as death, in people who have received a treatment or preventive intervention relative to those who have not. Thus, if the incidence rate among people who have received a vaccination was 0.02, and the incidence rate among people who have not is 0.1, the risk ratio would be 0.02/0.1 = 0.2. Referring to Equation 5.2 above, we see that the efficacy can also be defined as:

$$1 - \text{Risk Ratio}$$

Equation 5.5

Retrospective studies and studies that use logistic regression (a type of statistical test) cannot produce risk ratios as outcome measures. Instead, they produce **odds ratios.** The odds ratio is similar to the risk ratio when the risk of disease is rare (less than approximately 2 to 5 percent).

While risks are calculated using the total number of subjects in the denominator, odds are calculated using only the fraction of subjects in the denominator that are not represented in the numerator. Suppose that, for example, we conducted a survey of 100 people that were randomly sampled from the general population to determine the risk of having a cough at any point in time. The risk is defined as:

$$\frac{\text{number with cough}}{(\text{number with cough} + \text{number without cough})}$$

Equation 5.6

while the odds of having a cough would be defined as:

$$\frac{\text{number with cough}}{\text{number without cough}}$$

Equation 5.7

If 20 people have a cough, the *risk* of having a cough at any point in time would be 20/100 = 20 percent. The odds however, would be 20/80 = 25 percent.

In this instance, the *odds* of having a cough would not be a good estimator of the *risk* of having a cough. On the other hand, if only two people had a cough, the risk would be 2/100 = 2 percent, while the odds would be 2/98 = 2.04 percent—a number very close to the risk.

Attributable risk. Another commonly used measure of risk in cost-effectiveness analysis is the **attributable risk.** The attributable risk, which is also known as the **risk difference,** is the total risk that is attributable to a particular risk factor (or exposure) and is simply equal to the risk among those with the risk factor (exposed) minus the risk among those without the risk factor (unexposed). For example, if we were evaluating a smoking cessation program, the attributable risk would tell us how much of the risk of developing heart disease is due to smoking and how much is due to other risk factors (for example, high cholesterol). The attributable risk in this example would be calculated as:

$$\text{risk}_{\text{Smokers}} - \text{risk}_{\text{Non-smokers}}$$

Equation 5.8

The attributable risk and other measures of risk that are useful in cost-effectiveness analysis will be covered in more detail in Chapter Twelve.

Bias in Screening Interventions

Two common sources of bias that can arise with screening interventions are **lead-time bias** and **length bias,** each of which can erroneously make an intervention appear more efficacious than it really is. For example, consider the case of screening mammography; an intervention that is intended to detect breast cancer at an early stage and ultimately prolong the lives of women with the disease. In general, the duration of illness of breast cancer is measured from the time of diagnosis to the time of recovery or death (see "Duration of Illness" section above).

Consider a woman with early breast cancer who does not undergo screening mammography. It is likely that her cancer will grow until it eventually becomes apparent to her or her physician. At this point, she will likely undergo some diagnostic tests, which will confirm that she has breast cancer. If, after her diagnosis she chooses *not* to receive treatment, the time between her diagnosis and death might be three years.

Now, let us consider the same woman with early breast cancer. This time, however, let us assume that she undergoes regular screening mammograms. Under these circumstances, her breast cancer is detected two years earlier than it would have been had she not undergone screening mammography. However, once again she decides *not* to receive treatment, and because the diagnosis was made two years earlier, the time between her diagnosis and death would now be five years. If we were simply evaluating the efficacy of screening mammography, it would appear as though her life was prolonged by two years, even though she did not receive any treatment for her breast cancer. Moreover, she would have died at the same age, whether or not she underwent screening mammography. Under these circumstances, it *appears* as though her life was prolonged, even though the only difference is that her illness was detected earlier. This type of bias is referred to as lead-time bias.

Different types of breast cancer grow at different rates. While some breast cancers grow so slowly that women with the disease often die of other causes (and may never realize that they actually had breast cancer), other types can grow and progress rapidly, causing death within a period of months. If women were to receive screening mammograms every two years, rapidly growing cancers would have a chance to develop between screening exams and thus might not be detected by mammography. Instead, they would probably eventually be detected by the patient or the physician because of symptoms. On the other hand, slow-growing cancers would be detected more often by screening. Women with these slow-growing tumors would survive longer, because the tumors are less aggressive. Since the test primarily detects the less aggressive tumors, it would seem as if women who had received the screening mammogram would be more likely to live longer. The tendency for a test to primarily detect conditions that progress slowly compared to those that progress rapidly is called length bias. Like lead-time bias, length bias makes screening exams appear more effective at reducing mortality than they actually are.

Both lead-time bias and length bias must be accounted for in cost-effectiveness analyses examining screening interventions. While it is possible to correct for these types of bias, doing so usually requires modeling techniques that are beyond the scope of an introductory textbook.

Efficacy of Strategies to Prevent Influenza-Like Illness

Treanor and others (2000) examined the efficacy of oseltamivir in preventing influenza-like illness and its complications (see Appendix II). A number of authors have examined the efficacy of the influenza vaccine in preventing influenza-like illness. Additional information on the efficacy of the influenza vaccine and articles pertaining to influenza from the Centers for Disease Control and Prevention (CDC) may be found on the Internet at: http://www.cdc.gov/ncidod/diseases/flu/fluvirus.htm and http://aepo-xdv-www.epo.cdc.gov/wonder/PrevGuid/m0052500/m0052500.htm.

The Centers for Disease Control and Prevention estimates that influenza vaccines are usually between 70 and 90 percent effective. For example, about 10 to 30 percent of vaccinated persons will become ill with the influenza virus during a typical influenza season ("Prevention," 1998). The efficacy of the influenza vaccine depends on how well the vaccine was matched to the types of viruses in circulation in any given year. It is thought that the vaccine will be poorly matched to the circulating strains of virus about once in ten years (Bridges and others, 2000).

Unfortunately, these authors provide the only available estimate of the efficacy of the influenza vaccine in preventing influenza-like illness. Nichol and others (1995) estimated the efficacy of the influenza vaccine in preventing upper respiratory illness. We might either use the estimate obtained from Bridges and others (2000), 0.34, or attempt to adjust the efficacy of the vaccine from Nichol and others (1995) to reflect the efficacy of the vaccine at preventing influenza-like illness (see Table 5.3).

Tips and tricks. In their article, Bridges and others (2000) report that the efficacy of the vaccine against influenza-like illness was 33 percent and the efficacy of the vaccine against upper respiratory illness was 13 percent. Using Table 2 in the Bridges article or Table 5.3 in this book, you can calculate the efficacy of the vaccine based on the information provided. You will see that the efficacy of the vaccine they report against influenza-like illness and upper respiratory illness is erroneous (the actual values are 0.344 and 0.101, respectively). Students are encouraged to always recalculate reports of efficacy, risk, or other outcome measures reported in journal articles using the data the authors present in tables. Occasionally, misprints or mistakes occur.

TABLE 5.3. THE EFFICACY OF THE INFLUENZA VACCINE IN PREVENTING INFLUENZA-LIKE ILLNESS (ILI).

	Vaccinated	Unvaccinated	Efficacy
Bridges and others			
Episodes ILI (a, b)	14	21	0.34
Episodes URI (b)	24	26	0.1
Nichol and others			
Episodes URI	105	140	0.25
Episodes ILI (a)	61	113	0.46
Average for ILI			0.40

(a) Episodes of influenza-like illness per 100 persons.

(b) Data from Bridges and others (2000) are rounded.

Exercises 5.3–5.5

5.3. Calculate the efficacy of oseltamivir in reducing the duration of influenza-like illness using data from Treanor and others (2000).

5.4. Calculate the efficacy of the influenza vaccine in preventing influenza virus infection. Use data from Bridges and others (2000) and Wilde and others (1999) to obtain the mean efficacy.

5.5. Bridges and others (2000) found that the influenza vaccine was 10 percent effective at preventing upper respiratory illness, 34 percent effective at preventing influenza-like illness, and 86 percent effective at preventing influenza virus infection during the 1998–1999 influenza season. Nichol and others (1995) found that the influenza vaccine was 25 percent effective at preventing upper respiratory illness (over two times as effective as Bridges and others, 2000). What might account for the large difference in vaccine efficacy between these two studies?

Laboratory Test Data

When a patient receives a screening test for a disease (for example, a test for the influenza virus), the test does not always correctly identify the presence or absence of the disease it was designed to detect. The **sensitivity** of a test refers to the ability of a test to detect a disease when it is present. **Specificity** refers to the ability of a test to detect the absence of disease when disease is not present. If we are evaluating the cost-effectiveness of a laboratory test, a lot will hinge on how good the test is at telling people whether they do or do not have the disease. The accuracy of laboratory tests are often represented in a 2 × 2 grid (see Table 5.4).

If a disease is present and the test for the disease is positive, the result is said to be a **true positive.** Conversely, if the disease is present and the test result is negative, it is said to be a **false negative.** If the subject is disease-free, the laboratory test can produce either a **true negative** (a negative test when no

TABLE 5.4.   CLASSIC 4 × 4 GRID USED TO CLASSIFY LABORATORY TEST RESULTS.

	Disease Present	Disease Absent
Test positive	True positive	False positive
Test negative	False negative	True negative

disease exists) or a **false positive** (a positive test result when in fact no disease exists) result. The information in Table 5.4 can be used to calculate the sensitivity and specificity of a laboratory test. Let us see how this works mathematically.

Suppose that we have a hundred subjects with high cholesterol levels and a hundred subjects with normal cholesterol levels. If we set a cutoff point for high blood cholesterol levels, the test results might appear as they do in Table 5.5. The sensitivity of the test is represented as the number of true positives divided by the total number of people *with disease* or $90/(90 + 10) = 90$ percent. The specificity of the test is represented by the number of true negatives divided by the total number of people *without the disease* or $95/(95 + 5) = 95$ percent.

The sensitivity and specificity of laboratory tests are the most commonly reported values in the medical literature. These values can also be obtained from the manufacturer of the test. In cost-effectiveness analyses, though, we are sometimes interested in knowing how good the test is at detecting disease *in the general population*, rather than among people that have the disease, so the sensitivity of a test is not in of itself useful information.

In the real world, we usually do not know whether the patients actually have the disease when they are tested. To get an idea of how good the test will be at predicting disease among the 95 subjects who tested positive in the example in Table 5.5, we would divide the true positive test results by the total number of positive test results or $90/95 = 94.7$ percent. This is called the **positive predictive value** of a laboratory test. The positive predictive value of a laboratory test may be built into a decision analysis model in a number of ways and will be thoroughly discussed in Chapter Twelve.

Laboratory Testing for Influenza

In our analysis, we will not need to evaluate the influenza test because our research question examines the cost-effectiveness of presumptive treatment only. For those

TABLE 5.5. RESULTS OF A HYPOTHETICAL SAMPLE OF 100 PEOPLE WITH HIGH BLOOD CHOLESTEROL LEVELS AND 100 PEOPLE WITH NORMAL BLOOD CHOLESTEROL LEVELS.

	Disease Present	Disease Absent	Total
Test positive	90	5	**95**
Test negative	10	95	**105**
Total	**100**	**100**	

extra curious students, the sensitivity and specificity of influenza virus tests are listed on the Internet at: http://www.uhl.uiowa.edu/Publications/ Hotline/1999_11/rapid.html.

Distribution of Disease

For most diseases, the incidence rate, the severity of illness, and the mortality rate differ by age, gender, race, education level, and income. When conducting a cost-effectiveness analysis, it is important to account for these distributional effects.

Distribution by Age

While heart disease disproportionately affects older adults, asthma disproportionately affects children. It is therefore important to determine the age-specific incidence and mortality rates for the disease under study. It is also important to capture changes in disease severity for people of different ages. We will learn how to account for these changes in Chapter Nine.

Distribution by Stage

It is also important to capture the number of people in different **clinical stages** of a disease. Typically, chronic progressive diseases like cancer are divided into logical categories, each representing a different degree of disease severity. For example, breast cancer is sometimes staged as *in situ*, local, regional, or distant. *In situ* refers to cancer that is confined to a specific region within the breast, while local disease refers to cancer that is confined to the breast but may have spread within the breast tissue. Regional disease refers to cancer that has spread to nearby organs. Finally, distant disease includes cancer that has spread to distant parts of the body.

In cost-effectiveness analysis, we must keep track of the proportion of people in each stage at the time that a disease is diagnosed and consider how much time lapses as people progress from one stage to the next. Suppose we know that 30 percent of breast cancer patients are staged as *in situ*, 20 percent are staged as local, 30 percent are staged as regional, and 20 percent are staged as distant when breast cancer is diagnosed with screening mammography. Using this information, we will then be able to estimate a health-related quality of life (HRQL) score and mortality rate for each group of women in our hypothetical cohort. These changes are usually captured in a special type of decision analysis model called a **Markov model,** which will be discussed in Chapter Twelve.

With acute infectious diseases like influenza, patients' illnesses may range from mild to severe or life threatening. However, influenza usually is not staged like cancer is. Instead, influenza is often described by its complications, such as influenza pneumonia or secondary bacterial pneumonia.

Distribution by Gender, Race, and Socioeconomic Status

When obtaining data from the medical literature or other sources, it is important to keep a good record of the study subject's characteristics and demographics. Because disease incidence rates, prevalence rates, mortality rates, and HRQL scores vary greatly among men, women, people of different socioeconomic status, race, or country of birth, it is very important to keep these factors in mind when considering how the hypothetical cohort in your cost-effectiveness analysis compares to the cohort of the study you are examining.

In the Bridges and others (2000) study, the median income of the cohort is almost twice the median income of the United States population (U.S. Bureau of the Census, 1999). Because the affluent are much more likely to be healthy and are much less likely to visit a doctor than the average citizen, the medical utilization rates reported in this study will not likely reflect those we would expect in our hypothetical cohort (Lantz and others, 1998). Moreover, the population in this study was predominantly male, and males are known to seek medical care at lower rates than females (Schappert and Nelson, 1999).

When the cohort of a study differs demographically from your cohort, adjustments to study outcomes should only be made with the consultation of an experienced epidemiologist and should then be tested using a broad sensitivity analysis. Such adjustments require difficult assumptions. Suppose, for instance, that you have found a study that uses an insured cohort and wish to adjust the health status of the cohort to better reflect that of the U.S. population.

While the poor, racial minorities, and immigrants are less likely to have insurance than the average person, insurance status does not always predict the health of these populations. For instance, immigrants are more than twice as likely as non-immigrants to lack health insurance, but they are also generally healthier than the general United States population (Hendershot, 1988; Singh and Siahpush, 2001). Because it is very difficult to predict which factors account for health differences between men and women, different racial groups, or people of differing socioeconomic status, it is best to use studies that contain a cohort that is demographically similar to your hypothetical cohort, unless no alternative exists. When using electronic datasets, the characteristics of the subjects in the data should always be matched to the characteristics of your cohort.

FIGURE 5.2. PERCENTAGE OF FEMALES BY COUNTRY OF BIRTH IN NEW YORK CITY.

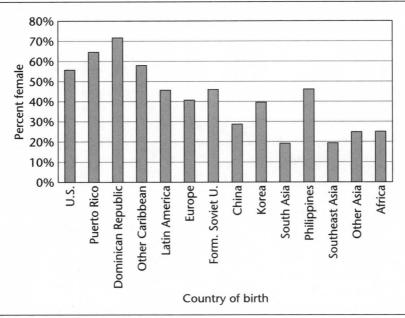

(*Source:* Housing and Vacancy Survey, 1996)

Figure 5.2 shows the variation in the percentage of females among different immigrant groups residing in New York City. Clearly, if we were interested in the incidence rate of certain thyroid diseases (some of which are more common among women) in immigrant groups, our results would be artificially influenced by the low proportion of females among South Asians and the high proportion of females among Dominicans.

Other Considerations Regarding the Distribution of Disease

There are a number of other factors to consider when thinking about how a disease is distributed within a society. Disease incidence rates are sometimes subject to seasonal and geographic variation, and the standard of medical care often varies substantially by geographic region. Moreover, health interventions are sometimes applied sporadically, making it difficult to determine who in society has received an intervention for a particular disease. For instance, if we wished to obtain a mean cholesterol value for the United States for a "no intervention" comparison, it would be difficult to find a representative sample of subjects that were not receiving cholesterol-lowering medications. All of these factors can affect your ability to generalize the data you obtain from a specific source to your hypothetical study cohort.

Variations in practice patterns can also affect the distribution of disease within society (Wennberg and Gittelsohn, 1982). Doctors often follow local trends in deciding which preventive interventions, medical treatments, or types of surgery they recommend for their patients. These variations in medical practice can have a significant impact on how the incidence rate of a disease, mortality rate of a disease, or even treatment side effects vary from one area of the country to the next. Finally, currently recommended medical screening tests and treatments do not always reach everyone in society.

Distribution of Influenza-Like Illness

In our sample cost-effectiveness analysis, we are interested in parameters pertaining to all healthy adults residing in the United States, so we must try to ensure that our data sources are representative of this population. In the "Incidence of Influenza-Like Illness" section above, we saw how the incidence rate of influenza-like illness varies by geographic region. We also learned how the healthy volunteer effect might affect our ability to apply existing disease incidence rates to our cohort. Fortunately, only the Bridges and others (2000) cohort differed markedly from the hypothetical cohort we wish to use. As we noted above, this cohort is disproportionately male and affluent, so we would expect that the rate of medical utilization would be somewhat lower than the general population. It is also possible that the lower incidence rate of influenza-like illness observed in that study, relative to the other studies we examined, was partly attributable to the demographics of the cohort. By using the median rate of influenza-like illness in the studies we found, the lower rate of illness observed in this study will not affect our estimate of this input. Because we are evaluating an acute disease, we do not have to worry about differences in disease staging.

We will be concerned with the distribution of disease by vaccine status, however. While the studies on vaccine efficacy contain only information on subjects that were either vaccinated or not vaccinated at all, most data derived from electronic databases or from cross-sectional population studies contain information on subjects in the general population (which includes both vaccinated and unvaccinated subjects). We should keep track of the vaccination status of the subjects in different data sources and make adjustments where necessary. To adjust for the vaccination status of a cohort, we can use data from the Behavioral Risk Factor Surveillance System (BRFSS), which is available online at: http://apps.nccd.cdc.gov/brfss/index.asp. This dataset contains information on the percentage of people in the United States that have been vaccinated against

TABLE 5.6.   AGE-SPECIFIC VACCINATION RATES, VACCINE EFFICACY, AND THE PREDICTED PERCENT CHANGE IN RATES OBTAINED FROM ELECTRONIC DATASETS.

Influenza Age Group	Coverage Rate	Vaccine Efficacy	Percent Non-Susceptible
15 to 24	16.6%	0.8	13.3%
25 to 34	15.3%	0.8	12.2%
35 to 44	18.4%	0.8	14.7%
45 to 54	25.9%	0.8	20.7%
54 to 64	38.0%	0.8	30.4%
Average	22.8%		18.3%

influenza. Table 5.6 summarizes the data from the Behavioral Risk Factor Surveillance System and the predicted changes in the incidence rates of hospitalization or mortality data obtained from electronic datasets.

The final column in Table 5.6 indicates the percentage of people who would have been susceptible to influenza virus infections had they not been vaccinated. In Exercise 5.4, we saw that the influenza vaccine was 80 percent effective at preventing influenza infections. To estimate the percentage of people who could have developed an influenza virus infection had they not been vaccinated, we simply multiply the percentage of people infected by the vaccine efficacy.

Because we are interested in the cost-effectiveness of vaccination or treatment relative to providing supportive care alone, we will need to adjust any data containing both vaccinated persons and unvaccinated persons so that they reflect rates of illness in persons that have not been vaccinated. Consider the hospitalization rate we calculated in Exercise 4.2. Many people in the United States received the influenza vaccine. If no one in the United States were vaccinated, we would expect the hospitalization rate to have been higher. We calculated the rate as follows:

$$\frac{\text{number of people hospitalized for influenza virus infection aged 18 to 65, 1997}}{\text{number of people aged 18 to 65 in the United States, 1997}}$$

Equation 5.9

However, referring to Equation 3.1, we see that the correct rate of influenza virus infection among unvaccinated people would be:

$$\frac{\text{number of people hospitalized for influenza virus infection aged 18 to 65}}{\text{number of } \textit{susceptible} \text{ people aged 18 to 65 in the United States}}$$

Equation 5.10

(Remember that we did not have data on fifteen- to sixty-five-year-olds, so we assumed that the rate among eighteen- to sixty-five-year-olds would be similar.)

Referring to Table 5.6, we see that about 18.3 percent of the population would not have been susceptible to the influenza virus and could not have been hospitalized that year. In other words, the population of people that could have developed an influenza virus infection would be 100 percent − 18.3 percent = 81.7 percent. In Exercise 4.4, we saw that there were 10,778 hospitalizations for influenza virus infections (Clinical Classification Software Code 123) among persons aged eighteen to sixty-five and 163,961,000 people aged eighteen to sixty-five residing in the United States. There were 163,961,000 · (0.817) = 133,956,137 people at risk of hospitalization in 1997. The hospitalization rate among the susceptible population (unvaccinated persons) would therefore be:

$$\frac{10,778 \text{ hospitalizations, persons 18 to 65}}{133,956,137 \text{ susceptible persons 18 to 65}} = 0.0000805$$

The incidence rate of influenza-like illness obtained from the National Health Interview Survey (NHIS) in the "Incidence of Influenza-Like Illness" section above also reflects rates of illness in the general population rather than among unvaccinated persons.

Secondary Complications of Illness

Many diseases place people at risk for developing secondary complications of illness. For example, diabetes mellitus increases the risk for heart disease, kidney disease, and blindness, among other illnesses. When diabetes mellitus is prevented through a proper diet and exercise, some heart attacks, cases of kidney disease, and so on will also be prevented. We must therefore be careful to include the costs and health effects of these secondary illnesses in our analysis as well. If the costs associated with secondary complications of illness are ignored, interventions that reduce the rate of the primary illness will be undervalued.

Secondary illness can also be caused by medications, surgical treatments, or diagnostic tests. Secondary illness sometimes arises in healthy people that are misdiagnosed with a disease and subsequently receive unnecessary treatment. For example, women who are screened with mammography may undergo unnecessary surgical biopsies if the test result is falsely positive.

Secondary Complications of Influenza-Like Illness

In our analysis, we will need to estimate the rate of secondary illness among people receiving the influenza vaccine, treatment with oseltamivir, and people receiving supportive care alone. Influenza is known to increase a person's risk for pneumonia, sinusitis, and otitis media (ear infection), and it can aggravate underlying chronic conditions (LaForce and others, 1994; Neuzil and others, 1999; Nichol and others, 1995; Sullivan and others, 1983). Because our hypothetical cohort consists of healthy adults, we will only be concerned with acute conditions arising from recent infections with the influenza virus. These secondary conditions may require treatment with antibiotics or lead to other events that might be relevant to our cost-effectiveness analysis.

Exercise 5.6

5.6. What is the probability that a subject with influenza-like illness will receive antibiotics? Use the data from Bridges and others (2000) listed in Table A2.1. Would you expect this finding? Why?

Medical Care Utilization

The chance of an ambulatory medical visit, hospital visit, or the need for long-term care may be obtained from the medical literature or from electronic datasets. The commonly used datasets are listed in Table 4.1.

Health interventions modify the chance of becoming ill or the severity of disease. In a cost-effectiveness analysis, it is generally necessary to obtain the rate of ambulatory care utilization and hospitalization when each intervention is applied. For debilitating diseases, it is also important to estimate changes in long-term care or hospice care utilization when each intervention is applied.

Measures of risk are usually used to determine the rate of medical care utilization for each intervention. For example, if we know that the annual rate of hospitalization for diabetes mellitus is ten hospitalizations per 1,000 people and that a particular treatment reduces the rate of hospitalization by 50 percent, the rate of hospitalization in the treatment group would be 10 hospitalizations per 1,000 people $\cdot$ 0.5 = 5 hospitalizations per 1,000 people.

Rates Obtained from Electronic Data

When using electronic data, it is important to ensure that the data are not subject to misclassification bias. Suppose, for example, that a diabetic person is treated for a foot ulcer resulting from his disease. The diagnosis recorded in the hospital or ambulatory care records might be either the foot ulcer or the diabetes.

Misclassification bias can be minimized by examining all of the conditions the patient had during the medical visit. The **primary diagnosis** represents what the doctor listed on the billing form (in an ambulatory care visit) or what the medical records listed as the reason for admission (in hospital records). Most electronic datasets also contain information on **secondary diagnoses** (other diagnoses that the patient had during the visit or hospital admission). In the case of the diabetic person seeking treatment for a foot ulcer, the foot ulcer will likely be listed as the principal diagnosis, while the diabetes mellitus will be listed as a secondary diagnosis.

Another problem that often arises with electronic data is that a particular disease may be associated with a number of different diagnosis codes (see Chapter Four). This is especially true when using International Classification for Disease (ICD) codes. For example, influenza virus infection with pneumonia (ICD-9 code 487.0) is associated with a different diagnosis code from influenza in general (ICD-9 code 487.1). It is important to ensure that all codes pertaining to a particular disease are included in the analysis. One way around this problem is to use Clinical Classification Software (CCS) codes rather than ICD codes when it is necessary to aggregate all conditions associated with a disease.

On a final note, it is also important to recognize that when using electronic data the number of outcomes (hospital admissions, clinic visits, and so on) that take place over the span of a year may not always equal the number of patients having that particular outcome. For example, a single patient may be hospitalized more than once or may see a clinician multiple times for a particular illness over the span of a year. Electronic data often capture all visits by diagnosis code over a year, regardless of whether a patient was seen or admitted more than once. For example, if the hospital data indicate that there were 1,000 hospitalizations for a chronic disease, it is possible that 500 people were admitted an average of two times for this condition.

Hospitalization Data for Influenza-Like Illness

There are a few issues to consider when using electronic data to estimate medical utilization rates for influenza-like illness. While subjects might visit their provider for an influenza-like illness, they are only likely to be hospitalized for influenza itself or secondary bacterial pneumonia. Other infections that comprise influenza-like illness are unlikely to be severe enough to require hospitalization. However, if we were to use hospitalization rates for influenza and secondary bacterial pneumonia, we would have to assume that the rate of hospitalization for influenza-like illness would be equal to the rate of hospitalization for influenza virus infections and secondary bacterial pneumonia among *healthy* adults. (See Exhibit 5.1 for a discussion of assumptions in cost-effectiveness analysis.)

Moreover, when examining the number of hospitalizations for bacterial pneumonia, there is no good way to determine whether the pneumonia was related to a recent influenza virus infection, occurred on its own, or occurred as a result of some other disease. If we were to use an electronic dataset (such as the National Hospital Discharge Survey) to estimate the number of hospitalizations for influenza virus infection, we would miss most secondary complications of these infections because this information will not be recorded in the patient's hospital billing data.

Finally, it is necessary to carefully match the data to the characteristics of our cohort and to reduce error introduced by seasonal variation. Let us see how these problems affected the rate of hospitalization we calculated in Exercise 4.4, 6.6 hospitalizations per 100,000 persons. In the "Distribution of Influenza-Like Illness" section above, we learned how to adjust this rate so that it would better reflect the rate of illness among unvaccinated persons (8.0 hospitalizations per 100,000 persons).

There are a number of problems associated with this estimate with which we must still contend. First, this rate does not include secondary complications of influenza virus infections. Second, it only represents one season of data. Third, it reflects the rate of hospitalization in all adults, rather than in healthy adults. As we learned in Chapter Two, people with chronic lung disease, heart disease, or diabetes are at increased risk of complications for influenza virus infections. We defined our cohort as all "healthy" adults (adults without chronic diseases that place them at risk of morbidity or mortality if they are infected with the influenza virus). Because adjusting the electronic data for all of these factors would be time-consuming and require assumptions, we should turn to the medical literature to see if there is a better estimate.

Evaluating the medical literature. The Centers for Disease Control and Prevention (CDC) estimated the probability of hospitalization for influenza-associated

EXHIBIT 5.1.   MAKING ASSUMPTIONS IN COST-EFFECTIVENESS ANALYSIS.

Oftentimes, assumptions about the course of an illness or the value of a parameter will be needed in a cost-effectiveness analysis. Any assumptions made by a researcher should be tested in a broad sensitivity analysis and clearly stated in any published report of the study findings. If the parameter is important, expert opinion should be solicited to better define the baseline value of that parameter.

conditions over many seasons for people aged fifteen to sixty-five without chronic medical conditions (twenty to forty hospitalizations per 100,000, "Prevention," 1999, which is available online at http://aepo-xdv-www.epo.cdc.gov/wonder/PrevGuid/m0052500/m0052500.htm). See Exhibit 5.2 for a discussion of the advantages of using a literature review conducted by the CDC.

This estimate was based on two studies of **excess hospitalizations** for influenza-associated conditions among healthy adults over a number of influenza seasons (Barker, 1986; Barker and Mullooly, 1980). Excess hospitalizations are defined as the number of hospitalizations for influenza-related conditions occurring during influenza season minus the number of hospitalizations occurring during the off-season. Note that the number of excess hospitalizations for conditions thought to be related to influenza virus infections is an imperfect estimator of the number of hospitalizations for influenza-like illness.

While influenza-like illness is a constellation of influenza virus infection along with other minor illnesses, influenza-associated conditions are those conditions that result in hospitalization or death that occur during influenza season. Influenza-associated conditions are very different from influenza-like illness. They include all conditions that are known to be worsened by an infection with the influenza virus or arise as a result of an infection with the influenza virus. For example, bacterial pneumonia is an influenza-associated condition. However, because the influenza virus is the only agent among influenza-like illnesses that is likely to cause a severe outcome, such as a hospitalization or a death, the rate of hospitalization for influenza-associated conditions should be similar to the rate of hospitalization for influenza-like illness.

The population weighted mean hospitalization rate for our cohort is approximately 24 hospitalizations per 100,000 persons. To convert this number into a

EXHIBIT 5.2.   CHOOSING BASELINE ESTIMATES IN COST-EFFECTIVENESS ANALYSES.

Generally, if there is a prevailing consensus regarding the baseline rate of a parameter, such as an official report from the Centers for Disease Control and Prevention (CDC), that estimate should be used (unless there is a good reason to believe that the estimate is out of date or is not applicable to your hypothetical cohort). When no consensus exists and data sources contain a high degree of error, it is best to present the data you have collected to medical experts. These experts can then weigh the different sources of error in your data and provide you with a more concrete estimate of the parameter you are interested in. When no data exist on a parameter, expert opinion can be used to generate an estimate of the parameter, however, when soliciting expert opinion, the Delphi process should be used (see Chapter Four).

probability, we simply divide 24 hospitalizations by 100,000 persons to obtain an overall probability of 0.00024.

At the time of publication, there had only been one recent study examining hospitalizations for influenza or related conditions among healthy adults (Neuzil and others, 1999). In this study, the authors examined excess hospitalizations that occurred due to influenza-related conditions among Medicaid recipients in Tennessee over nineteen influenza seasons. After averaging the data across all nineteen seasons, they found that the excess rate of hospitalization for influenza-related conditions among women without underlying chronic disease was 4 per 10,000 persons per year among women aged twenty-five to forty-five and 6 per 10,000 persons per year among women aged forty-five to sixty-five. Multiplying these rates by a factor of 10, we see that 40 excess hospitalizations per 100,000 healthy adults occurred among adults aged twenty-five to forty-five, and 60 excess hospitalizations per 100,000 healthy adults occurred among adults aged forty-five to sixty-five. The weighted probability of hospitalization in this study among healthy adults was approximately 0.00044, which is around ten times higher than the rate we calculated using HCUP-3 data and almost twice as high as the CDC estimate.

The primary limitation of this analysis was that Medicaid-insured patients tend to be poor and may therefore be at greater risk of complications of a disease (see the "Distribution of Disease" section above). Nonetheless, Neuzil and others (1999) data provide us with a high estimate of hospitalizations for influenza-associated conditions among healthy adults, and the calculations reaffirm that the CDC estimate is at least in the ballpark range of average hospitalization rates among healthy adults.

Ambulatory Care Data for Influenza-Like Illness

The National Ambulatory Medical Care Survey (NAMCS) and Medical Expenditure Panel Survey (MEPS) contain ambulatory care data for most diseases. Because influenza-like illness is a cluster of symptoms that may be induced by a number of diseases, it would be difficult to generate a list of diagnostic codes that encompassed this condition. Instead, we must attempt to estimate the rate of ambulatory care utilization for influenza-like illness from the medical literature. Estimates of the probability of a medical visit for vaccinated and unvaccinated persons are listed in Table 5.7.

Evaluating the medical literature. Recall that the data from Bridges and others (2000) were limited by lack of generalizability (external validity) because the study was 1) conducted at a single Ford Motors plant in southern Michigan, 2) used a relatively affluent cohort, and 3) used a predominantly male cohort. Nichol and others (1995) data were limited by 1) external validity and 2) a loose definition of

TABLE 5.7. PROBABILITY OF AN AMBULATORY CARE VISIT FOR INFLUENZA-LIKE ILLNESS FOR VACCINATED AND UNVACCINATED PERSONS FROM VARIOUS SOURCES IN THE MEDICAL LITERATURE.

Author	Vaccinated	Unvaccinated	Notes
Bridges and others	0.05	0.086	Definition = influenza-like illness.
Bridges and others	0.07	0.084	Definition = upper respiratory illness.
Nichol and others	0.31	0.55	Definition = upper respiratory illness.
Nichol and others	0.22	0.56	Upper respiratory illness rate adjusted to rate of influenza-like illness using data from Bridges and others.
Campbell and others	0.33	0.38	Non-randomized. Small sample.
Keech and others	—	0.32	Survey data of ill patients.

influenza-like illness. The Campbell and Rumly (1995) data were limited by 1) a small sample size, 2) external validity, and 3) the use of a non-randomized study design. Keech and others (1998) data were also limited because they obtained data by surveying people at the time of their illness and did not compare vaccinated subjects with nonvaccinated subjects.

The only data on ambulatory care medical utilization from randomized controlled trials are available from Nichol and others (1995) and Bridges and others (2000). The study by Campbell and Rumly (1995) used a non-randomized study design. The problem with comparing rates from a non-randomized cohort is that the subjects who chose to receive the influenza vaccine are likely to be different from subjects that did not. For instance, subjects who received the vaccine may be more conscientious or more concerned with their health than subjects who did not. It is difficult to predict whether such persons would be more or less likely to visit a physician if they fell ill than subjects that did not bother to receive the vaccine.

Adjusting estimates for the definition of illness. Males generally visit doctors less frequently than females and health status generally increases with income (National Center for Health Statistics, 1999; Schappert and Nelson, 1999). Because subjects in the Bridges and others (2000) cohort were relatively wealthy and predominantly male, medical utilization data in this study may not be representative of medical utilization among the average healthy adult in the United States. We should therefore attempt to generate a more representative estimate of medical utilization.

Recall that Bridges and others (2000) provide data for both influenza-like illness and upper respiratory illness. Using these dual definitions, we can adjust the Nichol and others (1995) data under the assumption that the proportionate number of ambulatory visits for upper respiratory illness and influenza-like illness would be consistent across these studies.

Because we are interested in the rate of ambulatory care visits in both vaccinated and unvaccinated subjects, we need to adjust two separate rates, one corrected for the definition of illness in the vaccine group and one corrected for the definition of illness in the placebo group (see Equation 5.1). The rate of medical visits among subjects who had an influenza-like illness in the Nichol and others (1995) study is approximately equal to:

$$\text{rate MD visits, } \cancel{\text{URI}} \text{ (Nichol and others, 1995)} \cdot \frac{\text{rate MD visits, ILI (Bridges and others, 2000)}}{\text{rate MD visits, } \cancel{\text{URI}} \text{ (Bridges and others, 2000)}}$$

Equation 5.11

Obtaining the number of medical visits during the 1998–1999 influenza seasons in the Bridges and others (2000) study (Appendix II, Table A2.1), we see that there were twenty-nine medical visits for influenza-like illness and forty-one medical visits for upper respiratory illness in the vaccine group. In the placebo group, there were fifty-one medical visits for influenza-like illness and fifty visits for upper respiratory illness. The adjusted rate of medical visits per 100 vaccinated subjects is approximately equal to:

$$31 \text{ visits, } \cancel{\text{URI}} \text{ (Nichol and others, 1995)} \cdot \frac{29 \text{ visits, ILI (Bridges and others, 2000)}}{41 \text{ visits, } \cancel{\text{URI}} \text{ (Bridges and others, 2000)}} = 22 \text{ visits ILI}$$

The adjusted rate of medical visits per 100 subjects in the placebo arm is approximately equal to:

$$55 \text{ visits, } \cancel{\text{URI}} \text{ (Nichol and others, 1995)} \cdot \frac{51 \text{ visits, ILI (Bridges and others, 2000)}}{50 \text{ visits, } \cancel{\text{URI}} \text{ (Bridges and others, 2000)}} = 56 \text{ visits ILI}$$

Effects of income. We may wish to consider what would happen to the number of ambulatory care visits if more low-income subjects were included in the analysis, because the Bridges and others (2000) cohort was more affluent than the Nichol and others (1995) cohort. While 75 percent of the subjects in the Bridges and others study earned more than $75,000 per year, only 36 percent of the patients in the Nichol and others study earned more than $39,000 per year. The National Health Interview Survey (NHIS) examines the number of physician contacts by income (Adams and others, 1996). Table 71 of the printed tabulation for the NHIS indicates that people with a total family income of less than $10,000 have about 1.6 times as many physician contacts as people with an income of more than $35,000 (Adams and others, 1999). These figures are summarized in Table 5.8 below.

Though it would be tempting to use the NHIS data presented in Table 5.8 to adjust the Bridges and others (2000) data, this would require difficult assumptions;

TABLE 5.8. ANNUAL RATE OF PHYSICIAN CONTACTS BY TOTAL FAMILY INCOME.

Income	Average Number Physician Contacts per Year
<$10,000	8.4
$10,000 to $20,000	7.1
$20,000 to $35,000	5.7
$>$35,000	5.4

we would have to assume that the increase in utilization rates would be equal in the placebo and control groups. While people with low income are more likely to have an illness than wealthy people, they are also less likely to be insured (National Center for Health Statistics, 1999). It is therefore difficult to determine whether uninsured people with influenza-like illness would be willing to pay for a medical visit for a relatively minor ailment. Moreover, the interaction between illness rates and disease is complex. Low-income people may be more likely than more affluent people to smoke and may therefore be at increased risk of influenza-like illness, but it is difficult to determine how much of an increase in rates we would be likely to observe, if any (Lantz and others, 1998).

Deciding which data to use. In the above sections, we saw that we have various limitations in sources of data on ambulatory care utilization for people who receive the influenza vaccine and people who receive a placebo injection. Two studies were based on randomized controlled trial study design. However, the cohort in the Bridges and others (2000) study differs demographically from the cohort we wish to include in our analysis. In the other randomized study, Nichol and others (1995), a separate definition of illness was used. A third study, Campbell and Rumly (1995), did not use a randomized design to determine vaccine efficacy. This study found only a small difference in the rate of ambulatory care utilization between the vaccine and the control group. In this textbook, we present average values from Nichol and others (1995) and Bridges and others (2000) for simplicity.

In Chapter Three, we discussed two possible approaches to managing multiple sources of error, meta-analysis, and the Delphi method. In meta-analysis, many studies are analyzed for their quality. Studies felt to be inappropriate for inclusion in the analysis are excluded. None of these studies would likely meet reasonable inclusion criteria. The best way to manage data with this degree of uncertainty is perhaps to present it to a panel of experts and attempt to generate a consensus opinion using the Delphi method (see Chapter Three). The experts should be presented with the three studies described here and evidence supporting potential differences in utilization by gender and income.

TABLE 5.9. PROBABILITY OF AN ILLNESS, A MEDICAL VISIT, AND A MEDICAL VISIT AMONG PERSONS WITH INFLUENZA-LIKE ILLNESS FROM BRIDGES AND OTHERS (2000) AND NICHOL AND OTHERS (1995).

	Vaccine	No Vaccine	Efficacy
Illnesses			
Bridges, URI	0.235	0.262	0.10
Bridges, ILI	0.141	0.215	0.34
Nichol, URI	1.05	1.4	0.25
Nichol, ILI	0.63	1.149	0.45
MD visits			
Bridges, URI	0.07	0.084	0.17
Bridges, ILI	0.05	0.086	0.42
Nichol, URI	0.31	0.55	0.44
Nichol, ILI	0.221	0.563	0.61
MD visits, ill			
Bridges, ILI	0.355	0.4	0.11
Nichol, ILI	0.351	0.49	0.28
Average	0.353	0.445	0.21

Some of the effects of gender and income may not be as apparent among subjects that actually become ill. While affluence may reduce one's chances of becoming ill in the first place, there may be less discrepancy in medical care utilization rates between rich and poor people who actually do become ill. In the next section, we will see that the rates of ambulatory medical care utilization among ill subjects in these studies are actually quite similar.

Adjusting for infection status. The data in Table 5.7 reflect the overall rates of ambulatory medical care utilization in the cohorts of each study. It will be useful to know the probability of a medical visit among persons who actually develop an influenza-like illness. The probability of a medical visit among persons with influenza-like illness is equal to:

$$\frac{\text{number of visits for influenza-like illness}}{\text{number of ill subjects}}$$

Equation 5.12

Applying this formula to the vaccine and placebo arms of the Bridges and others (2000) and Nichol and others (1995) studies, we may derive a mean rate of medical visits for vaccinated and unvaccinated persons with influenza-like illness (see Table 5.9). In this table, the probabilities of an illness, of a medical visit, and of a medical visit among subjects with influenza-like illness are listed by the definition of illness used in each of the studies.

Let us review the steps used to generate Table 5.9.

Step 1: Calculate the probability of an illness. The probability of developing an illness is equal to the number of subjects with influenza-like illness divided by the total number of subjects. Thus, the probability that vaccinated subjects will develop influenza-like illness in the Bridges and others (2000) study is: 82 ill subjects/582 subjects in total = 0.141 (see Table A2.1 in Appendix II or Table 2 in the Bridges and others (2000) study).

Step 2: Calculate the probability of a medical visit among all subjects. We calculated the probability of a medical visit among well subjects in the previous section (see Table 5.7).

Step 3: Adjust the illness rates from Nichol and others (1995) to reflect the probability of illness among subjects with influenza-like illness rather than upper respiratory illness. Applying Equation 5.12, divide the number of medical visits for influenza-like illness by the number of ill subjects. For example, among vaccinated subjects in Table A2.1, there were 29 physician visits and 82 ill subjects, yielding a probability of a medical visit of 29/82 = 0.355.

Step 4: Apply Equation 5.2 to each row value in Table 5.9 to calculate the efficacy of the influenza vaccine at preventing an influenza-like illness, a medical visit, and a medical visit among subjects who develop an influenza-like illness.

Thus, we have an average of 44.5 visits per 100 patients with influenza-like illness in the placebo group (a probability of 0.445) and 35.3 visits per 100 patients with influenza-like illness in the vaccine group (a probability of 0.353).

Notice that the influenza vaccine is more effective at preventing a medical visit than it is at preventing an influenza-like illness. For instance, in the Bridges and others (2000) study, we see that the efficacy of the vaccine in preventing an influenza-like illness is 0.34 and the efficacy of the vaccine at preventing an ambulatory medical visit for influenza-like illness is 0.42. This may occur because some vaccinated people who develop an influenza virus infection may be partially, but not completely, protected from the virus. Though they develop an illness, the illness is less severe than it might have been had the subject not been vaccinated, reducing the need for a medical visit.

Ambulatory visits for persons treated with oseltamivir. We are evaluating the cost-effectiveness of oseltamivir in reducing the duration and severity of influenza-like illness rather than its ability to prevent this illness. Therefore, we would not expect that oseltamivir would reduce the chance that people will initially visit a physician for influenza-like illness. However, this medication may reduce the chance of secondary complications of their illness and may therefore reduce the overall number of medical visits. Treanor and others (2000) examined the total number of secondary complications to influenza-like illness among subjects treated with oseltamivir. These secondary complications included otitis media, bronchitis, sinusitis, and bacterial pneumonia. (Be certain to remember that in measuring secondary complications to influenza-like illness, they are actually measuring secondary complications to influenza virus infection, because influenza is the only agent likely to result in a secondary complication. We will refer to secondary complications of influenza virus infection here so that students are able to distinguish the two disease categories.)

Since each of these complications required a separate medical visit in this study, we may assume that the rate of secondary complications is equal to the rate of ambulatory medical visits for secondary complications in the treatment arm of our analysis. However, we should note that all of the subjects in the study by Treanor and others (2000) were enrolled in a randomized controlled trial. Therefore, the rate of medical visits in this trial (efficacy data) may not reflect real-world conditions (effectiveness data). For instance, some people in the general United States population lack health insurance and may be less likely to see a doctor for secondary complications of influenza virus infections than subjects enrolled in this trial.

To calculate the probability of secondary complications among treated and untreated persons, we may apply Equation 5.13.

$$\frac{\text{number of subjects with secondary complications}}{\text{total number of subjects}}$$

Equation 5.13

Referring to Table A2.6 in Appendix II, we see that there were 11 secondary complications among the 124 subjects that received 75 mg of oseltamivir twice daily and 6 secondary complications among the 121 subjects that received 150 mg of oseltamivir twice daily. Although our subjects will only receive 75mg of oseltamivir twice daily, we may combine these two groups because there was no difference in treatment efficacy between them. By combining these two groups, we will be increasing the size of our statistical sample and will therefore be reducing random error. The overall rate of secondary complications among treated subjects was $(11 + 6)/(124 + 121) = 0.069$.

Among subjects in the placebo group, 19 of 129 or $19/129 = 0.147$ subjects experienced secondary complications to their illness. Conversely, approximately $1 - 0.147 = 0.853$, or 85.3 percent, of the visits for supportive care were due to influenza-like illness excluding secondary complications. The probability of a medical visit for influenza-like illness alone among subjects receiving supportive care is equal to the product of the total number of visits among people receiving supportive care, 0.445 (see Table 5.9) and the proportion of subjects who were infected with an influenza-like illness less subjects with secondary complications would be approximately $0.445 \cdot (1 - 0.147) = 0.379$. When we construct a decision analysis model in Chapter Seven, you will see how these values can be put to use. The overall rates of medical visits among subjects with influenza-like illness in each treatment arm are summarized in Table 5.10.

Side Effects

Virtually all invasive screening tests (diagnostic tests that require surgical procedures) and medical treatments are associated with side effects. Even treatments that are not associated with higher rates of side effects relative to the placebo group in randomized controlled trials may produce side effects in the real world. People who take pills often believe that the treatment is supposed to cause problems, so symptoms may arise via the placebo effect. In most double blind randomized controlled studies, some people receiving a placebo experience nausea, vomiting, headache, or other symptoms that they attribute to the medication.

Other medications can cause real side effects. Severe or long-term side effects should be captured in the denominator of the cost-effectiveness analysis (as QALYs). If the side effects from a medication are limited to minor complaints or short-term complaints, such as headache or nausea, the costs associated with any medical visits, medical treatments, and patient time need only be captured in the numerator of the cost-effectiveness ratio.

Side Effects Due to Vaccination or Treatment

Vaccination can cause arm soreness, and oseltamivir can cause nausea. However, neither of these interventions is likely to produce common side effects that require

TABLE 5.10. PROBABILITY OF AMBULATORY CARE VISITS FOR EACH OF THE HEALTH INTERVENTIONS UNDER STUDY.

	MD Visits per 100 Ill Persons
Supportive care	0.445
Treatment	0.379
Vaccination	0.353

follow-up visits to a doctor (Bridges and others, 2000; Nichol and others, 1995; Treanor and others, 2000). Nevertheless, we cannot rule out the possibility that subjects will experience side effects. To be on the safe side, we should include the possibility that side effects will arise in our sensitivity analysis. The cost associated with side effects will be discussed in the next chapter, and sensitivity analysis will be discussed in Chapter Ten.

Though it has not been found to produce common side effects, vaccination may rarely cause a neurological condition called the Guillian-Barré syndrome. People with the Guillian-Barré syndrome experience serious neurological problems, including partial or complete paralysis. Though most people will recover from this syndrome, occasionally some do not, and approximately 6 percent of all people will die from it or its complications. Fortunately, the probability of Guillian-Barré syndrome is on average about one in a million (Lasky and others, 1998). Because the condition has not been definitively shown to be associated with influenza vaccination (see Appendix II), is extremely rare, is usually of a short duration, and deaths only occur in 6 percent of those that develop this condition, we may safely exclude this condition from our QALY calculations. We will explore the potential cost of this condition in the next chapter.

Were we to include the data from Lasky and others (1998), we would utilize the range of values they provide in their study, 1 per 10 million to 9 per million, in our sensitivity analysis. This is the only study that we know of that examines the chance of Guillian-Barré syndrome among vaccinated people when current influenza vaccine is used. This study is included in Appendix II.

Health-Related Quality of Life Scores

In Chapter One, you learned that the health-related quality of life (HRQL) score is a valuation of life lived in a particular health state, where perfect health is assigned a score of one and death is assigned a score of zero, on a scale that ranges from zero to one. A year of life lived at an HRQL score of 0.5 is thus only worth half a year of life lived in perfect health. In this section, we will discuss ways in which HRQL scores may be obtained. Choosing the correct HRQL score for the disease you are studying can be challenging and will be discussed in greater detail in Chapter Eight. In this section, we will briefly discuss how HRQL scores are obtained.

To find HRQL scores for your analysis, you can either use published lists of HRQL scores (see Appendix IV for one such list) or derive the scores using special instruments.

Obtaining Scores from Published Lists

The use of published lists of HRQL scores is by far the easiest way to find the HRQL score you are looking for, but it is not always the best. One list of HRQL scores, derived from the Years of Healthy Life (YHL) measure, is currently available for most diseases (Gold and others, 1998). By using this measure, it is possible to obtain HRQL scores for different demographically defined groups. The problem with the YHL measure is that it may not capture all of the aspects of a disease that might be important for your analysis. For example, it is not useful for conditions that have a large psychological impact on a person or affect a person's ability to relate to others (Gold and others, 1996; Gold and others, 1998). Harvard University also maintains a list of HRQL scores that were extracted from the medical literature. These are available at www.hsph.harvard.edu/organizations/hcra/cuadatabase/intro.html.

Generating HRQL Scores Using Instruments

To derive scores on your own, you can administer special questionnaires designed to generate HRQL scores to health professionals or to patients. Alternatively, published information on the disease under study can be used to fill in the values. These questionnaires are formally known as **preference-weighted generic instruments.** Preference-weighted generic instruments contain a number of questions related to different aspects of the health-related quality of life called **health domains** (also known as **dimensions** or **attributes**). A person's ability to function normally in society, to perform daily activities, or to get from one place to the next are examples of health domains. Because each instrument captures different domains, it is important to try to match the domains captured by a given instrument with the domains particular to the disease under study. A description of the different diseases that might be studied using these instruments can be found in Table 5.11. The use of preference-weighted generic instruments will be discussed in detail in Chapter Eight.

Mortality Data

Mortality data are usually obtained from prospective studies or from electronic datasets. Virtually all electronic mortality data are maintained by the National Center for Health Statistics (NCHS). The NCHS is one of the "centers" among the Centers for Disease Control and Prevention (CDC). Local or state health departments collect mortality data. These data are then sent to the NCHS, which

TABLE 5.11. PREFERENCE-WEIGHTED GENERIC INSTRUMENTS USED TO DERIVE HRQL SCORES FOR COST-EFFECTIVENESS ANALYSIS.

- The EuroQol—useful for severe disease, painful disease, or diseases that lead to sensory loss. US scores will be available by mid-2003.
- The Health Utility Index—a widely used three-part index covering most aspects of health and disease.
- The Years of Healthy Life (YHL) measure—easy to use measure of chronic diseases. Less useful for mental illness or acute conditions.
- The Quality of Well-Being Scale—a widely used instrument covering sensory impairment, mental illness, and most other diseases. Good at capturing changes in health states over time.
- The Quality of Life and Health—useful for mental illness and other chronic diseases, especially good for interventions designed to prevent or treat cancer.

then compiles them and makes them available to the public in published and electronic formats.

The underlying causes of death in the United States are reported in an annual publication (usually about three years behind the current calendar year) that includes seventy-two selected conditions. Each condition is stratified by age, gender, and race. The electronic data include all conditions and underlying conditions reported in the United States.

Mortality data from the NCHS are not obtained from a statistical sample; they include all reported deaths nationwide. Though they are not subject to sampling error, they are susceptible to misclassification bias, which is a problem that arises when physicians filling out death certificates incorrectly or inconsistently record the cause of death on a reporting form. Imagine for example, that a particular patient develops heart disease as a result of long-standing, poorly controlled diabetes mellitus. If that patient later dies, the physician filling out the death certificate may be unsure whether to list diabetes or heart disease as the cause of death.

Prospective studies are generally more accurate with regard to cause of death. However, they may not be available for the disease you are interested in and rarely include sufficient information to determine the life expectancy of a cohort. In these studies, patients are often closely monitored, and thus the data are less susceptible to misclassification bias. These data are subject to sampling error, however, and prospective studies usually do not collect more than five years of data. Because cost-effectiveness analyses often consider the costs and benefits of health interventions over the lifetime of a hypothetical cohort, it is usually necessary to mathematically model mortality rates that extend beyond the endpoint of the study. This methodology will be briefly discussed in Chapter Twelve.

Mortality Among Persons with Influenza-Associated Conditions

Recall from the section on hospitalization data that excess hospitalizations were measured using influenza-associated conditions rather than influenza-like illness. Mortality due to influenza-virus infection is usually measured the same way. Among the various infectious agents that can cause influenza-like illness, only influenza virus infections or secondary bacterial pneumonia are likely to be fatal or to result in hospitalization. Therefore, if we assume that there will be very few deaths due to influenza-like illnesses other than influenza (such as sinusitis or otitis media), we can think of the number of deaths due to influenza-like illness and the number of deaths due to influenza-associated conditions as being approximately equal.

In the publication "Prevention and Control of Influenza: Recommendations of the Advisory Committee on Immunization Practices (ACIP)," the Centers for Disease Control and Prevention estimate that there are roughly 20,000 excess deaths due to influenza-associated conditions during the average year ("Prevention," 1999; Lui and Kendal, 1987).

The problem with this statistic is that it does not provide information on the distribution of these deaths by age or by health status. We will need to find a way to adjust this number so that it reflects only deaths among fifteen- to sixty-five-year-old persons without chronic disease.

We can estimate the proportion of deaths by age group using the age-specific mortality rates for influenza virus infections using published data. To accomplish this, we must open a spreadsheet program and laboriously type in the values for the age groups and the number of age-specific deaths due to influenza (Table 10 of the *Deaths, 1997* document discussed in Chapter Four, which is available online at http://www.cdc.gov/nchs/data/nvs47_19.pdf) (Hoyart and others, 1999). Once the age groups have been entered into the spreadsheet, we must calculate the percent distribution of deaths in each age group, then multiply this number by 20,000 (the average number of excess deaths due to influenza-associated conditions each year, see Table 5.12).

Thus, we know that there were about seventy-eight deaths recorded for influenza in 1997 among persons aged fifteen to sixty-five, and the predicted average number of deaths per year due to influenza-associated conditions is about 2,166. Though the CDC estimate does not provide us with all of the information we need, it is the only readily available estimate that contains data from many years.

By adjusting the CDC's estimate of excess deaths for age, we have reduced misclassification bias and virtually eliminated the year-to-year variation in deaths due to influenza. Our data are not ready for use just yet, however, as significant problems remain. Because the CDC data did not distinguish between deaths

TABLE 5.12.   ESTIMATING THE NUMBER OF DEATHS DUE TO INFLUENZA-ASSOCIATED CONDITIONS FOR PERSONS OF DIFFERENT AGES.

All ages	Actual *Influenza deaths*	Percent *Deaths (deaths age × total deaths)*	Predicted *Deaths percent deaths × 20,000*
<15	35	5 percent	972
15 to 24	4	1 percent	111
25 to 34	7	1 percent	194
35 to 44	18	3 percent	500
45 to 54	18	3 percent	500
54 to 64	31	4 percent	861
65+	607	84 percent	16,861
15 to 65	78	—	2,166
Total	720	100 percent	20,000

among healthy adults and deaths among adults with chronic illnesses, our current age-adjusted mortality figures would surely be overestimating the total number of deaths due to influenza-associated conditions that occur on an annual basis among healthy adults (it is likely that most of the deaths are actually among adults with chronic illnesses). We will return to this issue in Chapter Nine.

Exercise 5.7

5.7. Suppose that we knew the mortality rate from influenza-virus infection among people with chronic lung disease, diabetes, or heart disease. How might the total number of excess deaths due to influenza and secondary pneumonia estimated by the CDC be adjusted to reflect excess deaths among persons *without* these diseases?

CHAPTER SIX

WORKING WITH COSTS

Overview

Sandra Montero returned to her office after dropping off Sandra Jr. at daycare. Sandra always tried to incorporate exercise into her work routine, so after giving the security guard a friendly smile, she turned into the stairwell to make her usual four-flight climb up the stairs. After the first few stairs, she felt her thigh muscles ache and suddenly felt tired all over. She lumbered into her office, started to cough, and decided to visit the company physician.

After sitting for almost a half of an hour in the clinic, the doctor met her in the hallway, shook her hand, and informed her that he had reviewed her chart. He explained that it was an unusually busy day in the clinic, told her that she had the flu, and sent her home for the day with instructions to drink plenty of fluids and to take some over-the-counter medications. On her way home, she wearily picked up the medicines at a pharmacy near her house, then drove home and climbed in between her fresh linen sheets. Before dozing off to sleep, she remembered that Sandra Jr. would soon need a ride home, so she called her babysitter and asked him to pick her up from daycare.

When Sandra decided to see her physician, she set off a chain of events, each of which was associated with a cost. First, the receptionist, medical assistant, and the doctor each spent time seeing Sandra for her illness. Second, while sitting in the office waiting to see the physician, she unknowingly exposed the receptionist and an elderly file clerk to the influenza virus. While the receptionist developed a mild illness that kept her at home for a few days, the file clerk was hospitalized for secondary bacterial pneumonia. Third, Sandra decided to purchase some over-the-counter medications as recommended by her physician. Fourth, because of her illness, Sandra would stay home from work for the next three days. Finally, the babysitter had to leave his other job early to pick up Sandra Jr. from daycare.

So you can see how a relatively common illness can translate into a diverse range of medical and nonmedical costs. In our analysis, when thinking about the costs associated with an influenza-like illness, we must take all of these possible events into consideration.

Opportunity Costs

Recall from Chapter One that an opportunity cost is the value of goods and services in their best alternative use. In that chapter, we used the example of the opportunity cost of an MRI machine. An MRI machine is made up of steel and circuits, is built by engineers, and is operated by specially trained staff. All of these social resources could have been put to some other use. For example, the engineers might have been used to build a bridge, to improve the safety of a nuclear power plant, build a safer car, and so on. When we use these resources to build an MRI machine, we cannot use them for these other potentially important social uses. By thinking in terms of the resources used when a medical intervention is applied, we will be providing policymakers with better information on whether those resources should be spent elsewhere.

When the societal perspective is assumed, goods and services are generally thought of in terms of the social resources that are used rather than prices. Though at first it is difficult to think in terms of opportunity costs rather than the market price of an item or a service, there are many advantages to this approach. First, many of the goods and services consumed when a person becomes ill are not associated with a market price. If we think in terms of costs rather than resources, we might overlook some costs, such as the value of the time a doctor spends with a patient.

Second, the market does not always do a good job of placing a value on some items. In medicine, products and services sometimes cost considerably more than the resources that go into them. Moreover, the market value of a particular service in the United States varies depending on who is paying for it. For instance, one gynecologist in New York admitted that he charges uninsured patients $175 for a routine visit, but accepts payments of $25 from insurance companies for the same services (Kolata, 2001). If we were to use the $175 figure in our cost-effectiveness analysis, our estimate would be seven times higher than the standard fee paid by insurance companies. To estimate the cost of this gynecological visit, we might be better off considering the value of the resources that go into a gynecological visit. For instance, we might place a price on the amount of time the doctor spends with the patient, the number and types of laboratory tests the doctor would order, the overall time the patient spends in the clinic, and the amount the patient spends on transportation to and from the clinic.

Three Steps to Estimating Costs

So that we may come closer to estimating the opportunity cost of a medical intervention, the reference case scenario suggests that researchers should think of costs in three separate steps (Gold and others, 1996). First, as we create a flowchart outlining the events that typically occur throughout the course of an illness, we should try to identify all of the resources that are used when each event takes place. Because costs can be dramatically modified with the introduction of various interventions, we should consider costs separately for each arm of the study we are conducting. Second, we should measure the amount of each of these resources used. For example, when estimating hospitalization costs, we might estimate how many IV bags are used, as well as the amount of time a patient spends in the hospital. Finally, we should place a monetary value on these goods and services.

Step 1, identifying resources used. Once you have made a flowchart that outlines all of the different events in a cost-effectiveness analysis, you should identify the social resources used in each box in the flowchart (see Figure 6.1). For example, Sandra will remain at home in bed and will not drive to work while sick, whereas someone who remains well throughout influenza season will drive to work every day (or take a bus or train). Because the presence or absence of influenza-like illness causes a change in transportation usage, this should be counted as a cost.

Step 2, measuring the resources used. It is important to quantify the extent to which resources are used. For example, to estimate Sandra's transportation costs, we need to know how many miles she lives from her job, how much fuel she consumes, and so on.

Step 3, placing a monetary value on the resources used. The final step in determining a cost is to place a monetary value on each of the resources that were used. For instance, we might determine the market price of a gallon of gasoline and multiply this cost by the amount of gallons used in driving to work or to the clinic. For patient time costs, wages are applied to the number of hours spent receiving an intervention or treating a patient. In Sandra's case, she spent thirty minutes at the clinic before the doctor sent her home. If she made $30 per hour, the value of the time spent at the clinic would be 0.5 hours $\cdot$ $30 = $15.

FIGURE 6.1. PARTIAL FLOWCHART OF THE COURSE OF INFLUENZA-LIKE ILLNESS AND THE COSTS ASSOCIATED WITH EACH EVENT IN THE EVENT PATHWAY.

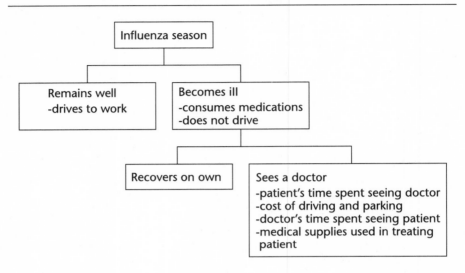

As you proceed through the sample cost-effectiveness analysis, you will learn how to identify relevant costs, measure the resources used, and place a monetary value on each of these resources. As we discuss each cost used in the sample analysis, each of these steps will be identified.

Micro-Costing and Gross-Costing

Though the reference case scenario recommends measuring all of the resources that were used to generate a cost before placing a monetary value on them, it is not always practical or necessary to do so. Suppose that we obtain a cost for ambulatory medical services from the medical literature or from an electronic dataset and that we are relatively certain that this cost is representative of the resources consumed in society. In this instance, we are essentially skipping steps 2 and 3 because the cost is provided for us. Aggregated costs obtained from electronic datasets or from the medical literature are called **gross costs.**

When using gross costs, we must still identify the resources used because the gross cost may not capture all costs in which we are interested. For instance, patient time costs are not included in the cost of a medical visit. Therefore, we must still estimate the amount of time a patient spends over the course of the visit.

Suppose that we were estimating the cost of Sandra's office visit using the three-step process of identification, measurement, and placing a value on each of the resources used. First, we would identify all of the resources used. These would include the cost of any medical supplies used, any tests performed, Sandra's time, the medical assistant's time, the secretary's time, and the physician's time. To measure the resources, we would estimate the type and number of medical supplies used and the amount of time each person spent treating, or receiving treatment for, the illness. If we were to measure these resources separately, we would assign a wage to each person's time, assign a cost to any tests that might have been performed or supplies used, and then add these costs together. The process of identifying each resource used, measuring these resources, valuing the resources, and adding them together is called **micro-costing.**

When to use gross-costs. Gross-costing is generally much easier and less time-consuming than micro-costing, especially when complex hospital costs are involved. As we saw in Chapter Four, it is possible to obtain a hospital charge and the average length of stay for a particular disease in a matter of minutes over the Internet.

Suppose we wanted to obtain the cost of the hospitalization for the poor elderly file clerk that Sandra exposed in the waiting room. The first step, identifying the resources used, is reduced to looking up the cost. In the second step, measuring the resources used, we only need to estimate the patient time cost, which is achieved by obtaining the average length of stay (ALOS) for the hospitalization. The final step, assigning values to the resources used, is achieved by adding the cost of the hospitalization to the product of the ALOS and the file clerk's wage to the overall cost.

The disadvantage of gross-costing in this circumstance is that hospital charges tend to overestimate the actual societal costs that are incurred. This happens because hospitals in the United States often charge more for their services than the actual costs of the resources that are consumed (especially if the hospital is a for-profit organization). In the "Using Cost-to-Charge Ratios" section below, we will see how to estimate the societal cost of a hospitalization using hospital charges. Although we have just outlined how convenient gross-costing can be, there are certain instances when it is important to itemize and valuate all of the goods and services used individually.

When to use micro-costing. In some hospitals, when a patient comes into the emergency room with a stroke, the doctors must order medications from the hospital pharmacy. The order is often written on the patient's chart and is subsequently sent to the pharmacy for review before it is dispensed. While this sequence of events is generally expedited in emergencies, it can still take considerable time because the pharmacy may be located in a different part of the hospital. It is conceivable that by the time the order is completely processed and the medication becomes available in the emergency room, the patient may have suffered serious damage from the stroke. One way around this problem is to simply make these lifesaving medications available in the emergency room. However, when medication dispensing is not tightly regulated and is administered emergently, it is easier for dosing errors to occur, and it is even possible that the wrong medication may be administered. A cost-effectiveness analysis examining this issue might assist hospital administrators in deciding whether it is better to keep these medications in the pharmacy, or have them available in the emergency room.

Now let us consider another example. If a doctor and a patient both agree that it is appropriate for the patient to receive a screening mammogram, in many clinics, the doctor will ask the patient to schedule a screening mammogram. One way to improve patient compliance with mammography and to reduce the patient's transportation costs is to have the patient undergo the mammogram immediately after the doctor's visit. A cost-effectiveness analysis on same-day mammography versus future scheduled appointments might help a clinic director make an informed decision about which choice is best.

In each of these examples, subtle changes occur in the way a product is delivered or a service is provided. If we were to use the gross-cost of an emergency room visit for stroke, we would not be able to distinguish the cost of requesting medications from the pharmacy from the cost of storing medication in the emergency room (because gross-costing would lump all of the costs associated with an emergency room visit together in one figure). Likewise, in the second example, we would also be unable to distinguish subtle changes in the costs of providing mammograms if we were to use gross-costs. In both of these examples, the central theme of the cost-effectiveness analysis centers around the cost of hospital services (in the first case) or ambulatory care services (in the second case).

Micro-costing, rather than a gross-cost estimate, should be used when the cost-effectiveness analysis is centered on changes in the way the resource is delivered (Gold and others, 1996). Micro-costing is also useful when a particular cost is not available in the medical literature or electronic data. For example, in our influenza study, we will see that no estimate of the cost of side effects to oseltamivir or vaccination is available, so we will need to micro-cost these events. As mentioned earlier, micro-costing may also more closely estimate the opportunity cost of medical goods and services.

The major disadvantages of micro-costing are that it requires a lot of work, costs can be missed, and the costs often lack external validity. Micro-costing is very resource intensive, especially when applied to complex costs, such as the cost of hospitalization. Unless administrative systems designed to measure resource consumption are used, it is also easy to miss important costs. Finally, because micro-costing is usually done at a local level, the costs may not be representative of overall national costs (Gold and others, 1996).

Measuring Changes in Costs

Because cost-effectiveness analyses only measure changes in costs (along with changes in the health-related quality of life and life expectancy), it is important to be able to identify which costs change when an intervention is undertaken and which costs do not. In this section, you will learn how to think about the dynamic and static properties of costs.

Fixed Costs and Variable Costs

In any given year, the average person makes about six physician contacts (see Table 5.9), misses a week or two of work, and so on. We are only concerned with those physician visits and days of work missed that change as a result of the interventions we are including in our cost-effectiveness analysis. Costs that change because a medical intervention is applied are referred to as **variable costs.**

When Sandra Montero visited the company clinic, she exposed a few people to the influenza virus and took up some of the secretary's time, the medical assistant's time, and the doctor's time. Her decision to visit the company clinic therefore consumed resources *that would not otherwise have been consumed,* and each of the resources is an example of a variable cost. **Fixed costs** are costs that do not change because of a health intervention. Whether she had visited the clinic or had gone directly home, the janitors would have to clean the clinic at the end of the day, the rent has to be paid, and so on. Administration, maintenance, medical equipment, computers, photocopiers, and the like are examples of fixed costs and should *not* be included in the analysis.

Of course, there are exceptions to this rule. Suppose that the company instituted an influenza vaccination policy that resulted in a dramatic drop in patient illnesses and visits to the clinic. The administration might choose to reduce the clinic's hours of operation to compensate for the lighter volume, or might even choose to close the clinic altogether. In this instance, the intervention (influenza vaccination) would have had a significant impact on the consumption of resources that might otherwise have been considered "fixed." If an intervention results in sufficient changes in patient volume to cause changes in staffing levels, changes in the wear and tear on medical equipment, or merits purchasing new equipment, these changes should be accounted for if they are likely to be relevant for the analysis.

Friction Costs and Transfer Payments

Within the context of cost-effectiveness analysis, **friction costs** are incurred when administration costs change for an employer, government agency, or some other entity because of an intervention or disease. When absenteeism or unemployment rates increase because of illness, for example, friction costs are incurred. For instance, in the last section, we saw that changes in patient volume can result in administrative costs that might otherwise be considered fixed costs. In general, such costs can be safely excluded from a cost-effectiveness analysis. In those rare instances in which an intervention is expected to have a very large impact on administrative costs at a worksite or in a government agency, researchers should consider including friction costs in their analysis.

Transfer payments are payments made from one entity to another as part of a social contract, such as welfare payments or social security payments. For instance, workers pay into the social security system with the expectation that the money will be returned to them when they retire. In this instance, the money is simply transferred from workers' paychecks to the government and is then transferred back from the government to the worker at a later date. The only resources consumed when transfer payments are made are the friction costs of administering such programs. Therefore, only the friction costs associated with transfer payments need to be included in a cost-effectiveness analysis.

Using Diagnosis Codes

In the "Using Data Extraction Tools" section of Chapter Four, we learned that diseases are categorized using a number of different systems. These systems include the International Classification for Disease (ICD), Diagnosis-Related Groups (DRGs), and the Clinical Classifications for Health Policy Research (CCHPR).

The ICD system is currently in its tenth revision and is often referred to by its revision number. For example, the ninth revision is still commonly used and is referred to as the ICD-9 system. Costs obtained from this system are very specific to a particular disease. For instance, using this system, it is possible to obtain costs for either influenza virus hospitalizations or for pneumonia secondary to influenza.

Sometimes, this system can be too specific. For example, diabetes mellitus can cause many different complications, each associated with its own ICD code. When examining diseases with a number of different complications, it can be difficult to determine which diseases are associated with which costs. For this reason, it is sometimes preferable to use a less specific system when examining costs associated with complex diseases.

The Clinical Classifications for Health Policy Research (CCHPR) system groups ICD codes specific to a particular disease. For example, CCHPR codes can be used to examine costs for five ICD codes that are related to diabetes mellitus without complications (CCS code 49) or thirty-eight conditions associated with complications for the disease—such as circulatory, neurological, or kidney problems associated with this disease (CCS code 50). They can also be used to examine each specific complication of the disease. For example, different kidney problems associated with the disease (ICD codes 25040–25043) are grouped together into diagnosis category 3.3.2.

While the CCS system aggregates codes for a particular illness, the Diagnosis-Related Groups coding system (DRGs) system aggregates diseases with similar costs. The DRG system is therefore the least disease-specific system. For example, costs related to diabetes mellitus mostly differ by the age of the patient and are listed as "Diabetes less than age thirty-five" and "Diabetes greater than age thirty-five." Other endocrine diseases are less common and are similar in cost, so those with an uncomplicated course in the hospital are grouped together under the general category "Endocrine disorders without complications." As we will see in a moment, DRGs are useful for adjusting hospital charges obtained from electronic sources.

Future Medical Costs

While future medical costs can be reduced by a successful health intervention, they can also be lowered as a result of a premature death. If an intervention is effective at reducing the severity of a disease, then future ambulatory care, hospitalization, and medication costs will all likely be lower among those who received the intervention (see Chapter One). However, this would also hold true if someone were to die prematurely from an accident or some other unfortunate event. This then raises the question, if premature death is associated with a reduction in future costs, should these savings be included in a cost-effectiveness analysis?

One of the cold facts of this world is that, while people benefit society in many ways, people also cost society something. When someone dies prematurely, his or her future health costs should theoretically be counted as savings in a cost-effectiveness analysis (Gold and others, 1996). Thus, while health interventions can potentially save money by reducing the severity of a disease, they may potentially increase societal costs by saving lives. For example, one study found that smokers actually saved society money because they tend to die at a relatively young age, while non-smokers tend to develop chronic diseases later in life and rack up huge medical bills (Barendregt and others, 1997).

Taking these considerations into account, the Panel on Cost-Effectiveness in Health and Medicine decided to put its theoretical concerns aside and allow researchers to exclude these future medical costs from the analysis. However, if future medical costs are likely to have a large impact on the analysis, the Panel recommends that these costs be tested in a sensitivity analysis. This way, the analysis can be compared with studies that do not include such costs. Future medical costs are available using electronic data sources, such as the Medical Expenditure Panel Survey (MEPS), or may be obtained from other research efforts that have included future medical costs in their analysis.

Adjusting Costs

When costs are obtained from the medical literature or from electronic datasets, they often require adjustment before they can be included in a cost-effectiveness analysis. Suppose that you have found a very good study on the cost of ambulatory care for influenza-like illness, but the study was conducted in 1997 and you have standardized your study to 1999 costs. Or suppose that you need to calculate hospitalization costs for your hypothetical cohort over the next forty years and have to determine the present value of these costs. Finally, imagine that you wish to use hospital charges from an electronic database. You wish to include these gross costs in your analysis but suspect that they do not reflect the opportunity cost of a hospitalization. In each case, you will need to adjust all of the costs reported in these data sources.

Adjusting for Inflation

When older cost data are used, they will underestimate the cost of medical care in present-day terms, unless they are adjusted for inflation. The methods section of most research papers will state the year in which all costs were obtained and electronic datasets always indicate the year for which the data were collected.

To inflate older cost data, visit the Bureau of Labor Statistics homepage (http://www.bls.gov) and click on the "Most requested series." Scroll down to the consumer price index headings and click on "All urban consumers" (the exact URL is: http://146.142.4.24/cgi-bin/surveymost?cu, or, for a more detailed query, http://146.142.4.24/labjava/ourside.jsp?survey-cu). You will be presented with a number of different price index options.

The type of data you wish to inflate should be matched with the relevant price index. For example, if you wish to inflate the cost of medical care, select "Medical care." Select the years for which you would like data for and click on the "Submit" button. You should be presented with a nice table listing the changes in the price of medical care over the years for which you would like the data (see Table 6.1). If you save these data with an ".htm" extension (regardless of your browser or operating system) and select the file type "html," you should be able to open the table in a spreadsheet program.

The annual changes in medical inflation between 1990 and 1999 appear in Table 6.1. In this table, "Index" refers to the medical price index, which is simply a ratio that refers to the price in a reference year relative to the price in the year represented in each row. Thus, the 1990 value, 162.8, indicates that prices have increased 162.8 percent since the reference year. The proportionate increase in prices may be calculated using the formula:

(high year index value − low year index value) / low year index value

Equation 6.1

Alternatively, the price may be inflated by simply multiplying it by:

high year index value / low year index value

Equation 6.2

For instance, to inflate $100 between 1990 and 1991, applying Equation 6.2, we get: $100 \cdot 177/162.8 = 108.7$.

It is always a good idea to examine trends in a particular disease. For example, new drugs that were introduced to the United States market in 1996 greatly reduced the mortality rates for HIV in developed countries and had a large impact on the cost of care. Thus, a study on the cost-effectiveness of an intervention to treat HIV that used 1998 data would likely produce a dramatically different result than if data from two years earlier were used, and simply adjusting these costs for inflation will not suffice.

TABLE 6.1. MEDICAL PORTION OF THE CONSUMER PRICE INDEX 1990–1999.

Year	Index	Percent Change
1990	162.8	—
1991	177	8.02
1992	190.1	6.89
1993	201.4	5.61
1994	211	4.55
1995	220.5	4.31
1996	228.2	3.37
1997	234.6	2.73
1998	242.1	3.10
1999	250.6	3.39

Exercise 6.1

6.1. Inflate the cost of an ambulatory medical visit from the Nichol and others (1995) (see Appendix II) study from 1994 to 1997 dollars.

Calculating Cost-to-Charge Ratios

Earlier, we mentioned that charges obtained from hospitalization datasets do not always reflect the true opportunity costs of the resources used. In fact, the reported hospital charges are sometimes more than twice the market value of the services and products provided during the hospitalization.

Data on hospitalization costs are obtained from hospital billing systems, which report the total charges that the patient incurred while in the hospital. A **charge** is the amount that a hospital, clinic, or pharmacy bills the patient or the patient's insurance company. Some of the goods and services hospitals charge for are inflated so that the hospital can generate profits or recover losses from investments that are unrelated to the billed admission. Hospital charges are therefore larger than the opportunity costs of the resources used.

Medicare conducts an extensive analysis of the actual costs of hospitalizing a patient to ensure that it is only paying for the services consumed by its patients. When a Medicare patient is hospitalized, Medicare generally does not pay the hospital what the patient was charged. Rather, it pays the hospital an amount that is roughly equal to the cost of the goods and services the hospital provides to the typical patient with a similar condition.

Medicare keeps tabs on what it was charged and what it actually paid for hospitalizations for each DRG code. These data are available through a system called medical provider analysis and review, or Medpar (http://www.hcfa.gov/stats/medpar.htm). In Medpar, each charge made to Medicare and each payment made by Medicare is listed by DRG.

One way to estimate the opportunity cost of hospitalization is to multiply the hospital charge for the disease under study by a **cost-to-charge ratio.** As the name implies, a cost-to-charge ratio adjusts hospital charges so that they better reflect the cost of the social resources used when a patient is hospitalized. We can exploit the information contained in the Medpar system to estimate cost-to-charge ratios. The cost of a hospitalization is estimated using the formula:

$$\text{charge for hospitalization} \cdot \frac{\text{amount reimbursed by medicare}}{\text{charge to medicare}}$$

Equation 6.3

If Medicare lists the amount it reimburses for each DRG, why not simply use this amount for the diagnosis under study? Though the reference case scenario suggests that it is acceptable to do so, there are two problems with this approach (Gold and others, 1996). First, charges to Medicare are applicable to people over the age of sixty-five or people with certain chronic conditions and may not be representative of charges for younger, healthier people. Second, because charges to Medicare are only reported by DRGs, the costs and charges are fairly nonspecific. For example, DRG 079 represents "infections and inflammations of the respiratory system," a group of widely different respiratory diseases. Though ICD-coded charges are much more specific than DRG-coded charges, cost-to-charge ratios generated using DRGs are generally acceptable for use in cost-effectiveness analysis.

Exercises 6.2–6.4

6.2. Obtain total hospital charges for DRG 079 and 080 (infectious and inflammatory respiratory conditions with and without complications) using Medicare's Medpar data (available at: http://www.hcfa.gov/stats/medpar.htm, see Chapter Four) and calculate a weighted cost-to-charge ratio.

6.3. Compare the charges you obtained from Medicare in Exercise 6.1 and the charges you obtained from HCUP-3 in Exercise 4.2. Why do these differ?

6.4. Multiply the HCUP-3 charges for ICD code 487 and CCS code 123 you obtained in Exercise 4.2 by the cost-to-charge ratio you calculated in Exercise 6.2.

Estimating the Cost of Ambulatory and Laboratory Services

Often, ambulatory care costs and the cost of medical tests will be artificially inflated relative to the amount of resources consumed. This is especially true of costs obtained from for-profit ventures. Technically speaking, profit should not be included in the valuation of a product or service because profit is, by definition, money earned in excess of the resources consumed. In practice, where profits are likely to be small, they can be ignored.

With the advent of health maintenance organizations, group practice providers, laboratories, and diagnostic services (such as catheterization laboratories and mammography suites) have tended to operate on thinner profit margins. Nonetheless, as we saw in the example of the private gynecologist in New York who charged uninsured patients seven times as much as insured patients, the reported charge for services can vary quite a bit, depending on whether the charges were obtained from the physician's charges or from the insurance company's reimbursement rate. The documentation that accompanies the electronic dataset will usually provide information on how the cost data were obtained. When using published data, it is often helpful to contact the authors of the study to determine how the cost data were obtained.

Discounting Future Costs

Medical interventions, especially preventive interventions, often result in decreased future medical costs that must be accounted for in present-day terms. Humans have a tendency to place a lower value on future events than on events that occur in the present. For example, if someone were to offer you $100 today or $103 dollars a year from now, you might forgo the extra three dollars to have the money in your pocket today.

If one waits for a payment, he or she may never get it. The person giving out the money might be able to pay it in a year, or the receiver might die before she has a chance to spend it. Of course, there are other reasons why people wish to have things immediately rather than in the future, one being simple human impatience. For all of these reasons, banks are willing to pay interest on the money people place in a savings account or certificate of deposit to provide customers with an incentive to keep it there.

If you were willing to wait one year to receive an extra $3 on an investment of $100, you would earn 3 percent by waiting ($100 · 1.03 per year = $103). Imagine that you were willing to accept *either* the $103 a year from now or $100 today. Imagine also that you were certain that you would *not* be willing to accept either $99 today instead of $103 a year from now *or* $102 a year from now rather than $100 today. In this case, your **time preference** is said to be three percent (Olsen and Bailey, 1981). Time preference refers to the **discount rate** that a person places on future expenditures.

In this case, the **net present value** of $103 spent in one year is equal to $100 today. The net present value of future earnings is the value of those earnings **discounted** into present terms. By discounting all future costs into their present-day terms, we are accounting for people's tendency to place a lower value on future earnings.

When to use discounting. Most health interventions result in changes in the amount of future resources consumed. For example, if hypertension is treated, patients may have to take a medication for the rest of their life. If they choose to do so, they will likely have fewer complications of their disease, such as heart attack and stroke, in the future. Suppose that we are evaluating the cost-effectiveness of a particular blood pressure medication relative to no intervention. In the treatment arm of the analysis, the cost of the medication in future years, the cost of any future disease related to hypertention, and all nonmedical costs (such as the cost of transportation) must be discounted into present terms. In the no intervention group, we would discount the costs of the untreated disease (and all of its complications) and nonmedical costs into present terms.

All future costs must be discounted into their net present value before they can be included in cost-effectiveness analysis (Gold and others, 1996). In Chapter Nine, we will see that future QALYs are also discounted in a cost-effectiveness analysis at the same rate of costs.

The reference case scenario bases the recommended discount rate on a technical valuation of public investments that is roughly equal to the real rate of return on government bonds (Gold and others, 1996). Because this rate varies over time, and the reference case is concerned with making all cost-effectiveness analyses comparable, the Panel on Cost-Effectiveness in Health and Medicine has settled on a rate of 3 percent until 2006. To maintain comparability with older cost-effectiveness analyses, and to make sure that the results of studies conducted in the present will still be useful in the future, the Panel also recommends that the study results be presented with no discount rate applied, with a rate of 5 percent applied, and with a sensitivity analysis conducted on rates between 0 and 7 percent (Gold and others, 1996).

Internationally, many studies utilize a discount rate of 5 percent (Drummond and others, 1997). When conducting a cost-effectiveness analysis outside of the United States, researchers may wish to use the discount rate most commonly applied in that country in the base-case analysis. However, results should be presented at a discount rate of 0 percent and 3 percent, and you should conduct a sensitivity analysis using a discount rate higher than the base-case value.

How to use discounting. The general formula for discounting future costs is:

$$\text{cost of future event} / (1 + \text{discount rate})^{\text{years}}$$

Equation 6.4

For example, if the hypertensive person in the example above were to suffer a stroke ten years into the future and was hospitalized at a cost of $10,000, the cost of the hospitalization in present-day terms at the standard discount rate of 3 percent would be:

$$\$10,000/(1.03)^{10} = \$7,440.94$$

Let us give a more practical example of how this formula is used. In cost-effectiveness analysis, we usually have to discount many costs over the average lifespan of people in the cohort, rather than over a single year into the future. Suppose our cohort consisted of 1,000 elderly people with high blood pressure, and the average person can be expected to survive ten years into the future. The number of survivors in each of these years and the total costs in each of these years might break down in a manner similar to Table 6.2.

In Table 6.2, the number of elderly persons with hypertension surviving over each year of the study is represented in Column 2. The total cost of the illness per person (including medications, ambulatory care visits, hospitalizations, and patient time costs) is represented in Column 3. The cost presented in Column 4 represents the total cost of the medical care in the cohort. This is equal to the product of the cost per person (Column 3) and the number of people remaining alive in that year (Column 2). Column 5 contains the total discounted cost for the entire cohort in each year.

In Table 6.2, we discounted costs on a year-to-year basis. However, it is also possible to discount all of the costs in the numerator of the average

TABLE 6.2. HYPOTHETICAL COST AND DISCOUNTED COST OF A COHORT OF 1,000 ELDERLY PERSONS OVER AN ELEVEN-YEAR PERIOD.

Year	Time	Number Surviving	Cost per Person	Total Cost	Discounted Cost
	1	2	3	4	5
				$C2 \cdot C3$	$C4/(1.03)^{C1}$
2002	1	1,000	$19,000	$19,000,000	$18,446,602
2003	2	990	$18,500	$18,315,000	$17,263,644
2004	3	910	$17,000	$15,470,000	$14,157,241
2005	4	840	$22,000	$18,480,000	$16,419,241
2006	5	750	$19,500	$14,625,000	$12,615,653
2007	6	605	$16,000	$9,680,000	$8,106,848
2008	7	500	$21,000	$10,500,000	$8,537,461
2009	8	380	$14,000	$5,320,000	$4,199,657
2010	9	170	$12,000	$2,040,000	$1,563,490
2011	10	90	$10,500	$945,000	$703,169
2012	11	40	$14,500	$580,000	$419,004
Total				$114,955,000	$102,432,010

cost-effectiveness ratio using the formula:

$$\sum_{1}^{T} \frac{(C_y)}{1.03^{y-1}}$$

Equation 6.5

where T is the mean number of years of life remaining in the cohort, and C_y is the cost for year y.

Discounting cost values obtained from the medical literature. When obtaining the total per person cost of a disease from the medical literature, it is important to make sure that the cost is representative of the resources used over a patient's lifetime, discounted to its net present value. When we find a global cost of a disease in the medical literature, we must ensure that 1) the cost of this disease was discounted into its net present value and 2) the discount rate the authors used is equal to the discount rate used in your analysis.

Assessing the "Relevancy" of Cost Data

While it is important to identify all costs included in a cost-effectiveness analysis, we need only measure, valuate, and include those costs that are likely to be "relevant" to our analysis (Gold and others, 1996). In this section, we will review some of the important things to consider when evaluating cost data for its relevancy using studies on the Guillian-Barré syndrome to illustrate our points.

In Chapter Five, we decided to exclude mortality estimates for the Guillian-Barré syndrome, because only one in a million people who receive the vaccine will develop this condition (if any), and only 6 percent of those people will die (Lasky and others, 1998). However, it is not clear whether the cost of this condition will be relevant, because it may require extended hospitalization and, in some cases, long-term care. The cost of the Guillian-Barré syndrome, $100,800 (range $70,000 to $130,000), is available from the medical literature (Meltzer and others, 1999, available at: http://www.cdc.gov/ncidod/eid/vol5no5/meltzer.htm).

The cost of Guillian-Barré is greatly affected by the probability of incurring this cost (1 in a million). The total cost is only 10 cents (1 per 1 million · $100,800 = $0.10), with a high cost of 9 per 1 million · $130,000 = $1.17 and a low cost of 1 per 10 million · $70,000 = $0.01. It is possible that the influenza vaccine does not cause this disease at all, so we might set the low value to zero in our sensitivity analysis, if we were to include this cost at all.

In this book, we will keep our analysis as simple as possible and exclude the cost and effects associated with the Guillain-Barre syndrome. We highlight this potential side effect because it illustrates a number of points to remember when deciding whether a cost you have identified should be included in the analysis. Students may encounter our published report on the sample analysis in the medical literature. The costs we present in that analysis differ from those presented here because of these simplifications.

First, it is often difficult to determine when a cost is likely to be large enough to merit inclusion in your analysis. Were we conducting a cost-effectiveness analysis for publication in the medical literature, we would include the cost of Guillian-Barré syndrome simply because we have the data. However, if these data were not available, we might exclude the cost based on the following criteria: 1) the disease is extremely rare and 2) the disease has not been definitively linked to recent influenza vaccines.

Second, the costs associated with this syndrome, like virtually all costs in a cost-effectiveness analysis, are determined by the probability that a patient will incur them. While Guillain-Barre syndrome is the most expensive disease, in terms of its absolute cost, that we might evaluate in our analysis, it would probably only add ten cents to the overall cost of vaccination because it is so rare. Extremely rare conditions generally need only be included if the costs associated with these conditions are potentially large.

Finally, the study by Lasky and others (1998) illustrates important concepts regarding the derivation of high and low values used in a sensitivity analysis. This study is our only known estimate of the range of probabilities that this syndrome might occur among vaccinated patients in our cohort. In the case of this disease, our baseline cost of ten cents is not likely to have much of an effect on the overall cost of the influenza vaccination strategy in our analysis. However, the high cost, $1.17, is fairly large. If we were to exclude this cost from a published study on strategies to treat or prevent influenza-like illness, our sensitivity analysis would not include this potentially relevant cost.

Determining Which Costs to Include

In this section, we will return to our sample cost-effectiveness analysis. We will apply the information you have learned thus far to obtaining cost data for strategies to treat or prevent influenza-like illness.

Because we are conducting our reference case cost-effectiveness analysis from the societal perspective, we will need to include every possible cost that is likely to be affected by each of the different interventions we are evaluating. To do so, we will have to identify all social resources that might be used, measure the resources that we think will affect the results of our analysis (either by micro-costing or gross-costing), and then value each of the resources that we think will be significant. So that all of our cost data are consistent, we will have to make certain that all costs are adjusted to 1997 U.S. dollars.

Cost-effectiveness analyses conducted from the societal perspective generally require costs for:

- Ambulatory care
- Hospitalization
- Medications
- Laboratory tests
- Transportation
- Long-term care
- Time the patient spends receiving the health intervention(s)
- The time spent by caregivers and others treating the ill person
- The effect of the intervention on nonmedical resources, such as environmental costs
- The effects of an intervention on the productivity of others or wear on machinery

Let us revisit the average cost-effectiveness ratio we described in Chapter One. The average cost-effectiveness ratio for the treatment arm of our analysis takes the form:

$$\frac{(\text{costs of treatment} - \text{costs averted by treatment})}{\text{QALYs gained by treatment}}$$

Equation 6.6

The left side of the numerator should include: 1) the cost of medical goods services, 2) the costs associated with resource utilization outside of the medical system (for example, costs associated with transportation, education, or the environment), 3) the costs associated with caregiving, and 4) the costs associated with the time it takes to receive an intervention or therapy for a disease. The right side of the numerator should include those resources in points 1–4 that will *not* be used when a patient is treated with oseltamivir.

Recall that all costs associated with pain, suffering (morbidity costs), and death (mortality costs) are captured in the denominator of the average cost-effectiveness ratio. Because the HRQL score is a valuation of morbidity, it implicitly captures all morbidity costs. This is convenient because we do not have to place a dollar value on morbidity or mortality costs.

Tips and tricks. The Health Utility index, a generic preference-weighted instrument used to generate HRQL scores, does not produce HRQL scores that value lost productivity. When this instrument is used, lost productivity due to illness must be added to the numerator of a cost-effectiveness ratio.

Table 6.3 outlines all of the costs we might include in our cost-effectiveness analysis. In this table, costs are broken down by the three health interventions we are studying. In addition to the medical costs associated with ambulatory care, hospital care, oseltamivir pills, and influenza vaccinations, patients might incur costs related to taking antibiotics or medications for symptom relief, such as over-the-counter flu medicines. Patient-specific costs include transportation costs (including the time spent traveling to and from the clinic or hospital), the time a patient spends receiving the health intervention, ambulatory care costs, and hospitalization costs. Additional costs might include those of caregiver time, the costs of future medical care averted, decreased crime, decreased pollution from

TABLE 6.3. COSTS TO CONSIDER FOR INCLUSION IN THE COST-EFFECTIVENESS ANALYSIS ON STRATEGIES FOR THE PREVENTION OR TREATMENT OF INFLUENZA-LIKE ILLNESS.

Health Costs	Patient Costs	Societal Costs

Supportive care
Medical care
• Hospitalization
• Ambulatory care
Secondary transmission
Secondary complications
OTC medications (a)
Antibiotics
	Time in treatment
	Lost time of caregivers
	Transportation to doctor
	  or hospital
	Transportation averted from
	  missed work
		Future medical costs
		Decreased crime
		Pollution from transportation
		Landfill from medical waste
		Missed school

Vaccination
Medical care
• Hospitalization
• Ambulatory care
Vaccine administration
Influenza vaccine
Side effects
• Fever
• Guillian-Barré
• Sore arm
	Time spent seeking and
	  receiving vaccine
	Transportation to receive
	  vaccine
	Time spent receiving
	  care for side effects
		Landfill from medical waste
		  (syringes and gauze)
		Pollution from transportation
		Resources used administering
		  vaccine at workplace

Treatment
Medical care
• Hospitalization
• Ambulatory care
Side effects
	Time spent receiving
	  treatment
	Transportation
	Caregiver time for
	  persons with side effects
		Landfill from medical waste
		Pollution from transportation
		Missed School
		Decreased crime
		Future medical costs

(a) OTC medications = over-the-counter medications.

transportation, environmental costs from medical waste, and costs associated with missing school when ill.

Compared to people in the supportive care arm of the study, people receiving vaccination or treatment with oseltamivir are likely to incur fewer future costs (either by averting the illness or by reducing complications of the illness). Some of the reduced or averted costs include those associated with medication, ambulatory care, hospitalization, transportation, and caregiving. However, people in each of these arms will spend additional time receiving the treatment or the vaccine. When subjects stay at home with influenza-like illness, they will not be driving as much. While they will incur fewer transportation costs, they may instead need caregiving, may need to visit a doctor, or may be hospitalized.

As alluded to above, the costs of future medical care can be averted in at least a couple of ways. First, as is often the case with the influenza vaccine, the illness itself can be averted altogether. Second, as is the case with both oseltamivir and the influenza vaccine, the severity or duration of the illness can be reduced. Finally, premature death itself can reduce future medical costs. As we discussed earlier, while it is theoretically sound to consider savings that occur as a result of premature death, this is rarely practiced.

Clearly, including all of the costs listed in Table 6.3 would be a monumental task. Fortunately, the reference case scenario allows us to exclude those costs that are not likely to have much of an impact on the outcomes of the analysis because they are small in magnitude. For example, it is not likely that many students will require additional tutoring due to missed classes, because influenza-like illness lasts only about ninety-seven hours on average, and only a small percentage of our eighteen- to sixty-five-year-old cohort is likely to be in school (Treanor and others, 2000).

While caregiver costs may be significant, caregiver costs for persons with side effects to medications will likely be negligible. Likewise, the cost of landfilling medical waste and the cost of pollution associated with transportation are likely to be small in magnitude.

Though criminals are as likely to get ill as anyone else, it would be difficult to determine the economic impact of reductions in crime due to influenza. For those so inclined, the Department of Justice maintains statistics on the number of crimes committed. It is possible that criminals will make up for their lost earnings when they get better, so including such costs might be counterproductive. Whatever the case, the costs are likely to be small.

Let us now examine each of the costs in Table 6.3 in more detail. In our discussion of each cost, we will outline whether micro- or gross-costing is typically used, and we will then identify the means used to identify, measure, and value each cost.

Hospital and Ambulatory Costs

Hospital and ambulatory care costs often constitute the largest proportion of the total cost in a cost-effectiveness analysis. While these costs are easy to identify, they are relatively difficult to measure and value. Again, consider the case of the elderly file clerk who was hospitalized after he came into contact with Sandra in the waiting room. While we could obtain information, using electronic datasets, on the length of time he might spend in the hospital, it would be fairly difficult to estimate how many tubes, bottles, and needles were used in caring for him. For these reasons, hospital and ambulatory care costs are usually obtained from the medical literature or from electronic datasets.

Some researchers attempt to micro-cost hospital and ambulatory care costs by using administrative data from individual hospitals or clinics. Hospitals carefully measure and value the resources that they use so that they know how much to bill for their services. However, the resources used from one hospital to the next are highly variable. Because cost-effectiveness researchers usually seek nationally representative data, information obtained from an individual hospital will not likely be externally valid. Because this process is time-consuming and may compromise the external validity of a study, gross-costing approaches are typically used. For those so inclined, Gold and others (1996) describe methods for micro-costing hospitalization costs.

Hospital charges relating to specific illnesses can be obtained from the Healthcare Cost and Utilization Project-3 (HCUP-3), from the Health Care Financing Administration (HCFA), from individual hospitals, or from the medical literature. Ambulatory care costs can be obtained from the Medical Expenditure Panel Survey (MEPS), the National Ambulatory Medical Care Survey (NAMCS), Medicaid, private sources, or medical providers.

Cost of hospitalization for the sample analysis. To obtain the cost of hospitalization in the sample analysis, we will use the gross cost we obtained from the HCUP-3 dataset in Exercise 6.4. In that exercise, we calculated the weighted mean hospital cost of influenza using CCS codes and ICD codes. Because the CCS coding system includes a broader array of influenza-related diseases than the ICD coding system, we should use the adjusted cost we obtained from the CCS system, $3,458.

Cost of ambulatory care for the sample analysis. To obtain the cost of ambulatory medical services, we will use the medical literature. Both Nichol and others (1995) and Bridges and others (2000) used gross-costing techniques to derive their estimates. In Exercise 6.1, we inflated the cost of ambulatory medical care in the Nichol and others (1995) study from $US 1994 to $US 1997. Though Nichol and others' (1995) data were obtained from multiple sources and represent the best cost estimate we have, the cost of prescription drugs is not disaggregated (listed separately) from other costs. Disaggregated costs are preferable because they will allow us to measure the cost of medications and side effects separately in our analysis.

Another option is to use data from Bridges and others (2000). They present cost data that are disaggregated by disease and present separate costs for prescription drugs and side effects. They used the MarketScan database to estimate these costs and then inflated the costs from 1996 to 1999 dollars (Medstat, 2001).

In Table A2.2 of Appendix II, we see that a co-payment of $10 was required for ambulatory care services. This payment is intended to discourage overutilization of ambulatory care services by the patient, and it is used to supplement the health insurance plan. Co-payments generally do not change much from year to year and are the same regardless of the ambulatory care services used, so they should not be deflated if they are included in the cost of a service. Whether they should be included as a cost in a cost-effectiveness analysis depends on an insurer's economic practices. Most insurance companies value a medical visit based on the expected overall cost of providing a particular service and merely require the patient to pay a fixed amount of that cost, so these costs should generally be included.

Exercises 6.5–6.6

6.5. Deflate ambulatory medical costs from Bridges and others (2000) to 1997 dollars (see Appendix II). Use the average inflationary rate between 1995 and 1997 to deflate these costs. Include, but do not deflate, the insurance co-payment in the overall cost of ambulatory care. (If you wish to impress your professor, you may obtain the medical portion of the CPI through the year 2000 to deflate these costs. They were not available at the time of publication.)

6.6. When they estimated ambulatory care costs, Nichol and others (1995) included the cost of medications in the cost of an ambulatory care visit. Bridges and others (2000), however, separated ambulatory costs from medication costs and co-payments. How does the estimated cost of ambulatory care compare between these studies when the cost of medications is added to the Bridges and others (2000) estimate?

Time Costs

Time costs are those costs associated with the time a patient spends receiving a medical intervention or spends receiving medical care. Likewise, if a caregiver or any other person must spend time away from day-to-day activities as a result of the intervention(s) or the disease under study, the time should also be included as a cost. The time a person spends receiving treatment for a disease is called the **time in treatment cost.** Recall from Chapter One that the time a person spends away from work or leisure activities as a result of an ongoing disease process should be included in the denominator of a cost-effectiveness ratio rather than the numerator. Thus, if we follow the rule that costs that are not associated with morbidity or mortality are included in the numerator, the identification of time costs is straightforward.

Time costs are almost always determined using micro-costing techniques. Therefore, the measurement and valuation of time costs is extremely important in cost-effectiveness analysis.

Measuring time costs. The time in transit to a medical clinic can be found in previously published cost-effectiveness analyses. The time in transit will be different for less serious conditions and diseases requiring specialty medical care. When people seek specialty care, such as care for cancer, they often want the best possible care available, so many people will travel long distances to visit well-known clinics (Secker-Walker, 1999).

The duration of physician contact by disease and physician specialty is available from the NAMCS (Schappert and Nelson, 1999); however, this does not include the time a patient spends waiting in the office. The mean contact time from averaged 1995–96 data was 19.2 minutes (Schappert and Nelson, 1999). The average length of stay (ALOS) is a good estimator of the time a patient spends in the hospital.

Valuing time costs. The reference case scenario assumes a societal perspective, so the time spent receiving medical care, a health intervention, or caring for another person should be valued as its opportunity cost. Practically speaking, the wage that a person earns provides a good estimate of the opportunity cost of a patient's time or a caregiver's time. When the wage earner is not paid, the wage of an equivalent job may be used. For instance, an unpaid parent's time may be valued at a housekeeper's wage. For a comprehensive list of earnings by profession, visit: http://www.bls.gov/oesnl/oes_alph.htm.

Problems arise in valuing a person's time when the study focuses on women or minority populations. African-Americans earn less than whites, and women to earn less than men, despite making similar contributions to society. Some economists argue that, because the value of the goods and services produced by women or African-Americans is similar to the value of goods and services produced by whites and men, the lower wages paid to these groups may not reflect the true opportunity cost of their labor. For this reason, interventions that are targeted toward African-Americans or other minority groups, or interventions that are targeted toward women (for example, screening mammography), should be calculated using both average wages and the wages of the group of interest. The difference in the wages between these groups can be seen as a type of systematic error in the way society values human labor, and this error can be tested in a sensitivity analysis.

While patients seeking medical care at a clinic generally miss time from work, patients admitted to a hospital will miss both work and leisure time. The time spent at work and leisure time are not technically valued in the same way. Theoretically, the market determines the value of the time that a person spends working. Both the employee and the employer agree that the wage adequately compensates for the time a person spends working and thus reflects the value of the services provided by the employee.

Time spent outside of the workplace, though, is not formally valuated. Therefore, if someone is hospitalized for seven days, we will only be able to estimate the value of the thirty-five hours of that time that would have been spent at work (theoretically, according to the Bureau of the Census, the workweek does not include lunch breaks). The reference case scenario suggests that all time-in-treatment costs should be valued at that person's wage, but it recommends that a sensitivity analysis be conducted on leisure time costs if they are likely to be relevant (Gold and others, 1996). The leisure time component of a time-in-treatment cost will only be relevant if hospitalization costs constitute a large portion of the overall cost of an illness. Remember, though, that the leisure time component of time spent ill (as opposed to the time spent in treatment) is captured in the HRQL score.

Time costs in the sample analysis. To identify the resources used, we must first consider which costs are included. The portion of lost productivity and leisure time captured in the HRQL score does not include the time a patient spends receiving a treatment, a health intervention, or medical care. Thus, the HRQL score does not capture the time a patient spends receiving the influenza vaccine, the time a patient spends at a medical clinic, the time a patient spends in the hospital, or the time spent in transit between a medical facility and home.

Because we are interested in the general population of the United States in the sample analysis, the wage of the average worker in the United States will roughly approximate the opportunity cost of an hour of time spent receiving a preventive intervention or treatment for subjects in our cohort. The hourly wage of the average person in the United States can be obtained from the United States Bureau of the Census (http://www.census.gov) (U.S. Bureau of the Census, 1999), and the hourly wage of workers in certain industries can be obtained from the Bureau of Labor Statistics (http://stats.bls.gov/oes/national/oes_nat.htm).

Exercises 6.7–6.9

6.7. Obtain the average wage in the United States using data from the United States Census. Be certain to include only the wages of people that are between the ages of fifteen and sixty-five, because this is the age range of our hypothetical cohort (Hint: follow the Internet links through to "Money Income in the United States" from the census homepage http://www.census.gov).

6.8. Assume that the time required to travel to and from a doctor's office, plus the time spent in the doctor's office, will consume approximately 1.5 hours of the patient's time per ambulatory medical visit. Add these costs to the cost of a medical visit you calculated in Exercise 6.5.

6.9. We obtained the average length of stay for influenza-related hospitalizations from the HCUP-3 dataset in Exercise 4.1. Add time-in-treatment costs to the cost of hospitalization.

Transportation Costs

The cost of transportation is usually obtained via micro-costing. When identifying the costs, the researcher should consider the mode of transportation, the amount of gasoline consumed, the time the patient spends driving, wear and tear on the car, and parking costs. When measuring the amount of resources consumed, the researcher might consider the number of gallons consumed and the amount of time it takes to get to the destination. When valuing these resources, the quantity and price of each resource are multiplied together, and these products are then summed. For example, a transportation cost estimate might take the form:

$$\text{cost of a gallon of gasoline} \cdot \text{the number of gallons consumed}$$
$$+ \text{ the hourly wage} \cdot \text{the number of hours patient spends in transit}$$

Equation 6.7

Transportation costs are almost always large enough to merit inclusion in a cost-effectiveness analysis. This is especially true in our study, because our hypothetical cohort is of working age and is likely to drive less when ill.

The pollution associated with transporting people to and from work, or to and from their medical clinic, may cause asthma, pneumonia, global warming, and a host of other problems. Though pollution is a major social problem in aggregate, it is rarely a big enough cost to include in a cost-effectiveness analysis.

There are few studies that measure the amount of time that a person spends traveling to or from a doctor's office, and transportation costs can vary quite a bit from one disease to the next. For example, breast cancer patients, who often seek highly specialized care and require a good deal of follow-up care, can travel eighty-nine hours or 369 miles throughout the course of their illness (Secker-Walker and others, 1999).

The Bureau of the Census collects information on the number of persons who commute to work and the average number of miles driven on this commute. This estimate is available at: http://www.census.gov/population/www/socdemo/journey.html. The market price of a gallon of gasoline does not reflect its opportunity cost. In addition to the environmental impact of burning gasoline, there are costs associated with constructing highways, subsidizing the United States petroleum industry, and the like. One group estimated the overall price of a gallon of gasoline to be between $5.60 and $15.14 (www.icta.org/progjects/trans/rlprexsm.htm) in 1998 ("The Real Price of Gas," 1998). Most cost-effectiveness analysts, though, simply use the price of gasoline paid at the pump when calculating transportation costs.

6.10. Assuming an average fuel efficiency of twenty-five miles to the gallon and an average public transportation cost of $1.50 each way, estimate the savings in transportation costs when someone remains in bed for one day with an influenza-like illness. Calculate the distance traveled using data from the Bureau of the Census (http://www.census.gov/population/www/socdemo/journey.html). The cost of a gallon of gasoline in 1997 was $1.25. Assume that most patients will not incur parking costs and that the wear and tear on a car is too small to merit inclusion.

6.11. In their study on the costs of influenza-like illness, Keech and others (1998) found that the average worker with influenza-like illness missed 2.8 days of work. How much money is saved when a person with influenza-like illness cannot travel to work? Should this cost be included in the reference cost-effectiveness analysis?

6.12. Assume that the average travel distance to work is similar to the average distance traveled for medical care. How would transportation costs affect our estimate of the cost of an ambulatory care visit or a hospitalization?

Side Effects

Side effects to a medication or treatment are commonly valued via micro-costing methods because there are not specific diagnostic codes for side effects to each possible treatment. One medication may produce multiple side effects, so it is necessary to identify all of the possible side effects, as well as the frequency at which they occur. Side effects to a test or treatment can be identified either through the medical literature or through information provided by the manufacturer of the medicine or device under study. Side effects are typically measured and valuated based on the ambulatory care or hospital resources used in treating them. For example, if a medication produces nausea, and nausea is known to be a common side effect to the medication, the patient may see a physician so that the medication or the dosage can be changed. As we saw in Chapter Five, it is not often easy to predict the frequency of medical visits for side effects, because most side effects are mild and will not require medical attention.

Though we have good information on the cost of rare side effects to the influenza vaccine, such as Guillian-Barré syndrome (Lasky and others, 1998), there is no published information on the cost of common side effects (such as fever or a sore arm). We can determine these costs by micro-costing or using electronic datasets. If we assume that a physician will provide only reassurance when a patient schedules a visit, we need not include the cost of antibiotics, laboratory tests, or other medical products as a part of these costs. The Medicaid rate of reimbursement for a fifteen-minute visit is a good estimator of such costs to society. The Medicaid rate for a standard medical visit was approximately $20 in 1997 (http://www.hcfa.gov/stats/carrpuf.htm). This rate may be used as an estimate for a medical visit for reassurance.

Alternatively, we can obtain the wages of physicians, medical assistants, and secretaries (which should roughly be equal to the wage of a receptionist) from the Bureau of Labor Statistics, available at: http://stats.bls.gov/oes/national/oes_nat. htm. If we assume that a patient will consume approximately 5 minutes of receptionist time ($10.71 per hour, $0.89 for 5 minutes), 5 minutes of medical assistant time ($10 per hour, $0.83 for 5 minutes), and 15 minutes of physician time ($65 per hour, $16.25 for 5 minutes), we can calculate the cost of a medical visit using micro-costing techniques. Adding these costs together, we obtain a figure of $18 (which is close to the Medicaid estimate). When micro-costing a medical visit, physician contact time can be obtained from the NAMCS, and laboratory test costs can be obtained from HCFA (see Table 4.1).

Regardless of which approach is used, we must add patient time costs for side effects. We might assume that the time required to drive to the doctor's office is similar to the time required to drive to work, and that patients will spend a total of approximately 45 minutes in the doctor's office (including the time spent waiting in the reception). Rounding our round-trip travel time of 44.8 minutes to 45 minutes, we can add the travel time to the time spent in the doctor's office to obtain a total time of 1.5 hours of patient time. This brings the total cost of a medical visit for side effects up to $1.5 \cdot \$16.74 + \$20 = \$45.11$.

Medication Costs

The discussion of micro-costing versus gross-costing is not relevant for medication costs, because they only represent one datum—the cost of the medication itself. The different medications consumed throughout the course of an illness must usually be identified using the medical literature or from clinical practice guidelines. The number of medications consumed can be obtained from the medical literature or from electronic datasets. Finally, the cost of medications can be obtained from the medical literature or from *Drug Topics Red Book* (2000). The *Red Book* lists the average wholesale price for virtually every medication prescribed, but this book must either be purchased or obtained from your local library.

To save you the trip to the library, we will provide the cost of various medications here. The cost of a five-day course of oseltamivir was $53 in 1999, the mean cost of five common over-the counter medications for influenza symptoms was $3.55, and the cost of the influenza vaccine was $5 for a preloaded syringe. Preloaded syringes are already filled with the influenza vaccine, reducing the time it takes to administer the vaccine.

Let us now turn to the medical literature to see how the estimates obtained from the *Red Book* compare with the estimates of others. Bridges and others (2000) surveyed patients with influenza-like illness to see how much they spent on over-the-counter medications. They found that the cost of over-the-counter medications was $8.63, and the cost of prescription medications was $49.38 (see Exercise 6.6). The most common prescription drug is likely to be an antibiotic for a presumed bacterial infection, so we may assume that this is a good estimate of the cost of antibiotics (the study predated the availability of neuraminidase inhibitors). Estimates of the total cost of vaccination are available from Bridges and others (2000) and Nichol and others (1995). Nichol and others estimated that the cost of vaccination was $10 in 1994. This cost estimate included both the cost of vaccination to public health clinics and one-half hour of patient time.

Bridges and others (2000) estimate that the vaccine and supplies would cost $2.66, that a patient would spend one half of an hour receiving the vaccine, and that a nurse would need fifteen minutes to administer the vaccine. We should assume that a vaccination would take about a third of this amount of time to administer (try timing this the next time you go in for a vaccine). While it seems like it takes forever for a practitioner to administer a vaccine, the process happens much more quickly than you might think.

The average wholesale price of an influenza vaccine in the *Red Book*, $5, differs from the cost reported by Bridges and others (2000), $2.66, because providers are able to purchase vaccines at bulk discount rates. From the societal perspective, we will want to include the discounted price of the vaccine, because this more closely reflects the opportunity cost of vaccination.

Exercises 6.13–6.16

6.13. Calculate the overall price of vaccination, using $2.66 as the price of a vaccine assuming one half hour of patient time and five minutes of time for injection by a registered nurse. The salary of a registered nurse is available at: http://www.bls.gov/oesnl/oes32502.htm.

6.14. How does this cost compare to the overall cost of vaccination estimated by Bridges and others (2000) and Nichol and others (1995)? Inflate or deflate these estimates before comparing them.

6.15. What is the cost of antibiotics and oseltamivir in constant 1997 U.S. dollars? Use data from Bridges and others (2000) to obtain the cost of antibiotics and data reported from the 2000 *Red Book* for the cost of oseltamivir (each contains costs in 1999 U.S. dollars).

6.16. Which of the treatments listed in this section will be associated with side effects?

Caregiver Costs

Caregiver costs are estimated using the mean number of hours a loved one or some hired stranger spends caring for a patient. These estimates are sometimes available in the medical literature. They can also be obtained from the Medicare Current Beneficiary Survey (http://www.hcfa.gov/surveys/mcbs/Default.htm). Unfortunately, these data are only available in electronic format and are costly. (This is why they are not listed in Chapter Four.) For some diseases, the time a caregiver spends with a patient must be estimated using the opinion of experts. When the person is a loved one taking time off from work, the time should be valued at the average wage of that person. When it is a home health aid or someone who does not earn a wage, the costs should be valued at the average wage of a home health aid. Because we have no information on the employment characteristics of those caring for influenza-like illness patients, the average wage will serve as an estimate of such costs.

Exercise 6.17

6.17. Keech and others (1998) found that the average worker with influenza-like illness required 0.4 days of caregiver support. What is the cost of caregiver support among persons with influenza-like illness?

CHAPTER SEVEN

CONSTRUCTING A MODEL

Introduction to Decision Analysis

Imagine that you have $100,000 to invest. You have always wanted to study public health, but you have also dreamed about writing a novel ever since you were in college. If you write a novel, you reason, you can simply invest the money in a mutual fund and earn interest, making small withdrawals as needed. Because you are undecided between the two options, you decide to examine which will be the better option financially. Decision analysis is a tool for making such decisions using statistical probabilities.

Decision analysis is based on a concept called **expected value,** in which the value of an uncertain event (such as making $10,000 in the stock market) is weighed against the chances that the event will occur. For example, if you know that the historical average increase in a particular mutual fund is 10 percent per year, then the expected value of the return on your $100,000 investment is $0.1 \cdot \$100,000 = \$10,000$.

If you know the expected value of various events, you will be in a better position to make your decision. You set your sights five years down the road and assume that, if you go to public health school, all of your money would be spent on your education, but you would be able to earn about $40,000 per year working in public health. Because school will consume two of the five years of this period, you will work for three years and earn $3 \cdot \$40,000 = \$120,000$ after graduation. You think that you might be able to save about $4,000 of this after taxes and living expenses over the three years. Therefore, the expected value of this decision is $4,000.

If you decide to write a novel, you will have spent your $100,000, along with the interest on the mutual fund over the five-year period, on living expenses. On the other hand, if you publish the novel, you could earn an additional $30,000. Your college English professor advises you that there is about a 1 percent chance that you will be published. Therefore, the "invest and write" option has an expected value of $\$30,000 \cdot 0.01 = \$300.00$.

You might not be satisfied with your calculations, because there is a chance that the mutual fund could do very well, but there is also a chance that you could lose money. If it does well, you could easily end up with $20,000 from your mutual fund investment at the end of five years, but if it loses money, you might not be able to finish your novel. There is also a chance that you will not find a job right out of public health school, or that the job you get will just barely pay your living expenses. Using a decision analysis model, it would be possible to calculate the expected value of each option and estimate the ranges of possible earnings at the end of the five-year period.

When applied to cost-effectiveness analysis, decision analysis models are ideally suited for calculating both the cost of an intervention and the effectiveness of an intervention, as well as a range of possible values for each. Technical types call the various decisions "competing alternatives." Decision analysis can thus be described as the process of "making an optimal choice among competing alternatives under conditions of uncertainty." In the case of cost-effectiveness analysis, the competing alternatives are the different medical interventions we are studying.

In the past, researchers performing a cost-effectiveness analysis had to write a computer program that would calculate the cost and effectiveness of different medical interventions, or attempt to calculate all of the costs and probabilities on a spreadsheet. Today, most cost-effectiveness analyses can be easily assembled using decision analysis software.

Project Map

1. Develop a research question.
2. Design your analysis.
3. Understand the sources of error in data.
4. Obtain data.
5. Organize data.
6. **Construct a decision analysis model.**
7. Calculate quality-adjusted life years.

8. Test and refine the decision analysis model.
9. Conduct a sensitivity analysis.
10. Prepare the study results for publication or presentation.

Throughout this chapter we will provide instructions for building a decision analysis model. In Chapter Ten, you will learn how to test this model by performing a sensitivity analysis. The basic functions of all decision analysis software packages are similar. If you choose to follow the examples provided here using decision analysis software, you will get a better feel for the concepts behind decision analysis. Tips on using different software packages are also provided throughout this book, and a list of software packages with online links is provided in Table 7.1. Many of these companies offer free trial versions of their software.

TABLE 7.1. DECISION ANALYSIS SOFTWARE PACKAGES AND INTERNET LINKS.

Software

Analytica (http://www.lumina.com). Not able to conduct Markov analyses, but otherwise powerful. Windows and Macintosh versions are available.

DATA (http://www.treeage.com). A powerful and easy to use program that is able to conduct Markov analyses and handle most complex research questions. Windows-based computers only (an older Macintosh version is available, however).

Decision Maker (http://www.nemc.org/medicine/cdm/dmaker1.htm). A powerful program that is able to conduct Markov analyses. Requires DOS.

Decision Pro (http://www.vanguardsw.com/). Not able to conduct Markov analyses, but otherwise powerful. Windows.

DPL (http://www.dpl.adainc.com). Not able to conduct Markov analyses, but otherwise powerful. Windows.

Precision Tree (http://www.palisade.com) and Crystal Ball. These programs require Microsoft Excel to run and are integrated into this spreadsheet program.

SMLTREE (no Web address). A powerful program that is able to conduct Markov analyses. Requires DOS. This program is no longer sold.

Internet resources

Star Office spreadsheet software may be obtained for free (subject to licensing agreement) from: http://www.sun.com/software/star/staroffice/get/get.html.

Decision Analysis Society (http://faculty.fuqua.duke.edu/daweb/). A site maintained by Duke University that contains useful information on the field of decision analysis as well as links to other resources.

Society for Medical Decision Making (http://www.gwu.edu/~smdm/). A site maintained by George Washington University that contains many resources on the field of decision making in medicine.

In this chapter, you will learn how to construct a decision analysis model for our sample cost-effectiveness analysis on strategies to prevent or treat influenza-like illness.

Types of Decision Analysis Models

There are a number of different types of decision analysis models. The most basic is a **simple decision tree.** Simple decision trees are usually employed to examine events that will occur in the near future. They are therefore best suited to evaluate interventions to prevent or treat illnesses of a short duration, such as acute infectious diseases. They may also be used to evaluate chronic diseases that may be cured (for example, by surgical intervention). When these trees are used to evaluate diseases that change over time, they sometimes become too unruly to be useful.

For chronic or complex diseases, it is best to use a **state transition model.** This type of model allows the researcher to incorporate changes in health states over time into the analysis. For example, if a person has cancer, there is a chance that the person will recover within a month or a year and then relapse. There is also a chance that the person will remain sick for some time or will die. With every passing month (or year), the chances of survival, recovery, or deterioration change. These models, which are also called **Markov models,** allow researchers to track changes in the quality of life, the quantity of life, and the cost of a disease over time when different health interventions are applied. Though they have become the most often used model for cost-effectiveness analysis, a clear understanding of simple decision analysis models is needed to understand how Markov models function. These latter models will be described in more detail in Chapter Twelve.

Some cost-effectiveness analyses, such as those piggybacked onto longitudinal studies or primary cost-effectiveness studies, do not require a decision analysis model. In these studies, data is collected as the study progresses, so they generally do not require a large number of probabilities that are derived from secondary sources of data. At the other extreme, very complex health interventions are sometimes studied using computer programs and complex mathematical formulas.

Constructing Simple Decision Analysis Models

In Chapter Two, we developed a flowchart that outlined the event pathway for the supportive care option (see Figure 2.2) in our sample analysis. Simple decision analysis models are constructed in almost the same way a flowchart outlines each health intervention you are studying. As you gain experience with cost-effectiveness analysis, you will be able to describe event pathways using decision analysis models rather than flowcharts, which will save you time when developing your research question.

In the sample cost-effectiveness analysis, we decided to evaluate two competing alternatives to providing supportive care in healthy adults: 1) vaccinating everyone at the beginning of influenza season or 2) treating people with an influenza-like illness with oseltamivir should they become symptomatic. If the choice between these options were obvious, there would be no reason to conduct a cost-effectiveness analysis. In the case of strategies for the prevention or treatment of influenza-like illness, the choices are not intuitive.

Though the vaccine is more effective at preventing hospitalization or death than treatment, it must be administered to every healthy adult in the population. Oseltamivir, on the other hand, is only given to those who actually develop an influenza-like illness, but it will only reduce the duration and severity of the illness, rather than prevent the illness altogether (Treanor and others, 2000). Because oseltamivir is only given to people who become ill, the cost and the number of side effects of this strategy may be lower than for vaccination. On the other hand, because vaccination prevents disease altogether, it may be the more effective strategy.

A decision analysis model will amalgamate the cost and effectiveness data pertaining to these strategies, analyze the effects of error in the data on the decision process, and ultimately identify interventions that are less costly or more effective.

Consider a very basic hypothetical situation. Suppose that vaccination and treatment of influenza each result in a gain of one year of life. Suppose further that vaccination is associated with an 80 percent success rate in preventing disease (and thus increasing life expectancy by one year), and treatment is associated with a 90 percent chance of increasing life expectancy by one year. If we wanted to construct a decision analysis tree to determine the average gain of life for each option, the model might appear as it does in Figure 7.1.

This tree has four components: 1) a decision node (box), 2) branches (lines), 3) chance nodes (circles), and 4) terminal nodes (triangles). The decision node indicates which choices we wish to evaluate, the chance node indicates the probabilities of two or more possible events, and the terminal node indicates the end points we wish to evaluate. In this case, if a patient is treated with oseltamivir, there

FIGURE 7.1. SIMPLE DECISION ANALYSIS MODEL EVALUATING GAINS IN LIFE EXPECTANCY FOR THE VACCINATION AND TREATMENT STRATEGIES.

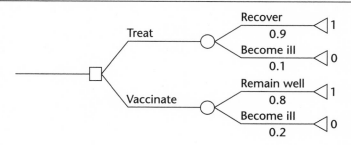

is a 90 percent chance that a year of life will be gained, and there is a 10 percent chance no additional years of life will be gained. In the Vaccinate arm, there is an 80 percent chance that the patient will gain one year of life.

There are basic rules governing the construction of decision trees that should be mentioned here.

- The total of the probabilities following a chance node must add up to 1.0. In the "treat" arm, if there is a 90 percent chance that the person will gain one year of life, there must be a 10 percent chance that the person will not.
- All of the possible outcomes must be represented at the terminal nodes. In this case, there are two outcomes: 1) a gain of one year of life, and 2) no gain in life. Each terminal node is assigned a value of 0 (no gain in life) or 1 (a gain of one year).
- Time moves from left to right. In other words, the model is constructed following the flow of events in the event pathway. (It is not necessary that each event perfectly follows another, however.)
- The tree is evaluated from right to left. When calculations are made, the value at each terminal node is multiplied by the probability of each branch to its left.

Let us see what happens when we complete the calculations by hand (see Figure 7.2).

In this hypothetical example, we see that treatment will save 0.9 years of life. We would thus choose this option over vaccination, which will save only 0.8 years of life. The process of multiplying each of the values at the terminal nodes

FIGURE 7.2.   WHEN EVALUATING EACH OPTION IN THE DECISION ANALYSIS MODEL, THE EXPECTED VALUE AT EACH TERMINAL NODE IS MULTIPLIED BY THE SUCCESSIVE PROBABILITIES OF EACH OPTION OF THE LEFT.

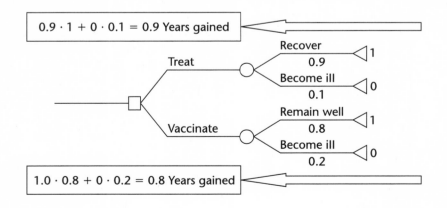

by all probabilities preceding it is called **rolling back** the decision analysis tree. This may seem like a silly evaluation, because we could have simply done the math in our heads. When decisions become increasingly complex, however, a decision tree not only helps you clearly see the event pathway but also greatly simplifies the calculations.

Building the Influenza Model

Trees have a tendency to grow on their own and, with proper pruning, a model can be built relatively quickly if you are well prepared and have done your research in advance. In this section, you will be given step-by-step instructions on how to construct a decision analysis model. If you choose to follow along with a decision analysis program, you may use the cost and probability values that you calculated in Chapters Five and Six. If you did not complete the exercises in these chapters but wish to construct the decision analysis model, follow the exercises but leave all of the probability and cost values blank. These may be filled in once the model is finished using the table of values provided at the end of this section.

Defining the Initial Branches

Because influenza-like illness is an acute infectious disease, we will construct a simple decision tree, rather than a more complex state transition model, for our cost-effectiveness analysis of strategies to prevent or treat influenza. The first step in building a tree is to outline the alternative interventions. Figure 7.3 illustrates the three interventions we are studying.

As mentioned above, the little box is called a "decision node," and the circles are called "chance nodes." The decision node forms the start point of a decision tree. At the decision node, we have three options to evaluate: to provide supportive care, to treat, or to vaccinate. We will refer to the branches emanating directly

FIGURE 7.3.   THE THREE STRATEGIES FOR PREVENTING OR TREATING INFLUENZA-LIKE ILLNESS ARE DEFINED AT THE DECISION NODE.

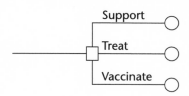

from the decision node as "arms," much the same way that a prospective trial refers to a treatment arm or a control arm.

The Support arm will evaluate health outcomes for subjects that are not treated or vaccinated. Subjects who develop influenza-like illness in this arm will be managed in the same way that anyone with this illness would. They may see a doctor, they may purchase over-the-counter medications, and so on. In the Treat arm, subjects will receive oseltamivir if they manage to see their primary care provider within forty-eight hours. In the Vaccinate arm, all subjects are vaccinated at the beginning of influenza season.

Recall that a tree is built following the event pathway, from left to right. As we move from the trunk of our tree to the branches, we come to the chance node. The chance node indicates that there are two or more possible events that could happen. In any given season, there is a chance that subjects will become ill with influenza-like illness, as well as a chance that they will make it through the season without becoming ill at all. This is true regardless of whether the person is to receive supportive care, is to be treated, or is to be vaccinated. It is important to keep in mind that vaccinated people may still become ill with an influenza-like illness because the vaccine is not 100 percent effective. After adding the chance of developing an influenza-like illness to each arm of the model, the decision analysis should look similar to Figure 7.4.

Tips and tricks. It is generally a good idea to limit the number of branches following a chance node to two. When a tree with three or more branches following a chance node is tested in a sensitivity analysis, the probabilities may sum to greater than one, causing an error message to be generated.

FIGURE 7.4.   THE FIRST EVENT IN THE EVENT PATHWAY IS ADDED TO THE FIRST CHANCE NODE IN THE DECISION ANALYSIS TREE.

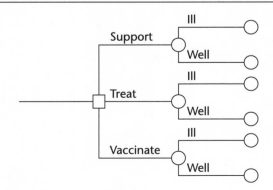

Defining Variables in the Decision Analysis Model

When we considered whether to invest money into public health school or the stock market, we wanted to know how we might fare in five years if our mutual fund fell in value. Just as we would want to assign different values to the growth of the mutual fund, we also want to have a way to assign different values to each probability we use in our decision analysis model. As discussed in Chapter Three, each number we use in our decision analysis model will have a baseline value, or most likely value, as well as high and low values. In our analyses we often want to change values and see how a range of values might affect the outcome of our model. If we were to use fixed values, we would have to manually change many numbers throughout our decision analysis tree each time we wanted to make a change. To make life easier, we work with variables rather than fixed numbers, which can be changed far more readily than fixed values.

Space in a decision analysis tree is precious, so we should aim to keep our tree pruned, manageable, and perhaps most importantly, easily understandable to ourselves and others. In decision analysis trees, variables are often named according to whether they represent a cost or a probability. To save space, the names of variables representing probabilities are usually preceded with a little "p," and the names of variables representing costs are preceded with a little "c." Thus, the variable representing the probability of becoming ill for people in the supportive care and treatment arms will be labeled "pIll," or the probability of becoming ill.

Now, let us input the chances of becoming ill into each branch of the decision analysis tree. For subjects in the Support and Treat arms of the analysis, the chance of becoming ill is equal to the incidence rate of influenza-like illness in unvaccinated people.

If we know the chance that a person will become ill, what is the chance that a person will remain well? This probability is calculated as:

$$1 - \text{probability of becoming ill}$$
$$\text{Equation 7.1}$$

Tips and tricks. Though we could enter Equation 7.1 into our decision analysis model, there is a shortcut common to most decision analysis software. The number sign, #, tells the computer to calculate the probability of the converse event $(1 - \text{the probability of interest})$. This function is built into many packages, because all of the probabilities at any chance node must add up to 1.0.

Estimating the probability of developing influenza-like illness among those who have been vaccinated is a little trickier. In this arm, the only people who become ill with influenza-like illness either: 1) had an illness caused by an agent other than the influenza virus, or 2) developed an illness due to the influenza virus because the vaccine failed. The probability of becoming ill among vaccinated people is defined as:

$$\text{incidence rate of influenza-like illness} \cdot (1 - \text{vaccine efficacy}_{ILI})$$
Equation 7.2

In Exercise 5.4, we calculated a vaccine efficacy of 0.40; thus, the probability is $0.45 \cdot (1 - 0.4) = 0.27$. The tree should now appear similar to the tree in Figure 7.5.

Entering Formulas into the Decision Analysis Model

As we saw in the last section, the probability of developing an influenza-like illness in the Vaccinate arm of the decision analysis tree is determined both by the efficacy of the vaccine at preventing influenza-like illness and by the incidence rate of influenza-like illness (Equation 7.2). If we were to vary either the efficacy of the influenza vaccine or the incidence of influenza-like illness, the probability of developing illness in the Vaccinate arm would change.

For example, suppose that the true mean incidence rate of influenza-like illness is 22 cases per 100 persons (0.22) from season to season, rather than the

FIGURE 7.5.   DECISION ANALYSIS TREE WITH THE CHANCES OF ILLNESS DEFINED AT EACH BRANCH EMANATING FORM THE DECISION NODE.

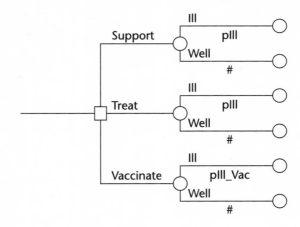

rate we estimated in Chapter Five (0.45). When the incidence rate of influenza-like illness is just 22 cases per 100 persons, the variable pILL_Vac (the chance of illness in the Vaccinate arm) assumes the value $0.22 \cdot (1 - 0.4) = 0.132$, rather than 0.27. Instead of calculating the high and low values for pILL_Vac by hand, we can define this variable using a formula. This way, when the incidence of influenza-like illness or the efficacy of the influenza vaccine is varied, the probability of becoming ill in the Vaccinate arm will also change automatically.

Let us create a new variable called Vac_Eff_ILI, which will define the efficacy of the influenza vaccine in preventing influenza-like illness. The final formula should take the form:

$$pIll\_Vac = pILL \cdot (1 - Vac\_Eff\_ILI)$$

Equation 7.3

Defining Terminal Nodes

So far, we have entered the probabilities that subjects will either become ill with influenza-like illness or remain well throughout the influenza season. We may now finish the Well branches of the decision analysis tree. Because wellness is an end point, we need to change these nodes to terminal nodes. However, we must still decide which costs should be included, if any, at these nodes.

In the Support and Treat arms, no costs are incurred if subjects remain well, so we can enter a zero at each terminal node. In the Vaccinate arm, all subjects will receive the vaccine, so vaccine costs should be added to all terminal nodes emanating from the Vaccinate arm. If we change the chance nodes in each Well branch of the decision analysis tree to a terminal node and then enter these values into the model, the tree should be similar to Figure 7.6.

Note that Figure 7.6 also contains the formula we have defined for the probability of illness in the Vaccinate arm. This formula is assigned to the Vaccinate arm of the decision analysis model alone but occurs before the variable pIll_Vac, which it defines. When the decision analysis model encounters the variable pIll_Vac in the Ill branch, it will look for the nearest definition of this variable (whether a formula or otherwise) that occurs to the left.

Defining Ambulatory Care Needs

When people become ill with influenza-like illness, they may or may not seek medical care. In Chapter Five, we estimated the probability that a person who

FIGURE 7.6.   DECISION ANALYSIS TREE AFTER ADDING THE COST OF THE VACCINE, THE PROBABILITY AND COST OF VACCINE SIDE EFFECTS, AND A FORMULA DEFINING THE PROBABILITY OF ILLNESS IN THE VACCINATE BRANCH.

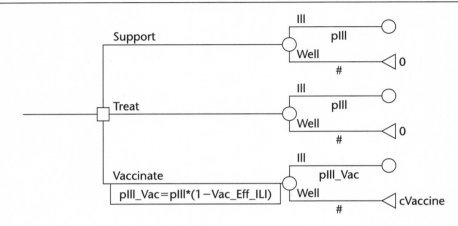

develops influenza-like illness will seek medical care for each arm of the decision analysis model (see the "Hospitalization and Ambulatory Medical Care Utilization" section).

Checking for conditional probabilities. Notice that the probability of a medical visit occurs in the Ill branch of each arm of the decision analysis model. Therefore, we must define the probability of a medical visit given that the subject has developed an influenza-like illness. Though it may seem logical that people will only see a doctor for influenza-like illness if they develop an illness, the rate of medical utilization obtained from a study often reflects the rate in the overall study cohort, rather than the rate among those people that actually become ill. We adjusted the rates we obtained in Chapter Five to reflect rates among ill people rather than among the general study cohort, so we may use these values without adjusting them in our model (see Table 5.9).

Each probability that is used in a decision analysis model is influenced by probabilities that occur to its left. Because of this, each probability entered into a decision analysis tree that falls to the right of a chance node is said to be a **conditional probability.** Conditional probabilities must be carefully defined in a decision analysis model. If we were to add a chance node defining the probability of hospitalization to each Doctor arm of the analysis in Figure 7.7, we would need to enter the probability of hospitalization given that the subject became ill *and* subsequently saw a doctor. We will return to this in the next section.

Adding branches. Let us add arms defining the chance of ambulatory medical care visits to all remaining chance nodes in the decision analysis tree (see Figure 7.7).

FIGURE 7.7. DECISION ANALYSIS MODEL AFTER THE PROBABILITY OF AN AMBULATORY MEDICAL VISIT (pMD) HAS BEEN ADDED AS A BRANCH TO EACH ARM OF THE TREE, AND THE COSTS OF A MEDICAL VISIT, OVER-THE-COUNTER MEDICATIONS (cOTC), AND CAREGIVING (cCARE) HAVE BEEN ADDED TO TERMINAL NODES OF THE SUPPORT AND VACCINATE ARMS.

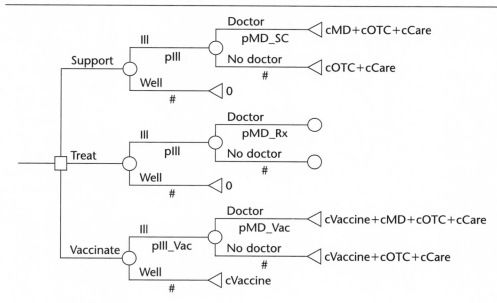

In this figure, the probability of an ambulatory care visit is defined separately in each arm of the tree, because the probability of a medical visit differs by the intervention administered. The variables pMD_SC and pMD_Rx indicate the probability of a medical visit among people who have developed an influenza-like illness in the supportive care and treatment arms, and the variable pMD_Vac indicates the probability of a medical visit among subjects who developed an influenza-like illness despite having been vaccinated. We will return to the differences between the probability of a medical visit for influenza-like illness in the Support and Treat arms in the next section. Note that the formula defining the variable pIll_Vac has been hidden to keep the presentation of the model simple.

Defining terminal nodes. Now, let us define the terminal nodes arising from the branches we have just added to our model. Subjects who become ill and see a doctor will incur the cost of an ambulatory medical visit (cMD). Subjects who do not see a doctor may still buy over-the-counter medications, so these costs must be added regardless of whether the patient sees a physician. They may also incur costs associated with over-the-counter medications (cOTC) and caregiving (cCare).

(Recall that the cost of caregiving was based on the mean number of days of caregiving received in a cohort of persons with influenza-like illness and therefore includes the probability of incurring this cost.) Because we have not finished defining events in the Treat arm of the model, these branches should be left as chance nodes.

Secondary Complications

The rates of ambulatory medical visits for influenza-like illness for vaccinated persons and persons receiving supportive care, which we calculated in Chapter Five, included secondary complications to influenza virus infections. Therefore, the variables pMD_SC and pMD_Vac in Figure 7.7 reflect the rate of medical visits for both primary infections with influenza-like illness and secondary infections with the influenza virus.

The benefits of treatment with oseltamivir include both improvements in subjects' health-related quality of life and reduced medical visits from secondary complications of oseltamivir. Because the reduction in secondary complications will be a major determinant of the overall cost of this strategy, we should add arms to our decision analysis model that indicates whether a subject is likely to require a second medical visit for secondary complications (see Figure 7.8).

In this figure, pMD_Rx should reflect the rate of ambulatory visits for influenza-like illness without secondary complications (see Table 5.10). The chance of secondary complications to influenza virus infection among treated persons, pSec_Rx, is equal to 0.069, and the chance of secondary complications among untreated persons, pSec_NoRx, is 0.147 (see "Ambulatory Visits for Persons Treated with Oseltamivir" in Chapter Five).

Defining terminal nodes. In our model, all subjects who see a doctor in the oseltamivir arm will be treated. Therefore, the cost of treatment and the cost of a medical visit should be included in terminal nodes emanating from the Doctor branch. Subjects who initially visited a medical clinic, received treatment, and developed a secondary complication of their illness incur the cost of two medical visits. Thus, the variable cMD is multiplied by two at this terminal node. One medical visit is assigned to subjects who initially receive treatment but experience no secondary complications of their illness, and one is assigned to subjects who experience secondary complications but do not initially see a doctor. All subjects are assigned the average cost of OTC medications and caregiving among ill persons.

Defining Antibiotic Use and Side Effects

Side effects will also occur as a result of vaccination, treatment with oseltamivir, and treatment with antibiotics administered to treat bacterial influenza-like illnesses and secondary complications of influenza virus infections. In Chapter Five,

FIGURE 7.8. TREAT ARM OF THE DECISION ANALYSIS MODEL AFTER THE PROBABILITY OF SECONDARY COMPLICATIONS TO INFLUENZA VIRUS INFECTION HAS BEEN ADDED AND THE TERMINAL NODES HAVE BEEN DEFINED.

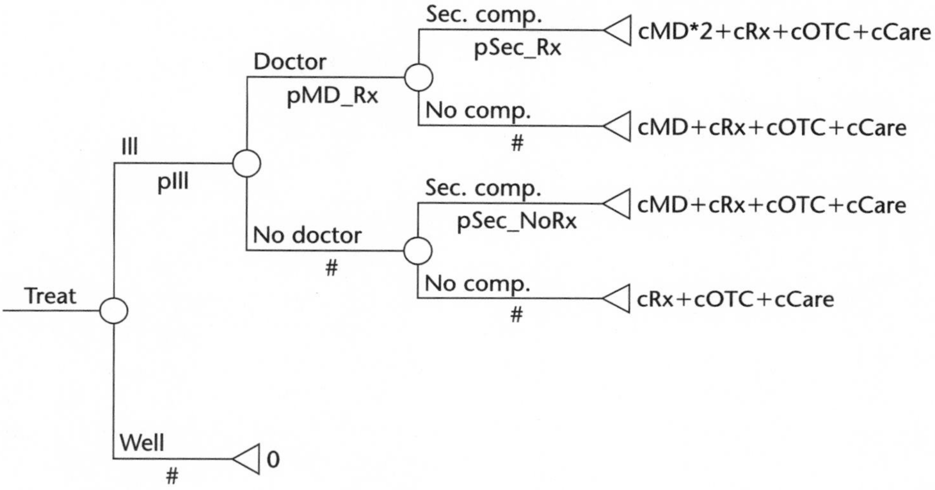

we learned that side effects to oseltamivir and vaccination were minimal, and additional medical visits or other costs due to side effects would only rarely occur. For this reason, we assumed that side effects requiring medical attention would only occur in one in a hundred people. We also assumed that they would only be associated with the cost of a medical visit for reassurance. To keep our model simple, we will add the same probability and cost of side effects whether a subject: 1) receives the influenza vaccine, 2) receives oseltamivir, or 3) receives antibiotics.

Defining the cost of antibiotics. The cost of antibiotics in each arm of the decision analysis model is equal to the product of the cost of antibiotics and proportion of subjects requiring antibiotics. We calculated the probability of antibiotic use for each arm of the analysis in Exercise 5.6 (see Table A1.4) and the cost of antibiotics, $46.42, in Exercise 6.15.

Because antibiotics may be associated with side effects, we should include the cost of side effects in the overall cost of antibiotics. The total cost of antibiotic use thus becomes:

$$pAbx \cdot (cAbx + pSE \cdot cSE)$$

Equation 7.4

where pAbx is the probability of antibiotics, and cAbx is the cost of antibiotics.

Checking for conditional probabilities. In Exercise 5.6, we calculated the chance that people with influenza-like illness will require treatment with antibiotics. In our model, we must go one step further and tabulate the probability that subjects will receive antibiotics *if* they visit a physician. Referring to Table A2.1, we can readily calculate the probability that a subject will receive antibiotics during a medical visit. The probability that a subject will receive antibiotics in the Support arm is 0.595, and the probability that a subject will receive antibiotics in the Vaccinate arm is 0.828.

In the Treat arm, the probability of receiving antibiotics is conditional upon having had secondary complications to illness. All subjects in the study by Treanor and others (2000) had influenza-like illness upon enrollment in that study. Therefore, the data obtained from that study reflect the probability of receiving antibiotics among ill persons. If we divide the number of subjects receiving antibiotics in that study by the number of subjects with any secondary complication (see Table A1.6), we obtain a value of approximately 0.7 regardless of whether the patient received a placebo or treatment.

Defining terminal nodes. In Figure 7.9, Equation 7.4 is added to the Support and Vaccinate arms, with a separate probability defined for the Support arm, pAbx_SC, and the Vaccinate arm, pAbx_Vac. The formula pSE · cSE is added twice to nodes emanating from the Treat branch for which subjects received both oseltamivir and antibiotics.

Defining Hospitalization Costs

Decision analysis models can become quite large and unruly, even when constructed to answer relatively straightforward research questions. To keep the model tidy, we can include the cost of hospitalization and the probability of hospitalization as a formula in the terminal nodes of our model, rather than add chance nodes to each arm of the model. We can also define events as cost formulas in the terminal nodes, so long as these events do not affect effectiveness outcomes. Figure 7.10 demonstrates the probability (pHosp) and cost (cHosp) of hospitalization added to all Ill branches of the decision analysis tree.

Notice, though, that the probability of hospitalization is a conditional probability. In Figure 7.10, the risk of hospitalization is therefore the same regardless of whether a patient becomes ill or sees a physician.

Probability of hospitalization among ill persons. In Chapter Five, we decided to use the estimated rate of hospitalization for persons without major medical conditions between the ages of fifteen and sixty-five from the Centers for Disease Control and Prevention (CDC). This rate, 24 per 100,000 persons, reflects the

FIGURE 7.9. DECISION ANALYSIS MODEL AFTER SIDE EFFECTS TO OSELTAMIVIR, VACCINATION, AND ANTIBIOTICS HAVE BEEN ADDED.

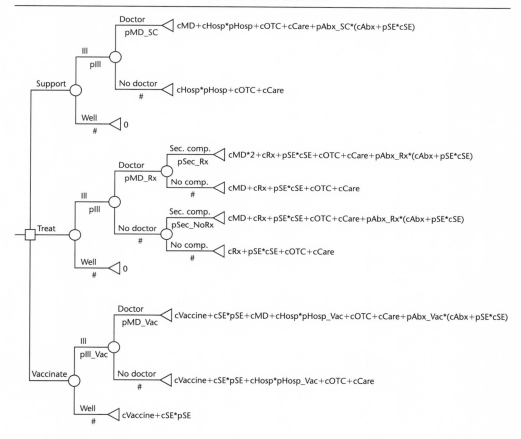

overall rate of hospitalization in the general population, or:

$$\frac{\text{total number of hospitalizations for influenza-like illness, healthy adults, 15 to 65}}{\text{total number of healthy adults, 15 to 65}}$$

Equation 7.5

In other words, this is the rate of hospitalization among all people, regardless of whether they saw a doctor and regardless of whether they developed an influenza-like illness.

If we added the probability of hospitalization to all terminal nodes emanating from a given arm in the decision analysis tree, including the Well node, we

FIGURE 7.10. DECISION ANALYSIS MODEL AFTER THE PROBABILITY OF HOSPITALIZATION HAS BEEN DEFINED AS A SEPARATE FORMULA IN EACH ARM AND THE COST OF HOSPITALIZATION HAS BEEN ENTERED INTO EACH TERMINAL NODE EMANATING FROM ILL BRANCHES.

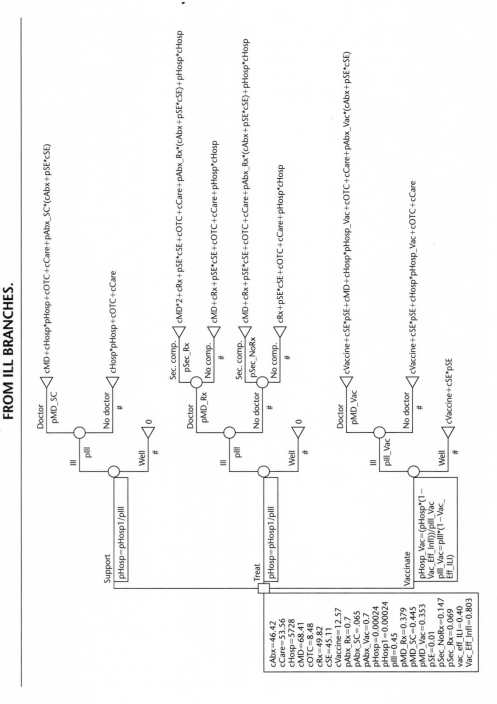

would be correctly tabulating the probability and the cost of hospitalization in the model. This is because the Ill nodes and the Well nodes in any given arm of the study encompass persons with and without an influenza-like illness (thus, the denominator in equal to the denominator in Equation 7.5). Because people who review the decision analysis tree would be confused by the presence of the variables pHosp and cHosp in the Well nodes of the decision analysis tree, we may simply adjust the probability of hospitalization so that it reflects the probability among ill persons alone. The probability of hospitalization among ill subjects is equal to:

$$\frac{\text{total number of hospitalizations for influenza-like illness}}{\text{total number of subjects with influenza-like illness}}$$

Equation 7.6

Unfortunately, the studies used to estimate the rate of hospitalization do not report the number of subjects who actually developed an influenza-like illness.

However, we can correct the variable pHosp to reflect only hospitalizations among persons who develop an influenza-like illness by dividing pHosp by the incidence rate of influenza-like illness. The chance of hospitalization among ill subjects in the Support and Treat arms becomes:

pHosp/pIll

Equation 7.7

By dividing pHsop by pIll, we are reversing the effect of multiplying these variables together at the Ill decision node as follows:

Value pHosp in Ill branches $=$ pHosp $\cdot$ pIll

Value of pHosp after dividing by pIll $=$ pHosp $\cdot$ ~~pIll~~/~~pIll~~ $=$ pHosp

Thus, we will hold the overall probability of hospitalization constant at 0.00024 regardless of the value pIll assumes in the decision analysis model.

Tips and tricks. Some software packages do not allow a variable to be placed on two sides of an equation as we did in Equation 7.7. Instead, it is necessary to create a separate variable with the same value.

Probability of hospitalization in the Treat arm. None of the randomized controlled trials examining oseltamivir has been large enough to determine whether this medication reduces hospitalization. Therefore, the risk of hospitalization among persons treated with oseltamivir is not known. In fact, it is possible that oseltamivir does not reduce a person's chances of hospitalization at all. In Chapter Five, we estimated the efficacy of oseltamivir in reducing the duration of influenza-like illness (see Table 7.2), however, reductions in the duration of illness will not likely

TABLE 7.2. PROPORTIONATE REDUCTION IN THE DURATION OF INFLUENZA-LIKE ILLNESS AMONG SUBJECTS TREATED WITH OSELTAMIVIR WITHIN 48 HOURS.

Measure of Improvement	Formula	Result
Duration of illness	1-76.3/97	0.2134
Severity of illness	1-686/887	0.2266
Return to full health	1-134/178	0.2472
Return to activity	1-173/230	0.2478

reflect reductions in hospitalizations. Our best bet would be to use expert opinion to estimate the risk ratio (see Chapter Five) of hospitalization among persons treated with oseltamivir and multiply this ratio by pHosp in the treatment arm. For simplicity, we will assume that oseltamivir does not reduce the risk of hospitalization and will leave this ratio out of our model.

Probability of hospitalization in the Vaccinate arm. The variable pIll_Vac has been defined to account for the efficacy of the vaccine in reducing influenza-like illness (see Equation 7.3). The actual chance of hospitalization among vaccinated subjects in the general population is:

$$pHosp\_Vac = pHosp \cdot (1 - Vac\_Eff\_Infl)$$

Equation 7.8

where Vac_Eff_Infl is the efficacy of the influenza vaccine in preventing influenza virus infections. In this formula, we use the efficacy of the influenza vaccine in preventing influenza virus infections rather than influenza-like illness, because people are only likely to be hospitalized for influenza virus infections or secondary complications of such infections, such as bacterial pneumonia. Note that, by subtracting the efficacy of the influenza vaccine from one in Equation 7.8, we are actually calculating the risk ratio of an influenza virus infection among vaccinated people (see Equation 5.5).

We should not insert this formula into our decision analysis model just yet. First, we must amend it to only include hospitalized patients in the Ill branch of our decision analysis model by dividing this probability by the probability of becoming ill, as we did in Equation 7.7. In the Vaccinate arm of the model, the chance of hospitalization is equal to:

$$pHosp\_Vac = (pHosp \cdot (1 - Vaccine\_Efficacy\_Influenza))/pIll\_Vac$$

Equation 7.9

Probability of hospitalization among persons with a previous medical visit. In the real world, people will generally visit a doctor before they are hospitalized. Those that do not visit a doctor are usually admitted to the hospital via the emergency room, incurring additional costs. It is not necessary to assign a different probability to hospitalizations occurring among subjects who saw a doctor before their hospitalization and subjects who did not; the cost of the ambulatory medical visit is counted separately, and the cost of an emergency room visit is counted in the overall cost of hospitalization. Moreover, if outside reviewers inspect the model, they will not be confused by the presence of the cost of hospitalization in the No Doctor node, because patients who fail to see a physician can still be hospitalized. Therefore, it is acceptable to simply add this cost to both the "Doctor" and the "No Doctor" branches of the model.

Patient Compliance

A final consideration for the treatment arm is whether the patients complete their courses of medication. In all studies examining oseltamivir, patient compliance was excellent. This might be expected, because patients with influenza-like illness are probably fairly motivated to get over their illness, the duration of treatment is reasonably short, and because the side effects associated with the medications are relatively insignificant. Because patient compliance is included in each of the outcomes of the study, this is effectively "built in" to the study results (if all of the patients had taken the medications, the results would have been better than they were). In real life, patients are rarely as compliant as they are during closely monitored clinical studies. Because we can assume that patient compliance is greater in these studies than it would be in the real world, patient compliance should be tested in a sensitivity analysis.

Final Costs

All of the costs and probabilities that we have calculated, along with a legend listing the abbreviations used in the decision analysis model, are presented in Table 7.3. Students who are building a decision analysis model should be certain that the values entered into the model match those in this table if they wish to verify that the model works. Also, do not forget to define the variables pIll, pIll_Vac, and pHosp_Vac as formulas. Failing to do so will affect the sensitivity analyses you will perform on the model in Chapter Ten.

We have now finalized our cost calculations and can reap the rewards of the first phase of all of our work by rolling back the decision tree. When a tree is rolled back, all of the outcomes at the terminal nodes are multiplied by their respective probabilities (see Figure 7.11).

Here, we see that vaccination is the least expensive option, and it is thus **cost-saving** relative to providing supportive care. For every person vaccinated, we

TABLE 7.3.   VARIABLES AND FORMULAS INCLUDED IN THE SAMPLE DECISION ANALYSIS MODEL.

Variable[a]	Name	Value
Cost of antibiotics	cAbx	46.42
Cost of caregiving	cCare	53.56
Cost of hospitalization	cHosp	5,728
Cost of medical visit	cMD	68.41
Cost of oseltamivir	cRx	49.82
Cost of over-the-counter medications	cOTC	8.48
Cost of side effects	cSE	45.11
Cost of vaccine	cVaccine	12.57
Incidence rate	pIll	0.45
Probability of antibiotics, support	pAbx_SC	0.595
Probability of antibiotics, treat	pAbx_Rx	0.7
Probability of antibiotics, vaccinate	pAbx_Vac	0.828
Probability of hospitalization	pHosp	0.00024
Probability of medical visit, support	pMD_SC	0.445
Probability of medical visit, treat	pMD_Rx	0.379
Probability of medical visit, vaccinate	pMD_Vac	0.353
Probability of secondary complications, treat	pSec_Rx	0.069
Probability of secondary complications, support	pSec_NoRx	0.147
Probability of side effects	pSE	0.01
Proportionate decrease illness (value)	pHealthy	0.213
Vaccine efficacy, ILI	Vac_eff_ILI	0.40
Vaccine efficacy, influenza	Vac_eff_Infl	0.803

Formula

Probability of hospitalization, support and treat	$pHosp = pHosp1/pIll$	
Probability of hospitalization, vaccinate	$pHosp\_Vac = (pHosp*(1 - Vac\_Eff\_Infl))/ Pill\_Vac$	
Incidence rate, vaccinate arm	$pIll*(1 - Vac\_Eff\_ILI)$	

[a]Some costs, such as the cost of transportation, have been left out for simplicity.

would expect to save $\$40.26 - \$48.58 = -\$8.32$. Furthermore, we see that we are off the hook for calculating secondary transmission costs (see Chapter Five). Still, we will require effectiveness information before we can compare the three interventions for cost-effectiveness. The next step in the analysis is to calculate effectiveness in the form of quality-adjusted life years.

FIGURE 7.11. COMPLETED DECISION ANALYSIS TREE SHOWING THE EXPECTED VALUE OF EACH STRATEGY (BOXES).

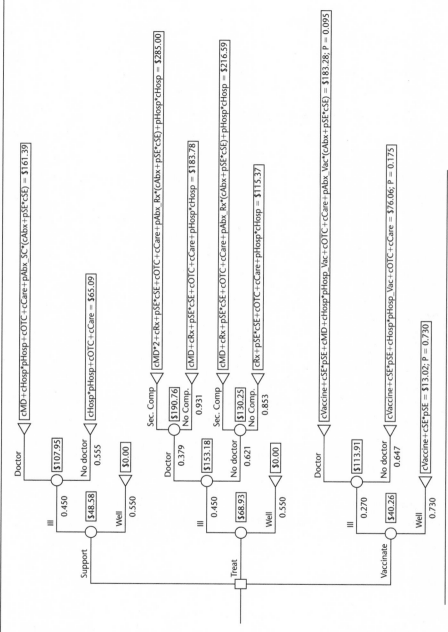

Note: These numbers will be slightly different if you populated your model with more recent data.

CHAPTER EIGHT

WORKING WITH QUALITY OF LIFE MEASURES

Overview

A quality-adjusted life year (QALY) may be thought of as a year of life that is lived in perfect health. Recall from Chapter One that HRQL scores assume a value between 0 and 1. This ratio may be simply thought of as a continuum of values representing the spectrum of quality of life ranging from perfect health to death. Thus, if a medical intervention adds 10 years of life, and each of these years is associated with an HRQL of 0.7, the medical intervention would have resulted in a gain of 7 years of perfect health (7 QALYs). This is graphically represented in Figure 1.3.

In this chapter, we will take the first step toward calculating QALYs as we learn the foundation of HRQL scores, learn how to obtain HRQL scores for cost-effectiveness analyses, and learn how to use HRQL scores in our sample analysis. In the next chapter, we will learn how to calculate and incorporate QALYs into our sample analysis.

Framework

In this section, we will briefly discuss the formal methods used to translate a person's perception of the quality of life in various health states into an HRQL score. Though every HRQL score in a reference case analysis is based on the methods presented in this section, it is not absolutely necessary to understand these methods to derive an HRQL score. Much like a computer hides all of the complicated programming code behind a point-and-click interface, preference-weighted generic instruments—the tools used to easily generate HRQL scores—hide this methodology behind a simple survey form. One such instrument, the EuroQol, is presented in Appendix VI.

In Chapter Five, we mentioned that these preference-weighted generic instruments may be completed using information from the medical literature. We will provide an example of how this is done in this chapter. HRQL scores can be completed by clinicians or alternatively, by patients with the disease under study (Gold and others, 1996). Once the instrument is completed, the researcher inputs the responses into a simple formula that produces an HRQL score suitable for use in a reference case cost-effectiveness analysis. In this section, we will discuss how these instruments are created. In the following sections, we will describe how they are used.

Preference-weighted generic instruments are designed using HRQL scores taken from a sample of subjects from the general population. This sample of people is subjected to a series of exercises based on **expected utility theory.** This may sound intimidating, but expected utility theory is little more than a way of turning concepts, such as quality of life, into a number (the HRQL score).

One method based on expected utility theory is called the **standard gamble** technique. Suppose you had an illness that required you to remain in bed for the rest of your life, and an evil magician appeared at the foot of your bed. Suppose that the magician told you that you could either remain as you are for the rest of your life or play a potentially deadly game. If you won this game, you would regain perfect health, but if you lost, you would die. To make an informed decision, you would want to know the chances of winning the game. The standard gamble technique is designed to estimate the risk of death that a patient would be willing to accept in a gamble for perfect health.

In this technique, subjects must choose between a health state (such as remaining in bed) and a gamble in which there is a chance of perfect health or death. The chance of death is changed until the decision between the health state and the gamble are perceived to be about equally desirable to the subject. For instance, suppose a subject is certain that she would be willing to risk a 50 percent chance of death in exchange for the opportunity to recover from her illness but would definitely not be willing to accept a 60 percent chance of death. The researcher would scale the probability of death up from 50 percent, until the patient is ambivalent about whether to take the gamble or to just remain in bed.

The probability at which the patient is ambivalent between taking the gamble and remaining in her hypothetical health state is the HRQL score for this health state. For instance, if she were completely undecided between remaining confined to bed or taking a gamble in which she had a 54 percent chance of death, the HRQL score for that health state would be $1 - 0.54 = 0.46$.

Another technique that uses expected utility theory is called the **time trade-off** method. Here, the patient is asked how much time in poor health she would be willing to trade for perfect health. Thus, the patient has to forgo future years of life in poor health in exchange for fewer years of life in perfect health. Once the subject has decided how much time she would be willing to sacrifice for better health, the HRQL score is obtained by dividing the life expectancy in perfect health by the life expectancy in the state of illness.

Preferences derived using the time trade-off and the standard gamble methods are formally called **utilities** (this is where the term "cost-utility analysis" comes from). We will not discuss the methods for deriving utilities in detail here. However, it is important to know that most preference-weighted generic health instruments and published lists of HRQL scores are estimated using exercises grounded in expected utility theory.

Who Should Valuate HRQL?

The Panel on Cost-Effectiveness in Health and Medicine recommends that HRQL scores be determined using preference-weighted instruments that are based on a representative sample of people within society (Gold and others, 1996). Others believe that these scores should be obtained from people who actually have the disease under study. People with a disease, it is argued, know what life is like with that disease and would thus be better at valuing the corresponding quality of life than the average person would.

The problem with deriving HRQL scores from people with the disease under study is that such scores are not consistent with the societal perspective. Remember that we are interested in valuing all inputs into our cost-effectiveness analysis from the perspective of everyone in society. Because not everyone in society has the disease we are interested in, deriving HRQL scores using only people with a particular disease betrays this principle. Instead, the scores should be representative of the value that the average person would assign to a particular health state (Gold and others, 1996).

How does the average person know what it is like to have a disease? To generate HRQL scores for health states, a sample of people will ideally go through a formal exercise in which they study different aspects of a health state. Once the person has an idea of what life might be like with the disease, the subject undergoes an exercise, such as the expected utility exercises described above, to generate an HRQL score.

When the scores are derived from a representative sample of people in a community, they are referred to as **community-derived preferences.** The word "preference" refers to an individual's perception of what life is like in a given health state. Consider a study that evaluates a medication used to treat arthritis. While eccentric old writers that sit around scrawling notes in smoky cafés all day would probably prefer arthritis in their knees, runners would probably prefer to have arthritis in their hands. Moreover, both writers and runners would be affected by the arthritis in different ways. For instance, if the writer was earning a living from writing, he may see arthritis as a more severe disease, which may lead to financial instability and depression. Therefore, a preference contains more information on the ways in which people's lives are affected by disease than other types of HRQL scores.

As mentioned above, the value a person places on a health state using established exercises is called a health utility. You will often hear the terms "preference" and "utility" used interchangeably in cost-effectiveness analyses. Because it is easy to mix these terms up, it is probably best to refer to preferences or utilities as HRQL scores because the term "HRQL score" is a catchall category (Drummond and others, 1997; Gold and others, 1996).

Deriving HRQL Scores

In the following sections, we will discuss how to obtain scores using preference-weighted generic instruments, how to use scores derived from published lists, and how to use HRQL scores in non-reference case measures, such as the disability-adjusted life year (DALY). Very large research efforts will sometimes also generate scores by taking a sample of subjects through a series of exercises based on expected utility theory so that they can generate HRQL scores from scratch.

Using Preference-Weighted Generic Instruments

Preference-weighted generic instruments are often used in cost-effectiveness analysis because the process of determining community-derived HRQL scores is costly and time-consuming, since it requires exposing large numbers of people to time-consuming exercises (Gold and others, 1996). There are a number of preference-weighted generic instruments available, and each has its strengths and weaknesses. Examples include the Quality of Well-Being (QWB) scale, the Health Utility Index, and the EuroQol. A complete list of instruments can be found at http://www.qlmed.org.

These instruments may be used to convert responses from physicians who have experience with the disease under study, or from patients who have the disease under study, into HRQL scores that estimate preferences derived from a representative community sample. Alternatively, researchers can obtain information about the disease from the medical literature and then use this information to fill in the blanks of a preference-weighted generic instrument. In other words, preference-weighted generic instruments are essentially tools that translate survey responses into HRQL scores. The resulting HRQL scores will be similar to those derived from a large representative community sample of people that have gone through exercises grounded in expected utility theory.

When a preference-weighted generic instrument is administered, respondents are asked a variety of questions about their perception of the quality of life in health states relating to the disease. Each question in the survey that refers to a particular aspect of the person's health-related quality of life is referred to as a **dimension** (also known as an **attribute** or **domain**). Preference-weighted generic instruments are more generally called **multi-attribute health status classification systems,** because they combine many different attributes of a disease into a single HRQL score (Drummond and others, 1997).

For example, people with influenza-like illness might have the following attributes (or dimensions of illness): fatigue, cough, and being confined to bed. Using one of these instruments, we can obtain a single HRQL score for all of these attributes of influenza-like illness.

The dimensions captured by an instrument can represent aspects of a disease beyond the biological symptoms the disease causes. For instance, diabetes can cause blindness or the inability to walk. These conditions may in turn affect the person's ability to function in society and may place strains on his relationships with others. Blindness, the inability to walk, a person's ability to function in society, a person's ability to relate to others, and a person's ability to work are all examples of health dimensions.

If we wished to generate an HRQL score that reflected the quality of life of people with diabetes, we would have to find an instrument that captured as many of the dimensions of this disease as possible. For example, the EuroQol (see Appendix VI) asks about people's ability to care for themselves, their ability to perform the activities they were able to perform when healthy, whether or not they have pain or discomfort, and whether or not they feel depressed (De Charro, 2001; EuroQol Group, 1990). Suppose that a woman with diabetes becomes depressed because she is no longer able to participate in social activities with her grandchildren. While the instrument would capture the extent to which the respondent was depressed, it will not capture the effect of the disease on her relationship with her grandchildren.

Some instruments will capture mobility limitations well, and others will capture emotional limitations well, but few will capture all of the attributes relevant to this disease. In the case of diabetes, the EuroQol would be a good instrument for capturing most of the relevant dimensions of this disease, even though it does not measure some of the more subtle effects the disease might have on a person's social life.

Let us consider another example. The Quality of Well-Being (QWB) scale measures mobility, physical activity, social activity, as well as the effect of various symptoms, such as fatigue, on HRQL (Kaplan and Anderson, 1988). If we were to use this instrument to obtain an HRQL score for diabetes, we would capture the impact diabetes might have on the woman's social life, but the instrument would still miss her depressed mood. Thus, while the EuroQol may be better at capturing the effect of diabetes on the woman's mood, the QWB may be better at capturing the social aspects of the disease.

Fortunately, both of these instruments are based on a representative sample of people's preferences for disease states. Because preferences reflect many people's subjective perception of what life would be like with a disease, it is not absolutely necessary to capture all dimensions of a disease in any given instrument. In the example of the runner and the writer with arthritis, we see that the use of preferences allows us to value different effects a health state might have on a person's overall HRQL. To understand this better, let us break down the various terms used in the names of these instruments, so that we may get a better idea of what they do and how they are used.

Preferences. The word "preference" is used to distinguish preference-weighted instruments from those that fail to take individual wishes or desires into account. While some HRQL scores are generated by having subjects rank a list of health states from best to worst, HRQL scores based on preferences allow people to better express how the disease would affect their lives. Consider the example of the cost-effectiveness analysis designed to evaluate a treatment for arthritis mentioned in the previous section. People who spend their days watching television may not be greatly bothered by arthritis, but both the writers and athletes will. While the eccentric writer would not be able to write at all, the runner might be able to switch to a less desired sport, such as swimming, and the television addict might merely have to learn how to switch hands when using the remote control. In the writer's case, the arthritic pain might lead to depression and interfere with his social activity. In the runner's case, the arthritis might interfere with her social activity, because she is not with her old running group and must swim alone, but this might not make her feel depressed. Therefore, by using preferences, we are able to compensate for the fact that the instrument we used failed to capture all domains relevant to the disease we are studying.

Weighting. Consider the EuroQol (De Charro, 2001, available at http://www. euroqol.org). Each category in Table 8.1 is assigned a weight using the time trade-off technique applied to a representative community sample of subjects. This weight reflects the preferences of these subjects for each of the health states listed in Table 8.1. When the instrument is filled out, each response is weighted according to the preferences of the representative community sample.

In the EuroQol, subjects are asked to check the categories in Table 8.1 that best describe the condition of interest. Recall that each of the three responses in each category is associated with a weight that was derived from a sample of patients using the time trade-off technique. To demonstrate how these weights are used, let us generate an HRQL score for influenza-like illness using this instrument and data we have already gathered from the medical literature. First, we must examine the different health states at different points in the illness. To do this, we will use information from Keech and others (1998) and Treanor and others (2000) to estimate the impact of the disease (see Appendix II for summaries of these articles). Though these articles do not provide all of the information we need to get the complete picture of influenza-like illness, we will use them to demonstrate how these instruments are used. In addition, because we are illustrating a point rather than conducting a formal study, we will round the numbers we obtain to keep the examples simple.

Let us round off Keech and others (1998) estimate of being confined to bed (see Chapter Six and Appendix II), from 2.4 days to 2 days. Keech and others (1998) also inform us that otherwise healthy workers with influenza-like illness need an average of 0.5 days of caregiver support. Let us round this up to 1 day

TABLE 8.1.   ABBREVIATED QUESTIONS CONTAINED IN THE EUROQOL (DE CHARRO, 2001).

Mobility (ability to walk or get around)

1. No problems	2. Some problems	3. Confined to bed

Self-care (ability to dress or wash)

1. No problems	2. Some problems	3. Unable to care for self

Usual activities (ability to work or study)

1. No problems	2. Some problems	3. Unable to perform

Pain

1. No pain	2. Moderate pain	3. Extreme pain

Anxiety/depression

1. Not anxious/depressed	2. Somewhat anxious/dep.	3. Extremely anxious/dep.

Note: For a complete version of this instrument, see Appendix Seven.

for the sake of simplicity. Finally, we know that the average worker will miss 2.8 days of work. Let us round this number up to 3. Now, let us assume that on days 1, 4, and 5 most patients with influenza-like illness will be able to get around, but that they will be confined to bed on days 2 through 3. Let us assume that people will generally have some self-care difficulties on day 3 for simplicity, and that people will miss work on days 2 through 4. Using the values from Table 8.1 and their respective preference weights, we will estimate the HRQL score of otherwise perfectly healthy people who develop influenza-like illness.

To obtain an HRQL score for any given day, simply subtract the preference weight values in Table 8.2 from 1.0. The only trick to calculating the HRQL score using this particular instrument is that a constant value (**0.081**), which is used to adjust the overall score, must be applied whenever the person is in less than perfect health. Thus, the HRQL of subjects on day 2 is $1.0 - \mathbf{0.081} - 0.314 - 0.094 = 0.511$. The mean HRQL over 5 days is calculated by adding up all of the values and dividing by 5, yielding a score of 0.7486.

If we were to apply the same values to the QWB scale, we would obtain an HRQL score of 0.605. The scores differ between these instruments for a number of reasons. First, the weights are based on a different sample of people. While the EuroQol was obtained from subjects living in Europe, the QWB scale was obtained using subjects in the United States. Second, each instrument captures different dimensions of the disease. Finally, each is based on a different method for estimating HRQL. If we were conducting our analysis in the Netherlands, it would be more appropriate to use the score obtained using the EuroQol than the score obtained using the QWB, because part of the difference in scores reflects the

TABLE 8.2. EXAMPLE OF HOW AN HRQL SCORE FOR INFLUENZA-LIKE ILLNESS MAY BE DERIVED USING THE EUROQOL.

	Day 1	Day 2	Day 3	Day 4	Day 5
Mobility	1 (0.000)	3 (0.314)	3 (0.314)	1 (0.000)	1 (0.000)
Self-care	1 (0.000)	1 (0.000)	2 (0.104)	1 (0.000)	1 (0.000)
Usual activity	1 (0.000)	3 (0.094)	3 (0.094)	3 (0.094)	1 (0.000)
Pain	1 (0.000)	1 (0.000)	1 (0.000)	1 (0.000)	1 (0.000)
Anxiety/depression	1 (0.000)	1 (0.000)	1 (0.000)	1 (0.000)	1 (0.000)
Score for day	1.0	0.511	0.407	0.825	1.0

Note: The severity rating for each day and each health state obtained from Table 8.1 is presented as a whole number, and weights for each state (obtained from the EuroQol instrument) appear in parentheses.

different cultural values of the subjects. On the other hand, the QWB scale allows us to capture specific symptoms of influenza, such as coughing and wheezing, so it may afford more specificity. Though the different weights used in each instrument can produce fairly wide ranges in HRQL scores, choosing an instrument that best matches the needs of your analysis can minimize this error (Gold and others, 1998).

Tips and tricks. Though the QWB scale is not based on expected utility theory, the Panel on Cost-Effectiveness in Health and Medicine has listed it as a QALY-compatible measure.

Generic versus disease-specific instruments. The term "generic" refers to the fact that these instruments can be applied to any disease. Some instruments have been developed to generate scores for specific diseases, such as cancer. In practice, it does not matter whether the instrument was designed for a particular disease or is generic in nature, so long as the instrument: 1) is preference-weighted, 2) captures aspects of the respondent's overall health status, 3) captures aspects of the effect of disease on the respondent's productivity and leisure, and 4) is based on a representative community sample of people (Gold and others, 1996).

Identifying attributes. Because different attributes (or domains) of different diseases are captured by different instruments, it is important to identify the attributes of interest to your study. A complete list of instruments used in health and medicine research can be found at http://www.qlmed.org. This web site has a search engine that allows the user to enter specific diseases or attributes of interest to better facilitate a match between the disease under study and an appropriate instrument. Note that not all of these instruments meet the criteria outlined by the Panel on Cost-Effectiveness in Health and Medicine for use in reference case cost-effectiveness analyses. In addition, any instrument you choose should meet the four criteria outlined in the subsection above, "Generic Versus Disease-Specific Instruments." A broad overview of some of the currently available instruments is presented in Table 5.11.

HRQL Scores Generated from Large Health Surveys

It is also possible to use large national health surveys that contain questions similar to those in preference-weighted generic instruments to generate complete lists of HRQL scores for different diseases. To generate lists of health scores, responses from large health surveys are assigned different preference weights. Using a computer program, the responses from the national survey in question are then essentially matched to responses on the generic instrument and lists of HRQL scores are generated for each disease the surveyed subjects had.

This method for deriving HRQL scores is more controversial than directly using generic instruments, because many feel that it has not been rigorously tested and is somewhat theoretical. The controversy arises because the responses on the national survey under study have to be fit into the framework of the instrument using mathematical techniques. Nonetheless, lists of HRQL scores are acceptable for use in a reference case analysis so long as appropriate health domains are captured.

Because national health surveys are generally very large and are often representative of a nation's population, it is possible to generate HRQL scores for any specific group within that population (or nation). For example, one might be interested in estimating the HRQL scores in certain ethnic minority groups or among people with low income. A partial list of HRQL scores derived from the National Health Interview Survey (NHIS) by Gold and others (1998), which is called the Years of Healthy Life (YHL) measure, is provided in Appendix II. These HRQL scores were based on only two dimensions of health, rather than four or more. The YHL measure is therefore less specific than other health instruments.

If we wished to use the YHL measure to derive the HRQL of people with and without influenza-like illness, it would be a less than perfect measure for a number of reasons. First, peoples' perception of their health status may not reflect how frustrated they are that they must stay in bed all day, feel lethargic, and have sore throats. In fact, the YHL measure, which collects data from the National Health Interview Survey (NHIS) is not very useful for acute diseases at all, because the data are collected on an annual basis, and subjects who had influenza some months ago may consequently not think of themselves as ill at all.

At the time of publication, the YHL measure was the only available comprehensive list of HRQL scores for different diseases or conditions. The YHL measure is based on the subject's perception of his or her health status and the subject's role function (Erickson and others, 1995). However, the Agency for Health Research and Quality has incorporated questions specific to the EuroQol into its Medical Expenditure Panel Survey. Once community weights have been obtained for people in the United States and applied to this instrument, a much more comprehensive list of HRQL scores should be available. Likewise, once national surveys in European countries that the EuroQol presently has representative community weights for are developed, lists of HRQL scores should become available in these countries.

While the health of U.S. citizens is generally inferior to citizens of most other industrialized countries (for example, Japan or the nations of Western Europe), it is generally much better than the health of citizens of most developing countries. Therefore, the YHL is not appropriate for use outside the United States. One measure that is available, but is not compatible with the reference case scenario, is the disability-adjusted life year (DALY). A final source of HRQL scores is a compiled list of values that has been prepared by Harvard University. These scores are listed according to their compatability with the reference case scenario and are available at www.hsph.harvard.edu/organizations/hcra/cuadatabase/ intro.html.

Using Disability-Adjusted Life Years

One last method that should be mentioned, but is not accepted by many health economists, is the practice of deriving HRQL scores from experts rather than a representative community sample. The scores associated with the DALY were derived using experts in part because it was necessary to generate many scores and in part because the scores were to be applied to people in distinct geographic regions of the world (Murray and Lopez, 1996).

The disability-adjusted life year is a QALY in reverse. It measures the years of healthy life lost to disease, rather than the years of healthy life gained by an intervention. Because of this, the HRQL scores associated with the DALY vary on a scale where 0 is equal to perfect health and 1 is equal to death (the opposite of HRQL scores associated with QALYs). To convert a DALY score, which is called a disability weight, into a standard HRQL score, the score must be subtracted from 1.0.

It is generally acceptable to have either patients or physicians fill out generic preference-weighted instruments to obtain HRQL scores, because the responses are preference-weighted and based on a community sample. However, when physicians or patients are used to generate HRQL scores from scratch, the responses they provide will be colored by their perspectives on the disease they are evaluating. The results may therefore be different from those derived from a representative community sample (Gold and others, 1996). For example, physicians may be likely to overrate the physical aspects of an illness but underrate the psychological aspects of illness. Since DALY scores are generated by professionals, they likely differ from those derived from a community sample.

Things to Consider Regarding HRQL Scores

Though HRQL scores used to calculate QALYs should always be obtained from a representative community sample, it is important to ensure that the sample from which the scores were generated is also representative of your hypothetical cohort. This is crucial, because the severity and manifestations of a disease (and the perception of quality of life with a disease) vary depending on age, gender mix, and racial composition. They also vary by the distribution of disease, by the stage of illness, and whether subjects have undergone health interventions for the condition. Whether you are generating HRQL scores using preference-weighted generic health instruments, are using a published list of HRQL scores, or are employing exercises based on expected utility theory, the scores derived must correlate with the severity and distribution of the disease in your cohort. In this section, we will briefly describe how the demographic characteristics or the characteristics of a particular disease might affect the HRQL score you use.

The Effect of Age on HRQL

In general, younger people tend to think about health very differently than older people. While an elderly person may not place a high value on sexual function, a younger person almost certainly will. Moreover, because younger people on average are in better health than older people, they tend to have higher average HRQL scores and tend to place very different values on different health states (this is apparent in the quality-adjusted life table published by Erickson and others, 1995, in Appendix V). For these reasons, it is important to ensure that the HRQL scores that you are using are derived from people similar in age to your hypothetical cohort.

The Effect of Disease Stage on HRQL

It is also important to obtain HRQL scores specific to different stages of a disease. Let us consider diabetes as an example. Adult onset diabetes is usually asymptomatic in its early stages; however, various aspects of a diabetic's health tend to deteriorate over time. These changes include the loss of sensation in limbs, loss of vision, repeated hospitalizations, as well as a number of other problems. As time goes on, more and more of these conditions may develop. They also tend to develop concurrent to one another, complicating a diabetic's overall health state. Thus the HRQL of a person who has had the disease for ten years will be very different from the HRQL of someone who has had the disease for twenty years, regardless of that person's age.

The event pathway used to construct your flowchart or decision analysis model can be used to guide cost-effectiveness researchers in categorizing different health states for different stages of disease. Regardless of how HRQL scores are obtained, changes in health states must be carefully accounted for over time.

The Effect of an Intervention on HRQL

If diabetes is appropriately managed, the likelihood of developing future complications is reduced, and thus the general health status of treated persons will be improved relative to those who are untreated. On the other hand, the treatment itself can be associated with side effects that can have an impact on a person's health.

Because a cost-effectiveness analysis must evaluate the differences between people who have and have not received a particular intervention, such as medications used to treat diabetes mellitus, scores must be estimated for subjects in the intervention and non-intervention groups. These scores can often be obtained using the disease-specific HRQL score and a measure of risk among persons who have received the intervention (see Chapter Five for a discussion of different measures of risk). We will learn how to adjust scores using measures of risk in Chapters Nine and Twelve.

Use of HRQL Scores in Diverse Populations

Health-related quality of life scores for a disease may be different for men and women, persons of different social classes, and so on. Some care should be taken when applying HRQL scores to a group that differs demographically from the general population (for example, African-Americans).

Direct Versus Indirect HRQL Scores

Many cost-effectiveness students become lost in the jargon associated with HRQL scores. One of the more confusing aspects is the use of the terms **"directly derived"** and **"indirectly derived"** HRQL scores. While some authors use the word "direct" to describe HRQL scores that are derived directly from people rather than from multi-attribute utility models (like the Years of Healthy Life measure), others use it to refer to HRQL scores that were derived directly from ill persons rather than healthy ones. At the end of the day, the cost-effectiveness researcher can simply ignore such semantic problems and have a nice warm cup of tea.

CHAPTER NINE

CALCULATING QUALITY-ADJUSTED LIFE YEARS

Overview

Project Map

1. Develop a research question.
2. Design your analysis.
3. Understand the sources of error in data.
4. Obtain data.
5. Organize data.
6. Construct a decision analysis model.
7. **Calculate quality-adjusted life years.**
8. Test and refine the decision analysis model.
9. Conduct a sensitivity analysis.
10. Prepare the study results for publication or presentation.

This chapter demonstrates three approaches to calculating health-adjusted life years. Each of these approaches provides a unique perspective on what QALYs are, how they are used, and how they are calculated. We will call these methods: 1) the "life table method," 2) the "summation method," and 3) the "disability-adjusted life year (DALY) method." In the life table method, the number of people in a hypothetical cohort who survive from one year to the next is entered into a table. The quality of life of each survivor is then accounted for, and the total number of years lived in perfect health is added together (Erickson and others, 1995; Muennig and Gold, 2001). In the summation method, changes in the number of QALYs over time are added together (Drummond and others, 1997). This method is similar to the life table method but does not require the construction of complicated life tables. In the disability-adjusted life year (DALY) method, the total number of healthy years of life lost to a disease is added to the total years of health lost to that disease (Murray and Lopez, 1996). This method requires students to think about the total number of years lost to disease rather than the gains in quality life.

Any of these methods can be used to calculate QALYs (or DALYs) using either a spreadsheet program or a decision analysis program. Decision analysis programs can also be used to mathematically model life expectancy in a hypothetical cohort using formulas. In this chapter, we will demonstrate how QALYs are calculated by hand or through the use of a spreadsheet program. In Chapter Twelve, we will discuss how QALYs can be calculated using a state transition (or Markov) model, which was introduced in Chapter Seven.

We will begin this chapter with an introduction to the life table method. We will then explore how to calculate the incremental number of QALYs gained by summation. This will be followed by a discussion of how the incremental number of DALYs averted are calculated. Finally, we will apply the summation method to calculating QALYs gained for each of the interventions in our sample cost-effectiveness analysis.

Using the Life Table Method

Life expectancy is calculated using life tables. To estimate how long a person will live at birth, we must consider all causes of mortality together. If we were to examine the cost-effectiveness of an oral medication used to treat congestive heart failure (CHF) using life tables, we would examine the life expectancy of people given the oral medication and the life expectancy of people receiving the current standard of care. The group receiving treatment and the group receiving the standard of care would each have the same risk of dying of causes unrelated to CHF, such as traffic accidents. However, one group would have a lower risk of dying of CHF-related conditions. The differences in the rate of mortality from CHF-related conditions would account for the incremental differences in life expectancy between each group.

Life expectancy may be calculated using a **standard life table** or an **abridged life table.** While a standard life table calculates life expectancy for a group of people based on the mortality rate over one-year age intervals, an abridged life table uses five-year (or larger) age intervals. Thus, while an abridged life table is easier to construct, a standard life table is slightly more accurate. Appendix V contains abridged life tables and quality-adjusted life tables for the United States population for 1997.

Adding a measure of quality. Quality-adjusted life expectancy (QALE) is the number of years of perfect health one can expect to live at birth. Quality-adjusted life expectancy is equal to the product of the life expectancy at birth and the average health-related quality of life (HRQL) score. It therefore accounts for the effect of disease on both the quantity of life and the quality of life (or either the quality of life or the quantity of life alone.) For example, the life expectancy of the average person was 76.1 years in 1996, and the average HRQL was 0.854 (National Center for Health Statistics, 1999). The QALE was therefore 76.1 years · 0.854 = 64 years. Quality-adjusted life expectancy is shorter than life expectancy because it estimates the number of years of perfect health rather than the total number of years the person would be expected to live.

Of course, a person's QALE changes when disease is present. It also changes when different medical interventions are administered, because interventions have an effect on the quality and quantity of life (or either the quality of life or the quantity of life alone). The number of QALYs gained when a medical intervention is implemented is calculated using the equation $QALE_{intervention\ 1}$ − $QALE_{intervention\ 2}$, where Intervention 1 is the more effective intervention. In the case of our sample analysis, Intervention 2 might be supportive care, because it is presumably the least effective of the three interventions we are evaluating.

If we were to break QALE down into its components, we would have:

$$\text{life expectancy}_{intervention\ 1} \cdot \text{HRQL}_{intervention\ 1} - $$
$$\text{life expectancy}_{intervention\ 2} \cdot \text{HRQL}_{intervention\ 2}$$
$$= \text{total QALYs gained by intervention}$$

Equation 9.1

Figure 9.1 illustrates the calculation of QALYs gained when the quality of subjects' lives is improved, but life expectancy is unchanged. Consider the case of a congenital joint deformity that can be surgically corrected at birth and that is not responsible for any reduction of life expectancy. If the average HRQL score for people who are not treated for this deformity is 0.66 and the HRQL score for persons who are treated with surgery is 0.71, the number of QALYs gained from treatment is:

$$76.5 \cdot 0.71 - 76.5 \cdot 0.66 = 3.8$$

FIGURE 9.1.   GAIN IN QUALITY-ADJUSTED LIFE EXPECTANCY FOR CONGENITAL JOINT DEFORMITY TREATED AT BIRTH RELATIVE TO AN UNTREATED CONGENITAL JOINT DEFORMITY.

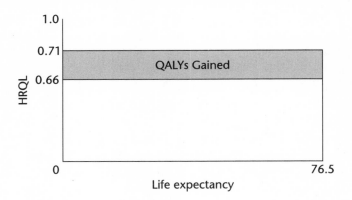

In real life, a person's HRQL changes from year to year, so an average life-time score, such as the 0.66 value used in this example, will not perfectly reflect the year-to-year changes in a person's health status. Let us return to the sample cost-effectiveness analysis and explore how changes in both quality and quantity of life are measured in a cost-effectiveness analysis. Figure 9.2 illustrates changes in both the quality and quantity of life that might occur when subjects are vaccinated before the start of a single influenza season.

Changes in life expectancy. Notice that the life expectancy at age fifteen is 82.2 years, while the life expectancy at birth is 76.5 years. One of the good things about growing older is that your life expectancy grows with you. This reflects the adage, "If you've made it this far, you'll make it all the way." This phenomenon occurs because as we grow older, the risk of death at younger years is behind us. Thus, when we reach seventy-five years of age, we will have an average of 12.5 years ahead of us rather than a measly 1.65 years.

Changes in quality of life. Notice, too, that the mean HRQL is not 1.0, but 0.87, because no one is always in a perfect state of health. In fact, as we saw above, the average HRQL of all people in the United States is just 0.854. Cost-effectiveness analyses should measure gains in the cohort's *average* health status rather than the cohort's *ideal* health status (Gold and others, 1996). In Figure 9.2, we see that each added year of life gained (the shaded area on the far right of the diagram) is lived in less than perfect health. Notice, too, that the life gained is lived at an HRQL of 0.87. Any future years of life gained by an intervention must also be adjusted to reflect the health status of the cohort under study.

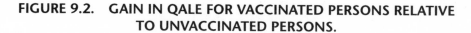

FIGURE 9.2. GAIN IN QALE FOR VACCINATED PERSONS RELATIVE TO UNVACCINATED PERSONS.

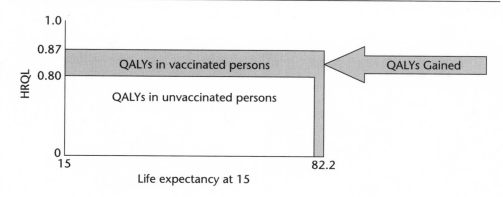

Charting the Lifetime Health Path of Your Cohort

In the life table section above, we saw that QALE is calculated by multiplying the average life expectancy of your cohort by the average HRQL score for your cohort. In reality, QALY diagrams will not be nice and square like those in Figures 9.1 and 9.2. In these figures, the patient lives at a constant HRQL, then "drops dead." In fact, most diseases result in large fluctuations in the quality of life of an individual as a person's health deteriorates. The changes in the health status of a cohort over time are sometimes referred to as a **lifetime health path** (Gold and others, 1996).

Regardless of whether the life table method, the summation method, or the DALY method is used, a lifetime health path should be generated for your hypothetical cohort (see Figure 9.3). There are three steps researchers must take before they are able to generate a lifetime health path.

Step 1. Identify the different health states of the cohort and how they change over time.

Step 2. Calculate the time spent in each health state.

Step 3. Obtain the HRQL score associated with each health state.

The changes in health states are usually obtained from the medical literature. For instance, people with a particular type of heart disease may be classified into five categories: 1) well, 2) mild disease, 3) moderate disease, 4) severe disease, and 5) dead. Likewise, the time spent in each state is usually obtained from the medical literature. For instance, people with this disease may have a mean age of onset at sixty-two years, spend five years with mild disease, spend three years with

FIGURE 9.3.   LIFETIME HEALTH PATH FOR PERSON WITH A HYPOTHETICAL HEART DISEASE.

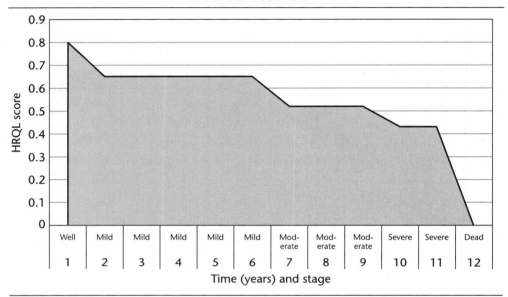

Note: The shaded area represents the total number of QALYs over this twelve-year period.

moderate disease, and spend two years with severe disease before dying at a mean age of seventy.

Finally, to calculate the HRQL score associated with each of the health states, the researcher must choose a preference-weighted generic instrument that best captures the attributes of the disease under study and assign an HRQL score to each state. These steps will be presented with various concrete examples throughout this chapter.

If you follow each of these steps, you will have created a lifetime health path. The lifetime health path of your cohort is similar to the event pathway we generated to construct our decision analysis model in the sample cost-effectiveness analysis. However, as you will see throughout this chapter, a lifetime health path is much easier to generate than an event pathway.

Using the Summation Method

The summation method is much simpler than the life table method (Drummond and others, 1997). To construct a quality-adjusted life table, the researcher must consider *all* causes of morbidity and mortality together, even though cost-effectiveness analyses only include *changes* in costs, quality of life, and length of life when a health intervention is applied. If we have published information on the extent to which an intervention prolongs life and affects the quality of life, the changes in quality of life from year to year can simply be summed together.

Let us return to the example illustrated in Figure 9.1 and explore another way of thinking about changes in the quality of life from year to year. Recall that the QALYs gained were calculated by subtracting QALE for untreated people from the QALE for treated people. Let us look at another way of calculating the total number of QALYs gained. In this example, each person receiving the intervention would realize a gain of $0.71 - 0.66 = 0.05$ QALYs per year for 76.5 years. The overall gain in QALYs may also be calculated by adding the change in the HRQL score for each year (0.05) over the life span of the average person in the cohort (76.5 years). The total improvement in HRQL is: $0.05 \cdot 76.5 = 3.8$ QALYs gained (or 0.05 QALYs gained for each of the 76.5 years).

Though the result is the same regardless of the method used, the framework of the problem is different. Rather than estimate changes in QALE, it estimates the annual change in the HRQL of one intervention relative to another and adds up these incremental changes in HRQL over the duration of time for which the intervention benefits the cohort.

There are five steps in the summation method. The first three steps are common to each of the methods we describe in this chapter.

Step 1. Detail the changes in the health status of your cohort.

Step 2. Calculate the time spent in each health state.

Step 3. Calculate the HRQL score associated with each health state.

Step 4. Multiply the incremental change in the HRQL score associated with each health state by the time spent in each health state.

Step 5. Add up each of the products you obtained in Step 4.

Calculating differences in life expectancy. When interventions result in changes in life expectancy, this method takes advantage of the fact that the HRQL score for death is equal to zero (Drummond and others, 1997). For instance, suppose that a new treatment for congestive heart failure (CHF) has no impact on the overall quality of life, but improves life expectancy by one year. Suppose further that the average HRQL of people with CHF is 0.5, and the average untreated life expectancy is three years. The two interventions would accrue the following QALYs:

$$
\begin{array}{lll}
\text{Treatment:} & 0.5 + 0.5 + 0.5 + 0.5 & = 2.0 \text{ QALYs} \\
\text{No treatment:} & 0.5 + 0.5 + 0.5 + 0 & = 1.5 \text{ QALYs}
\end{array}
$$

The total number of QALYs gained by treatment is: $2 - 1.5 = 0.5$

Calculating incremental QALYs gained. Now let's look at a slightly more sophisti-cated example. Suppose that we are evaluating a hypothetical treatment that is 50 percent effective at preventing death from an infectious disease. We apply Steps 1–3 listed above and determine that the mean HRQL of treated subjects is 0.75 over the course of a year, and the mean HRQL of untreated people is 0.74 over the course of a year. The overall incremental increase in HRQL is simply:

$$\text{duration of illness} \cdot (\text{HRQL}_{\text{treated}} - \text{HRQL}_{\text{untreated}})$$
$$\text{or } 1 \cdot (0.75 - 0.74) = 0.01$$

We search the medical literature and find that people with the disease live two years less than people without the disease. Because the efficacy of the drug is 0.5, treated people would be expected to live $0.5 \cdot 2$ years $= 1$ calendar year longer than untreated people on average. However, this year would not have been lived in perfect health, so the incremental gain in life must be quality adjusted. The in-cremental gain in quality-adjusted life is:

$$\text{years gained} \cdot \text{mean HRQL}$$
$$\text{or}$$
$$(2 - 1) \cdot 0.75 = 0.75$$

We can thus add the incremental gain in quality of life from the intervention, 0.01, to the incremental gain in quantity of life lived in perfect health, 0.75, to obtain a total incremental effectiveness of $0.01 + 0.75 = 0.76$ QALYs. The entire equa-tion takes the form:

$$\text{duration of illness} \cdot (\text{HRQL}_{\text{treated}} - \text{HRQL}_{\text{untreated}}) + \text{years gained} \cdot \text{mean HRQL}$$
Equation 9.2

Now let us go one step further still and consider the lifetime health pathway for people with the hypothetical heart disease depicted in Figure 9.3. In this ex-ample, the sum of HRQL scores is equal to the area under the curve. In other words, the area under the curve is equal to the sum of people's QALYs over each of the last twelve years of their lives. Now let us consider what would hap-pen if a group of people were given a treatment that would prolong their lives by one year and improve their HRQL by 10 percent for each year they were alive (see Figure 9.4). The dark shaded curve represents their QALE if untreated and

FIGURE 9.4. LIFETIME HEALTH PATH OF A COHORT WITH TREATED DISEASE (TOTAL AREA) AND A COHORT WITH UNTREATED DISEASE (LIGHT AREA).

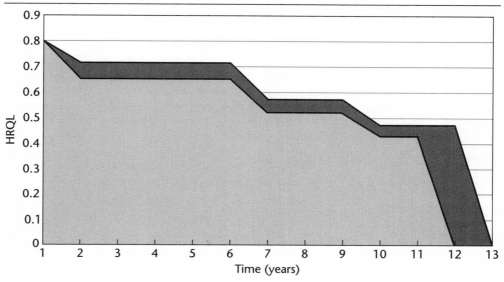

Note: The difference between these two curves (dark area) is equal to the incremental QALYs gained.

the light shaded curve represents their average QALE if treated. In this case, the incremental gain in QALYs is equal to the area under the dark shaded curve minus the area under the light shaded curve.

Notice that this figure differs from Figure 9.2 in that the QALYs in each intervention arm are tabulated starting at the age in which the intervention is applied rather than at birth. Because the summation method only includes incremental QALYs (QALYs gained), we do not need to bother with any event that happens prior to the intervention.

Exercises 9.1–9.2

Suppose that we were investigating the cost-effectiveness of a medication to treat congestive heart failure (CHF) and were comparing this to the current standard of care. We find that the medication has no side effects (and therefore does not lower the HRQL of people who take it), but it does nothing to improve the overall quality of life. Among untreated patients, the average life expectancy with CHF is five years. Among treated patients, the average life expectancy is six years. Using the Health Utilities Index (HUI), we find that the average HRQL of a person with CHF is 0.48.

9.1. How many QALYs are gained by the treatment we are evaluating?

9.2. Once we have finished our analysis, the food and drug administration releases a warning that, in post-marketing surveillance, some people on this medication experience severe and debilitating abdominal pain. We recalculate our HRQL scores by adding the fraction of patients with abdominal pain to our HUI score and find that patients with CHF in the treatment arm have a mean HRQL score of 0.45. How many QALYs are gained in the treatment arm of the study?

Using the DALY Method

An alternative way of thinking about changes in QALYs, when different medical interventions are applied, is to consider the total number of QALYs that are lost when each intervention is applied (Murray and Lopez, 1996). When calculated this way, the outcome is referred to as a disability-adjusted life year (DALY) rather than a QALY. The DALY is used extensively in international cost-effectiveness analyses, so we will describe it here. It also serves to illustrate an alternative way of thinking about QALYs.

QALYs gained versus DALYs lost. In reality, interventions in health and medicine reduce the loss of life and reduce the total morbidity caused by a disease, rather than result in gains in health or gains in longevity. In fact, when we speak of a QALY "gained," we are making a relative comparison between two interventions; if untreated patients die ten years prematurely and treated patients die five years prematurely, the treatment results in an incremental "gain" of five years of life, but only relative to untreated patients. The formula for calculating the total DALYs due to a particular disease is:

the years of life lost (YLL) + the years lost to disability (YLD)

Equation 9.3

In the DALY, "health lost" is referred to as "disability," which most people associate with a physical handicap, but it is meant to refer to disease in this measure. The years of health lost in the DALY is equal to the product of the disability weight for the disease (the DALY form of an HRQL score) and the time with the disease. The disability weight is equal to $1 - HRQL$. Thus, if the HRQL is 0.9, the disability weight is $1 - 0.9 = 0.1$.

To calculate incremental differences in DALYs, we simply subtract the DALYs in one intervention from the DALYs in the competing intervention to obtain the total number of DALYs averted. For example, if we were comparing treatment to no treatment, the number of DALYs averted would be:

$$DALYs_{treatment} - DALYs_{no\ treatment}$$

Equation 9.4

Suppose patients receiving the current standard care for diabetes mellitus suffered the loss of ten years of life, and their HRQL was reduced by 0.1 for the final ten years of their life. People without diabetes mellitus can expect to live 76.5 years of life at birth. Thus, in this example, people with diabetes mellitus would be expected to live to 76.5 years − 10 Years = 66.5 years on average (YLL = 10). They also experience a loss in HRQL of 0.1 for 10 years and thus lose the equivalent of $0.1 \cdot 10$ years = 1 year of healthy life (YLD = 1). The DALYs lost to disease are:

$$YLL + YLD$$

$$= 10 + 1$$

$$= 11\ DALYs$$

Their QALE (which, when calculated this way, is officially called disability-adjusted life expectancy, or DALE) is thus 76.5 years − 11 years = 65.5 years.

If a new treatment for diabetes mellitus prolonged life by 1 year (YLL = 9) and stemmed losses in HRQL to 0.05 over the last 10 years of life (YLD = $10 \cdot 0.5 = 0.5$ years), the DALYs lost to disease in the treated group would then be:

$$= 9 + 0.5$$

$$= 9.5\ DALYs$$

Their DALE is 76.5 years − 9.5 years = 67 years. To calculate the total DALYs averted (the equivalent of the total QALYs gained), we would simply subtract 11 DALYs − 9.5 = 1.5 DALYs averted using Equation 9.4. If we were to apply Equation 9.1, the result would be the same (67 years − 65.5 years = 1.5 DALYs).

If we were to calculate the total number of years gained for the hypothetical new treatment for diabetes mellitus described in the previous section using QALYs, we would need to twist our brains once more and think of the scenario in a slightly different way. Recall that untreated patients lose an average of

10 years of life and experience a loss of 0.1 in HRQL during their last 10 years of life. Also recall that the treatment results in a net gain of 1 year of life and a net improvement in HRQL of 0.05. The incremental gain in QALYs with treatment is:

$$\text{duration of illness} \cdot (\text{HRQL}_{treated} - \text{HRQL}_{untreated}) + \text{years gained} \cdot \text{mean HRQL}$$
Equation 9.2

or

$$10 \text{ years} \cdot (0.95 - 0.9) + 1 \text{ year} \cdot 0.95 \text{ HRQL}$$
$$= 0.5 + 0.95$$
$$= 1.45 \text{ QALYs}$$

Notice something fishy here? The incremental gain in DALE, 1.5 DALYs, and the incremental gain in QALE, 1.45 QALYs, are not equal. This discrepancy results from the way that DALE is conceptualized; the difference between Equation 9.2 and Equation 9.3 is that the years of life lost are not quality adjusted in Equation 9.3. While QALYs count lost time at the average HRQL of the cohort, DALYs count lost time at an HRQL of 1.0. When using DALYs in cost-effectiveness analyses, be certain to quality adjust the final year of life lost or simply use Equation 9.2. The DALY is scheduled to undergo revision in 2004 (Arnesen and Nord, 1999).

Calculating QALYs in the Sample Analysis

In this section, we will illustrate how to calculate the number of QALYs gained by vaccination and treatment, relative to supportive care. To do this, we will use the summation method. We will estimate the average HRQL score of our cohort using the Quality of Well-Being (QWB) scale, one of the measures acceptable for use in cost-effectiveness analysis.

In Chapter Five, we learned that hospitalization and mortality rates for influenza virus infection are typically estimated using excess hospitalizations and deaths due to influenza-associated conditions. The number of excess deaths due to influenza-associated conditions serves as a good estimator of the mortality rate due to influenza-like illness because only influenza and its secondary complications are likely to be fatal.

To calculate the number of QALYs gained when influenza-like illness is treated, or when people are vaccinated at the beginning of the influenza season, we will need the following information:

1. The HRQL score for the average healthy person, persons with influenza-like illness, and persons without influenza-like illness between the ages of fifteen and sixty-five in the United States.
2. The number of QALYs lost when subjects in our cohort die from influenza-associated conditions.

In the following sections, you will learn how to calculate HRQL scores for persons with and without influenza-like illness. You will also learn how to estimate the total number of lives lost to influenza-associated conditions. Next, you will learn how to calculate the QALYs gained in each arm of the sample analysis by hand. Finally, you will learn how to calculate the QALYs gained using the decision analysis model you constructed in Chapter Seven.

Calculating HRQL Scores for Influenza-Like Illness

Influenza-like illness affects many attributes of health. When people are confined to bed, it affects their mobility and ability to take care of themselves (Keech and others, 1998). It also contains a social component because people often miss work and occasionally need caregiving. Finally, it causes physical discomfort. Ideally, we would choose to utilize a preference-weighted generic instrument that captures all of these attributes (or dimensions) of a person's health. In Chapter Eight, we saw that the EuroQol captures all of these attributes; however, it may be biased because the community samples used to derive the results were of European origin (our cohort resides in the United States). Also of consideration is the QWB scale, which captures each of these attributes, as does the Health Utility Index (HUI) (Feeney and others, 1995). The Years of Healthy Life (YHL) measure, which is based in part on the Health Utilities Index, captures the social domain of health as well as a person's perception of how healthy he or she is (Gold and others, 1998). Based on this information, it seems that the QWB scale would be the best measure for our analysis. Not only was it based on a cohort of people living in the United States, it captures all of the domains that are relevant to our analysis.

Let us apply the three initial steps to calculating QALYs we described earlier to our analysis.

Step 1. Identify the relevant health states of influenza-like illness. In Chapter Eight, when we generated an HRQL score from the EuroQol instrument, we saw how we might use the studies by Keech and others (1998) to identify the relevant health states of influenza-like illness. If we were to calculate HRQL scores in earnest, we would want to incorporate other studies from the medical literature to incorporate all significant health events. However, this would require lengthy descriptions of these studies, so we will not do this here.

Step 2. Estimate the duration of each health state. Treanor and others (2000) found that influenza-like illness lasts around ninety-seven hours when untreated. In Chapter Eight, we saw how differences in the severity of the disease can be estimated on a day-to-day basis to estimate the average HRQL score for this illness.

Step 3. Calculate the HRQL score for each of the interventions. Instructions on obtaining HRQL scores from preference-weighted generic instruments are provided in Chapter Eight, so we will not repeat those steps here.

There are two important things to consider when determining the HRQL score for influenza-like illness. This disease is self-limited and of a short duration so we must decide how we will value future years of life gained when subjects are vaccinated. We must also determine how to average the HRQL of influenza-like illness, which typically lasts just ninety-seven hours, over the time frame of our analysis, which we decided in Chapter Two would be one year.

HRQL of future years of life. Future years of life gained will not be in perfect health and should thus generally be counted at a value less than 1.0 (Gold and others, 1996). In other words, if a treatment for diabetes results in a gain of ten years of life, those ten years would be lived at a mean HRQL for diabetics, say 0.7, rather than the mean HRQL for healthy people, 1.0. Thus, in the case of diabetes, subjects would gain $0.7 \cdot 10$ years $= 7$ QALYs.

When examining a chronic disease such as diabetes, the HRQL for the disease alone is used even though subjects may have diseases other than diabetes that would affect their HRQL, because the impact of the disease on the quality of life usually far outweighs the effect of other illnesses on the overall HRQL. In our analysis, though, people will be in good (but not perfect) health after influenza season. The question then arises, Should future years of life gained by vaccination or treatment be valued in perfect health (an HRQL score of 1.0) or should they be valued using the average health of healthy adults (an HRQL score of less than 1.0)?

We could estimate the average HRQL of our cohort using the mean HRQL for people in the general United States population. This can easily be done using the YHL measure, because this measure incorporates the HRQL of the average person in the United States. A mean HRQL score cannot easily be obtained with any other measure. If we were to attempt this using the QWB or EuroQol, we would have to administer these instruments to a representative sample of the United States population and this would not be feasible in most research efforts. The problem with using the QWB to determine the HRQL score for influenza-like illness and the YHL measure to determine the average HRQL score for the general population is that the approach involves using two separate measures whose scores may not match perfectly.

The second approach would be to simply assume that our cohort would have an HRQL of 1.0 for every future year of life gained by an intervention. Using the YHL measure to estimate the baseline HRQL of our cohort will bring us closer to a real-world estimate of the QALYs gained by vaccination, so we will take this approach.

Tips and tricks. The average YHL scores are listed by age interval in the QALE table in Appendix V, and the YHL scores are listed by disease in Appendix IV. Students with additional interest in the calculation of YHL scores may wish to calculate age-specific mean scores using these two appendices. See Erickson and others (1995) and Gold and others (1998) for further readings.

Averaging HRQL over one year. The HRQL score for influenza-like illness derived from the QWB scale is 0.61 and the average HRQL of healthy adults obtained from the YHL measure is 0.875. We must calculate the average HRQL for persons with influenza-like illness over one year:

$$(\text{HRQL}_{\text{ILI}} \cdot \text{duration of illness} + \text{HRQL}_{\text{average health}} \cdot \text{duration wellness}) / \text{total hours}$$

Equation 9.5

$$= (0.61 \cdot 97 \text{ hours} + 0.875 \cdot 8{,}663 \text{ hours}) / 8{,}760 \text{ hours} = 0.872$$

The age-specific HRQL scores generated using the QWB scale and YHL measure are listed in Table 9.1. (Because the actual difference in HRQL between these categories is very small, the numbers presented here have been widened for teaching purposes.)

Calculating Years of Life Lost

Let us first estimate the years of life lost when a subject dies from an influenza-associated condition. In Chapter Five, we learned that the CDC estimates that approximately 20,000 people die from influenza-associated conditions each year. In that chapter, we estimated age-specific mortality rates using the annual number

TABLE 9.1.   AGE-SPECIFIC AND MEAN HRQL SCORES FOR THE AVERAGE SUBJECT, SUBJECTS WITH INFLUENZA-LIKE ILLNESS (ILI), AND NO INFLUENZA-LIKE ILLNESS.

	HRQL Score		
Age Group	Average	ILI	No ILI
15 to 24	0.92	0.91	0.93
25 to 34	0.91	0.9	0.92
35 to 44	0.89	0.88	0.9
45 to 54	0.85	0.84	0.86
54 to 64	0.79	0.78	0.8
Mean	0.872	0.862	0.882

of excess deaths and the proportion of persons dying from influenza-associated conditions by age group. We left that section of Chapter Five with a caveat: we accounted for mortality among all adults, rather than among adults without chronic diseases that place them at risk for complications of influenza virus infection. In this section, we will adjust our data to better reflect the mortality from influenza-associated conditions among healthy adults.

To begin estimating the number of life years lost to influenza-associated conditions, first refer to the mortality spreadsheet created in the "Mortality Data" section of Chapter Five (see Table 5.12), which contains the number of deaths in ten-year intervals for persons aged fifteen to sixty-five. Next, create a new column indicating the midpoint of each age interval (for example, the midpoint for 15 to 24 would be $(15 + 25)/2 = 20$).

Tips and tricks. The last age in an interval may be reported as a rounded number or a number that represents the person's calendar age. For example, a ten-year age interval may be reported as fifteen to twenty-five or fifteen to twenty-four. The latter includes all persons aged fifteen years and zero days to twenty-four years and 364 days. Both of these age intervals are equivalent.

Finally, create a column representing years of life lost at the midpoint of each age interval. This can readily be obtained from a life table (see Appendix V, Column 7). For example, the number of years of life lost to death at age twenty is equal to the life expectancy at age twenty, which was 57.5 years in 1997 (remember, your life expectancy grows with you, so at age twenty, you can expect to live to be 77.5 years of age). Your spreadsheet should look something like Table 9.2.

Now, add a column representing the total number of years lost for each age interval (number of deaths · years lost), and in the bottom row, total the column values (see Table 9.3).

TABLE 9.2. YEARS OF LIFE LOST TO INFLUENZA BY AGE INTERVAL.

Age Group	1 #Deaths	2 (Age1 + Age2)/2 Midpoint	3 Life Expectancy at Age Years Lost
15 to 24	111	20	57.5
25 to 34	194	30	48.1
35 to 44	500	40	38.7
45 to 54	500	50	29.7
54 to 64	861	60	21.4
Total	2,167	—	

TABLE 9.3. TOTAL YEARS OF LIFE LOST TO INFLUENZA FOR THE UNITED STATES COHORT.

Age Group	1 #Deaths	2 (Age1 + Age2)/2 Midpoint	3 Life expectancy Years Lost	4 Column 1 · Column 3 Total Years Lost
15 to 24	111	20	57.5	6,389
25 to 34	194	30	48.1	9,353
35 to 44	500	40	38.7	19,350
45 to 54	500	50	29.7	14,850
54 to 64	861	60	21.4	18,428
Total	2,167	—		68,369

The total number of years lost in persons aged fifteen to sixty-four to influenza-like illness is thus 68,369.

Discounting future years of life. Like money, people have a tendency to place a lower value on health events that take place in the future when compared to the present. For example, people tend to be more motivated to prevent illness in the immediate future (for example, putting on a seat belt), than they are to prevent illness in the distant future (for example, to start an exercise program with the goal of preventing future heart attacks). This philosophy is prevalent throughout society and the field of medicine. For example, the health care system places far more resources toward treatment than it does toward prevention, in part because patients, physicians, and health care institutions value health in the present more than they do health in the distant future.

To keep numerator and denominator values consistent (among other, more technical reasons), the reference case scenario recommends that the 3 percent discount rate be applied to both future costs and future QALYs gained. *Any health outcome or health cost that occurs in the future must be discounted into present-day terms at the same rate that costs are discounted* (Gold and others, 1996). As with costs, the discount rate applied to effectiveness should be tested in a sensitivity analysis.

Recall from Chapter Six that the general formula for discounting is:

$$\text{future event}/(1 + \text{discount rate})^{\text{time}}$$

Equation 6.4

where "time" is the number of years into the future at which the event occurs.

In our sample analysis, the costs occur in the immediate future, and we will not need to discount them. On the other hand, when people die in the analysis, we must account for all of the future years of life that they would have lived had they not developed an influenza-associated condition. In your spreadsheet, add a column that discounts all future years of life lost (see Table 9.4).

Incorporating HRQL. So far, you have learned how to calculate the total number of years of life lost to influenza-like illness and its complications. You have also learned how to discount those future years of life lost to their net present value. Because these years would not have been lived in perfect health, we still have to adjust them for quality.

On your spreadsheet, insert two blank columns between Column 4 and Column 5. Next, type in the mean HRQL scores for persons in each age interval in the first blank column from Table 9.1. Finally, multiply values from Column 4 by the values you typed in for Column 5 (see Table 9.5).

TABLE 9.4. DISCOUNTED YEARS OF LIFE LOST TO INFLUENZA FOR THE UNITED STATES COHORT.

Column	1	2	3	4	5
		(Age 1 + Age 2)/2	*LE − Column 2*	*Column 1 · Column 3*	*Column 4/ $(1.03)^{Column\ 3}$*
Age Group	**#Deaths**	**Midpoint**	**Years Lost**	**Total Years**	**Discounted Years Lost**
15 to 24	111	20	57.5	6,389	1,168
25 to 34	194	30	48.1	9,353	2,257
35 to 44	500	40	38.7	19,350	6,164
45 to 54	500	50	29.7	14,850	6,172
54 to 64	861	60	21.4	18,428	9,789
Total	2,167	—		68,369	25,550

TABLE 9.5. DISCOUNTED QALYs LOST TO INFLUENZA FOR THE UNITED STATES COHORT.

Column	1	2	3	4	5	6	7
		$(Age\ 1 + Age\ 2)/2$	$LE - Column\ 2$	$Column\ 1 \cdot Column\ 3$	Copy Values	$Column\ 4 \cdot Column\ 5$	$Column\ 6/(1.03)^{Column\ 3}$
Age Group	Number Deaths	Midpoint	Years Lost	Total Years Lost	HRQL	QALYs Lost	Discounted QALYs Lost
15 to 24	111	20	57.5	6,389	0.92	5,846	1,068
25 to 34	194	30	48.1	9,353	0.91	8,464	2,042
35 to 44	500	40	38.7	19,350	0.89	17,125	5,456
45 to 54	500	50	29.7	14,850	0.85	12,550	5,217
54 to 64	861	60	21.4	18,428	0.79	14,567	7,738
Total						58,791	21,594

Adjusting for vaccine status and chronic disease. The mortality rates we obtained from the CDC and NCHS were obtained from the general United States population. Recall from the "Distribution of Disease" section of Chapter Five that some of the people between aged fifteen and sixty-five in the United States were vaccinated. In this section, we calculated the predicted increase in events (such as deaths) that would have occurred had no one been vaccinated in the United States. Because subjects in the supportive care and treatment arms of the analysis will not receive the influenza vaccine, we must adjust the total number of excess deaths from influenza-associated conditions among persons aged fifteen to sixty-five in the United States to reflect the deaths that would have occurred had no one been vaccinated.

Neuzil and others (1999) calculated the number of excess deaths due to influenza-associated conditions among Medicaid-insured women in Tennessee over a nineteen-year period. They examined the mortality rate for women with a variety of chronic diseases, including chronic lung disease, heart disease, diabetes, HIV, and renal disease, as well as the mortality rate for women who were otherwise healthy. They found that women with chronic diseases had an excess death rate of 1.1 deaths per 10,000 person-months, while women that were in good health had an excess death rate of 0.02 deaths per 10,000 person-months. Because our hypothetical cohort is composed of healthy adults, we shall have to adjust our mortality data to reflect the predicted number of deaths among healthy adults rather than among the population in general.

Exercises 9.3–9.5

9.3. Calculate the predicted number of discounted QALYs lost to death from influenza-like illness if no one between the ages of fifteen and sixty-five were vaccinated.

9.4. Adjust the total number of deaths obtained in Exercise 9.3 to reflect mortality rates among healthy adults using data from Neuzil and others (1999).

Calculating QALYs in the Vaccination Arm

Let us summarize the data that we have collected and analyzed that we will need to estimate the number of QALYs in the vaccination arm of our analysis. First, after adjusting for vaccine status and the presence of chronic disease in Exercises 9.3 and 9.4, we estimated that 472 QALYs are lost to death from influenza-associated conditions among healthy adults each year. Second, we assumed that, in the vaccination arm, the probability of death will be reduced by a proportion equal to the vaccine efficacy at preventing influenza virus infection (0.803). Finally, we learned that the probability of developing influenza-like illness will be reduced by a proportion equal to the efficacy of the vaccine in preventing influenza-like illness (0.40). We must now use this information to combine data on the reduction in years of life lost to influenza-associated conditions with the changes in morbidity due to influenza-like illness to calculate the number of QALYs gained by vaccination.

Calculating changes in morbidity. In Table 9.1, we presented mean HRQL scores for influenza-like illness. We must now adjust these scores so that they reflect the HRQL of people who have received the influenza vaccine. We will use the efficacy of the influenza vaccine at preventing influenza-like illness (0.40) to calculate the mean improvement in HRQL (see Table 9.6) when people receive the influenza vaccine. (This assumes that vaccination will only improve the HRQL of the cohort by reducing the total number of influenza-like illness cases. In fact, vaccination should produce greater improvements in HRQL by eliminating most cases of influenza virus infection and secondary bacterial pneumonia, which are much more severe than other influenza-like illnesses.) The mean HRQL of subjects in the vaccination arm is calculated using the formula:

$$\text{average HRQL}_{\text{cohort}} \cdot (1 - \text{vaccine efficacy}_{\text{ILI}}) + \text{HRQL}_{\text{no ILI}} \cdot (\text{vaccine efficacy}_{\text{ILI}})$$

Equation 9.6

TABLE 9.6.   AGE-SPECIFIC AND MEAN HRQL SCORES FOR THE AVERAGE SUBJECT, SUBJECTS WITH NO INFLUENZA-LIKE ILLNESS (ILI), AND HRQL ADJUSTED FOR THE EFFICACY OF THE INFLUENZA VACCINE.

Age Group	HRQL Score		
	Average	No ILI	Adjusted
15 to 24	0.92	0.93	0.924
25 to 34	0.91	0.92	0.914
35 to 44	0.89	0.9	0.894
45 to 54	0.85	0.86	0.854
54 to 64	0.79	0.8	0.794
Mean	0.872	0.882	0.876

Keep in mind that, by using the efficacy of the influenza vaccine at preventing influenza-like illness, we are assuming that the vaccine is as effective at reducing the severity of disease as it is at preventing the disease. This assumption should be stated in the published report of our sample analysis and tested using a sensitivity analysis.

Calculating changes in mortality. The number of deaths prevented by vaccination is equal to:

efficacy, influenza vaccine · number of deaths, influenza-associated conditions

We must therefore assume that the influenza vaccine to prevent 0.803 of all deaths due to influenza-associated conditions. Using the data we calculated in Exercise 9.4, we can estimate the number of years of life lost to influenza-associated conditions among vaccinated persons (see Table 9.7).

Exercises 9.5–9.7

9.5. Using data on heart disease, lung disease, and diabetes obtained from the National Health Interview Survey (NHIS) and data from the U.S. Bureau of the Census (see Appendix III), we estimate that the total number of healthy adults aged fifteen to sixty-four was 174,955,000 in 1997. Among those with influenza virus infection, we would expect there to be 1,471 years of life lost during the average influenza season, resulting in a loss of 472 discounted QALYs. How many QALYs are there in the vaccination arm?

9.6. How many QALYs do we assign subjects in the supportive care arm?

9.7. What is the incremental cost-effectiveness of vaccination relative to supportive care per person (see Figure 7.11 for cost values)?

Calculating QALYs in the Treatment Arm

As with vaccination, the gain in HRQL must be determined by averaging the HRQL score for persons without influenza-like illness with the HRQL score for persons with influenza-like illness using the efficacy of oseltamivir at reducing the severity of illness using Equation 9.6. In Chapter Five, we calculated the efficacy of oseltamivir in reducing the duration of influenza-like illness using data from Treanor and others (2000). These researchers also determined the efficacy of oseltamivir in reducing the time required to return to normal health, the time required to return to normal activity, and a self-rated measure of the severity of illness.

TABLE 9.7. QALYs LOST TO INFLUENZA-ASSOCIATED CONDITIONS IN THE VACCINE ARM OF THE SAMPLE COST-EFFECTIVENESS ANALYSIS.

	6	7	8	9	10	11
					1 − Vaccine Efficacy	*Column 9 · Column 10*
Age Group	Total Years Lost	Discounted Years Lost	HRQL	QALYs Lost	Reduction in QALYs	Adjusted ALYs Lost
15 to 24	130	24	0.92	22	0.197	4
25 to 34	188	45	0.91	41	0.197	8
35 to 44	398	127	0.89	113	0.197	22
45 to 54	322	134	0.85	114	0.197	22
54 to 64	433	230	0.79	182	0.197	36
Total	1,471			472		93

Note: Columns 1 through 5 from previous tables have been removed.

If we are interested in determining the effect of oseltamivir on the changes in the HRQL of persons with influenza-like illness, we will want to use the efficacy of this medication in reducing the severity of illness, because this outcome best reflects subjective changes in pain and suffering. Table 7.2 lists the efficacy of oseltamivir in reducing the severity of influenza-like illness, 0.2266.

The number of future years of quality-adjusted life lost in the treatment arm is equal to the product of the number of future years of quality-adjusted life lost in the supportive care arm, the average HRQL score, and the efficacy of oseltamivir in preventing mortality due to influenza. None of this is relevant to our analysis, of course, because the gains in life for healthy adults is so minimal that it adds up to little more than a rounding difference in the QALYs due to morbidity (see Exercise 9.5).

Exercises 9.8–9.9

9.8. Calculate the mean HRQL for subjects in the oseltamivir arm of the analysis.

9.9. Calculate the total number of QALYs lost to death from the influenza virus in the oseltamivir arm of the analysis, assuming a treatment efficacy of 50 percent.

Incremental Cost-Effectiveness of Each Intervention

In Chapter One, we learned that the incremental cost-effectiveness ratio is calculated using the formula:

$$\frac{(\text{total cost of intervention } 1 - \text{total cost of intervention } 2)}{(\text{QALYs, intervention } 1 - \text{QALYs, intervention } 2)}$$

Equation 1.2

When multiple interventions are compared, a cost-effectiveness table is generated, listing the least effective intervention first and the most effective intervention last. The incremental cost and the incremental effectiveness are subtracted from top to bottom (see Table 9.8).

Of the three interventions under study, vaccination is the most effective, so it is listed last in the table. The next most effective intervention is treatment, which is listed second, and the least effective is supportive care, which is listed first. The first row in the table lists the total cost and the total effectiveness of supportive care alone. The incremental cost of treatment is equal to the total cost of

TABLE 9.8. INCREMENTAL COST EFFECTIVENESS TABLE FOR THE THREE INTERVENTIONS UNDER STUDY.

	Total Cost	Total Effectiveness	Incremental Cost	Incremental Effectiveness	Incremental Cost Effectiveness
Support	$48.58	0.872	—	—	
Treat	$68.93	0.874	$20.35	0.002	$10,175
Vaccinate	$40.26	0.876	($28.67)	0.002	Saving

treatment—the total cost of supportive care. Likewise, the incremental effectiveness of treatment is equal to the total effectiveness of treatment—the total effectiveness of supportive care. The incremental cost-effectiveness is equal to the incremental cost divided by the incremental effectiveness. Because Table 9.8 lists the average HRQL score over an entire year rather than 97 hours of illness, these values may confuse readers of the analysis. For this reason, when it came time to publish the sample analysis, we presented HRQL scores over the duration of influenza-like illness. Both methods will produce equivalent incremental HRQL values, however.

Typically, the incremental cost-effectiveness of the most effective intervention is only calculated relative to the next most effective intervention. Therefore, the incremental cost of vaccination is equal to the total cost of vaccination minus the total cost of treatment. Likewise, the incremental effectiveness of treatment is equal to the total effectiveness of vaccination minus the total effectiveness of treatment.

Using QALYs in Decision Analysis Models

In the section above, we calculated the total number of QALYs in each arm of the analysis using the efficacy of the influenza vaccine or oseltamivir in preventing or treating influenza-like illness. We walked you through the laborious task of calculating QALYs by hand so that you could better understand how they work. However, your labors were not necessary; the decision analysis model will do the work of calculating the total QALYs for you. Most software can also calculate the incremental cost and the incremental number of QALYs gained when each intervention is applied and will generate a table similar to Table 9.8.

The decision analysis model apportions subjects based on whether they are ill or well. Therefore, all branches labeled "Well" or "Healthy" should have an HRQL of 0.882 entered into the terminal node (see Table 9.1), and all branches labeled "Ill" should have an HRQL of 0.862 entered into them. If you do this and roll back the tree, you should obtain the same values you calculated in Exercises 9.3–9.11.

Recall that we apportioned cost events in the treatment arm using the efficacy of oseltamivir in reducing the duration of illness, and we apportioned QALYs using the severity of illness. You will not notice the difference between the total QALYs in the treatment arm that we calculated by hand and the total QALYs produced when rolling back the tree, because the difference is so small. However, researchers should always be mindful of when the event pathway for costs differs from the event pathway for effectiveness. Adjustments should be made to the decision analysis tree where necessary. The advantage to entering the Ill and Well HRQL scores into the decision analysis tree is that it requires less work and we can conduct a sensitivity analysis on these values.

## CHAPTER TEN

CONDUCTING A SENSITIVITY ANALYSIS

Overview

At various points in this book, we have seen how the value of some variables in our analysis can be very difficult to establish with absolute certainty. More often, we find that we are able to determine a plausible range of values from different articles in the medical literature or from different datasets, in which we believe the true value lies. In this chapter, you will learn how to test the effect of this uncertainty on the output of the decision analysis model.

There are many different ways of testing variables in a sensitivity analysis. These include a **one-way (univariate) sensitivity analysis,** in which a single variable is tested over its range of plausible values while all other variables are held at a constant value; a **two-way (bivariate) sensitivity analysis,** in which two variables are simultaneously tested over their range of plausible values while all others are held constant; a **multi-way sensitivity analysis,** in which more than two variables are tested; and a **tornado analysis** (or **influence analysis**), in which each variable is sequentially tested in a one-way sensitivity analysis. The tornado analysis is used to rank order the different variables in order of their overall influence on the magnitude of the model outputs.

Sensitivity analyses can also be used to test for errors in the decision analysis model. By showing how a variable affects the output of a model over a range of values, a sensitivity analysis will bring to light inconsistencies in the model's design. This chapter will conclude with a discussion of a **Monte Carlo analysis,** which allows the researcher to treat the hypothetical cohort in a cost-effectiveness analysis as if it consisted of real people rather than a bunch of probabilities, costs, and QALYs.

Project Map

1. Develop a research question.
2. Design your analysis.
3. Understand the sources of error in data.
4. Obtain data.
5. Organize data.
6. Construct a decision analysis model.
7. Calculate quality-adjusted life years.
8. **Test and refine the decision analysis model.**
9. **Conduct a sensitivity analysis.**
10. Prepare the study results for publication or presentation.

Consider the incidence rate of influenza-like illness. Not only were we unable to find a good estimate of this rate in electronic datasets or the medical literature, this rate can change dramatically from one season to the next. It is therefore important to know how the vaccination strategy would compare with the treatment or supportive care strategies if the incidence rate of influenza-like illness were set at the very low or very high values.

Suppose that we decided to use 0.3 (or 30 cases per 100 persons) as a low value and 0.6 (or 60 cases per 100 persons) as a high value. To see how the results of the analysis might change when the incidence of influenza-like illness is very low, we could simply enter 0.3 into our decision analysis model and roll it back. We might then enter 0.6 into our decision analysis model and again roll it back to see what effect a very high rate would have on each of the three strategies we are evaluating. Needless to say, it would be very inconvenient if we had to do this for every variable we included in the model.

Fortunately, decision analysis programs have much easier (and much more sophisticated) ways of testing the effect of **parameter uncertainty** on the model outcomes. Recall from Chapter Three that there is a true mean value of each parameter used in any cost-effectiveness model. Only an omniscient being would know the true values of all of the parameters we wish to use, so we have to compensate for our human frailty and conduct a sensitivity analysis on the inputs we are uncertain about. The inputs we are least likely to be certain about are the assumptions we have made (for example, the amount of time it takes for a nurse to administer the vaccine). We also included parameters in our model that may have contained bias, such as the incidence rate of influenza-like illness. Finally, there were some values that we were fairly confident about, such as the cost of the influenza vaccine itself.

The parameters we are least certain about should be tested over the widest range of values (because it is plausible that the values are much higher or much lower than our baseline estimate). Parameters that we are somewhat more confident about can be tested over a narrower range of values. When a particular strategy remains dominant over the range of plausible values for the inputs that we are uncertain about, the model is said to be **robust.**

One-Way Sensitivity Analysis

There are a number of techniques for conducting a sensitivity analysis. The simplest is called a one-way sensitivity analysis. In this type of sensitivity analysis, a single variable is tested over its plausible range of values, while every other variable is held constant. If we were to test the incidence of influenza-like illness at the highest and lowest likely values, we would have conducted a one-way sensitivity analysis. In addition to testing the effect of uncertainty on the decision analysis model outcomes, one-way sensitivity analyses can be used to answer certain research questions and help ensure that the decision analysis model was constructed properly.

Let us see what happens when we vary the cost of vaccination between $6.99 and $48.79. (We will return to these values in the next section.) In Figure 10.1, the y-axis indicates the expected value (overall cost) of each strategy, while the x-axis indicates the different vaccine costs at which the model was tested. The expected value refers to the cost of each arm of the decision analysis tree when a variable assumes a specific value. For example, if the cost of the vaccine were $6.99, the expected cost of the Vaccinate arm would be about $31 per person, while the Support and Treat arms would cost around $44 and $49 per person, respectively.

If the cost of the vaccine were $20.92, our model predicts that the strategy of vaccinating all subjects would cost about the same amount as providing only supportive care. When a variable is set to a value that changes the dominance of one intervention relative to another (the point at which one intervention becomes more cost-effective than another), the value is called the **threshold value** of that variable, and it is equal to the x-axis value at the point at which two lines in a one-way sensitivity analysis cross.

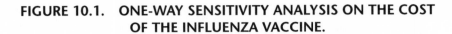

FIGURE 10.1.   ONE-WAY SENSITIVITY ANALYSIS ON THE COST
OF THE INFLUENZA VACCINE.

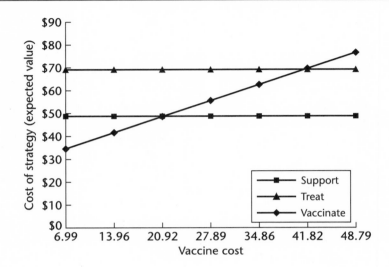

If the cost of the vaccine were $48.79, our model predicts that the strategy of vaccinating all persons in our cohort would cost around $77—about $28 more than the cost of providing supportive care alone and $7 more than the cost of providing oseltamivir. Remember, this is only an analysis of cost values. Therefore, if the cost of the vaccine is $48.79 in the real world, vaccination may still be a cost-effective strategy relative to oseltamivir, but it will not be a cost-saving strategy.

Using One-Way Sensitivity Analyses to Validate a Model

When examining the results of a one-way sensitivity analysis, you should always ask yourself whether the expected value of a strategy changes in a predictable way. For example, in Figure 10.1, we would expect that the vaccination strategy would become increasingly less attractive as the cost of the vaccine increases (in other words, the expected value of vaccination strategy would increase at a faster rate than the expected value of the other strategies).

In fact, the expected value of the Support or Treat arms should remain constant as the cost of the vaccine increases, because neither of these arms of the decision analysis model includes the variable cVaccine (the cost of the vaccine). If the expected value of the Support or Treat options did increase, we would know that there is a problem with the way that the model was assembled. (Specifically, cVaccinate would have been erroneously entered as a variable in another arm of the decision analysis model.) Thus, a one-way sensitivity analysis can also be used to test for errors in the decision analysis model.

The easiest way to test that the model has no glaring errors is to consider how you might expect changes in a particular cost or probability to affect a model, and then to vary that cost or probability over a wide range of values. Varying a probability from zero to one, or a cost from zero to a very large number, allows you to see the relationship between the strategies under study at predictable end points. For example, if we test the incidence rate of influenza-like illness from an incidence rate of zero percent to an incidence rate of 100 percent, we would expect the cost of supportive care or treatment to be zero when the incidence rate is zero because no costs would be incurred by healthy people in our model (see Figure 10.2). We would also expect vaccination to be more costly relative to the other interventions at low incidence rates and less costly than the other interventions at high incidence rates. This type of testing is called **model validation.**

Tips and tricks. You will not be able to set the incidence rate of influenza-like illness to a value of zero because we have entered an equation, pHosp = pHosp/pIll, that contains this variable in the denominator. If you perform a sensitivity analysis from a probability of zero to a probability of one on this variable, your software will give you a division by zero error when it tests the value at zero.

FIGURE 10.2. ONE-WAY SENSITIVITY ANALYSIS ON THE INCIDENCE RATE (PER PERSON) OF INFLUENZA-LIKE ILLNESS.

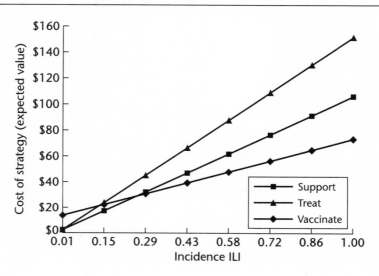

Exercises 10.1–10.2

10.1. In Figure 10.2, we see that the line representing the cost of treatment is very close to the line representing the cost of supportive care at low incidence rates of influenza-like illness. As the incidence rate increases, these lines grow further apart. Is this what we would expect?

10.2. How would we expect the cost of the vaccination arm of our decision analysis model to compare to the supportive care arm when the incidence rate of influenza-like illness is zero?

Answering Secondary Questions Using One-Way Sensitivity Analyses

One-way sensitivity analyses are frequently employed to address clinical or policy questions that are not directly related to the primary research question. For instance, in our research question we examined whether it would be cost-effective for people to receive an influenza vaccination at work, as part of a medical visit for some other reason, or in an institutional setting (such as schools or prisons). In the real world, though, if the government were to recommend the influenza vaccine for healthy adults in one of these settings, some people would make special trips to their doctors just to get the vaccine. Policymakers may be interested in knowing how much vaccination would cost in the real world if they made a formal recommendation to vaccinate people in the workplace, or as part of a medical visit for some other reason.

It might also be helpful to provide readers with information on other possibilities unrelated to our primary research question. For instance, we might wish to conduct a broad one-way sensitivity analysis on the cost of oseltamivir. If we demonstrate that there is a price point for this medication that renders it cost-effective relative to vaccination, it is possible that our analysis will be used to determine the market price of the medication.

Exercises 10.3–10.4

10.3. What is the threshold of value for the treatment option relative to the supportive care option when the cost of oseltamivir is tested in a one-way sensitivity analysis?

10.4. Would it be necessary to set the cost of oseltamivir to the threshold value for cost-savings for it to be perceived as cost-effective?

Determining "Plausible" High and Low Values

Rather than test the highest and lowest *possible* values of each parameter used in a decision analysis model, a sensitivity analysis should test the *plausible* range of values of each parameter to see how it might impact the cost or effectiveness of each strategy. Consider our estimate of the cost of vaccination, $12.57 (see Exercise 6.13). To generate this value, we added the cost of patient time (thirty minutes to receive the vaccine) and the cost of administering the vaccine (five minutes of time for a registered nurse) to the cost of the vaccine itself. Because we are interested in the cost of administering the vaccine in the patients' workplace or as part of a medical visit for routine care, we do not need to add other costs, such as the cost of transportation, to the cost of the vaccine itself.

In the real world, though, if the government or some other agency recommends that all healthy adults receive the influenza vaccine at work, some people who do not have a work-based vaccination program will nevertheless rush out to their doctor, even if this is not recommended. If everyone were to go to his or her doctor just to get a vaccine, our estimate of the cost of the vaccine would be much too low, because we did not include transportation costs or the additional patient time costs required for a trip to a health clinic.

Let us consider the highest and lowest possible costs for the vaccine. Both Nichol and others (1995) and Bridges and others (2000) estimated the cost of vaccination using an estimate of the cost of the vaccine itself and then added thirty minutes of patient time to this cost. Neither study included the cost of transportation nor other costs associated with a medical visit. Instead, they assumed that these vaccines would be administered in the workplace, or as part of a routine medical exam.

In some workplaces, practitioners stop by workers' cubicles and offer the influenza vaccine, while in others, employees simply visit their occupational health office. After getting the vaccine, employees usually head back to work. Under these circumstances, patients might spend ten minutes waiting to get their vaccination, which would result in a vaccination cost of about $6.99. On the other hand, if people were to drive to their doctors' offices specifically for an influenza vaccination, they would incur transportation costs and might consume an hour and a half of their valuable time, bringing the cost of vaccination up to $48.79.

It is unlikely that everyone would go to his or her doctor to receive the vaccination, so $48.79 is not a plausible value for the cost of vaccination. On the other hand, some people will, so $6.99 is much too low, and so it is also not a reasonable estimate. If $6.99 is not a plausible value and $48.79 is not a plausible value, how do we know where to draw the line between plausible and implausible? Let us build a model to see what would happen if some people decided to go to their doctors just to receive a influenza vaccination, while others received the vaccine at their workplaces over an average time of ten minutes (see Figure 10.3). In this model, the variable pYes represents the probability that people will drive to their doctors' offices to receive the influenza vaccine. If everyone drove, the cost of the influenza vaccine

FIGURE 10.3.   A SIMPLE DECISION ANALYSIS MODEL DESIGNED TO TEST THE OVERALL COST OF THE INFLUENZA VACCINE WHEN SOME PATIENTS INCUR THE HIGHEST POSSIBLE COST AND OTHERS INCUR THE LOWEST POSSIBLE COST OF THE INFLUENZA VACCINE.

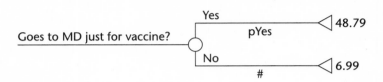

would be approximately $48.79, and if everyone received the vaccine at work in just ten minutes, the cost of the vaccine would be approximately $6.99.

Figure 10.4 illustrates a one-way sensitivity analysis of this model over a broad range of probabilities for pYes. Suppose we found a study indicating that 15 to 25 percent of adults vaccinated over the previous season made a special trip to their doctor to receive the vaccine. The expected value of the decision analysis model is about $15 when pYes is equal to 25 percent (the solid line in Figure 10.4).

If we were interested in recommending influenza vaccination to everyone, regardless of whether he or she had to go to a physician, the highest plausible value for the cost of the influenza vaccine might be around $15. We should note, too, that the vaccine would cost approximately $28 (the threshold value for dominance of the vaccination strategy in Figure 10.1) if 50 percent of all healthy adult vaccine recipients went to their doctors or to vaccination clinics just for an influenza vaccination (the dashed line in Figure 10.4). Thus, we know that vaccination would remain the dominant strategy, even if close to 50 percent of all subjects were to make special trips to their physicians. In considering both 1) the threshold value of the overall cost of the vaccination strategy relative to treatment and supportive care, and 2) the overall cost of the influenza vaccine required to reach this threshold value, we conducted a two-way sensitivity analysis.

Two-Way Sensitivity Analysis

To understand the relationship between the chance that people would visit their doctors just to receive a vaccination and the cost of the vaccine, we had to conduct two one-way sensitivity analyses. To do this, it was necessary to first examine the threshold value of the cost of the vaccine (about $28) and to then examine the

FIGURE 10.4.   ONE-WAY SENSITIVITY ANALYSIS ON THE PROBABILITY THAT PATIENTS WILL VISIT THEIR DOCTOR JUST TO RECEIVE THE INFLUENZA VACCINE.

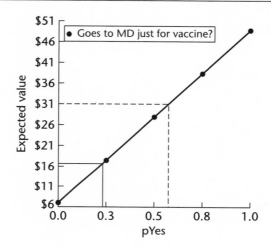

proportion of subjects visiting their doctors for the vaccine required to drive the cost of vaccination to $28 (about 50 percent). We could have captured both of these events at once if we had conducted a two-way sensitivity analysis. A two-way sensitivity analysis indicates how simultaneous changes in two variables affect the cost-effectiveness of a given intervention when all other variables are held at a constant value.

Many variables in a cost-effectiveness analysis are interdependent and small changes in two variables can therefore have a large effect on the expected value of a given strategy. For example, the effectiveness of influenza vaccination is dependent on both the incidence rate of influenza-like illness and the efficacy of the vaccine in preventing influenza-like illness in any given season. If we had overestimated the mean efficacy of the influenza vaccine from season to season in the United States, vaccination might still have been cost-saving so long as the overestimation was not large. On the other hand, if both our estimate of the incidence rate of influenza-like illness and our estimate of vaccine efficacy were too high, the cost-savings that we found to be associated with vaccination might not be real.

In Figure 10.5, any intersection of values on the x-axis and y-axis will fall into one of two zones, solid or clear. Each zone indicates which arm will be dominant with respect to costs. For example, if the efficacy of the influenza vaccine at preventing influenza-like illness were 0.4, and the incidence rate of influenza-like

FIGURE 10.5.   TWO-WAY SENSITIVITY ANALYSIS ON THE EFFICACY OF THE VACCINE AT PREVENTING INFLUENZA-LIKE ILLNESS AND THE INCIDENCE OF INFLUENZA-LIKE ILLNESS.

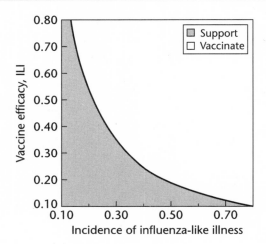

illness were 40 cases per 100 persons, the vaccination strategy will be dominant with respect to cost (because the intersection of these two values falls in the clear zone). However, if the actual efficacy of the influenza vaccine were 0.3 and the actual average annual incidence rate of influenza were 20 cases per 100 persons, then supportive care would be dominant with respect to cost.

Analysis of Influence

Conducting sensitivity analyses may seem like a lot of fun the first few times you do it, but no researcher would want to spend an entire week conducting one-way sensitivity analyses on all of the variables used in the model. If we knew which variables had the most influence on the relative cost (or effectiveness) of each intervention, we could focus on just those variables.

However, the overall influence of a variable on the cost or effectiveness of a particular strategy is not easy to predict. The extent to which a variable can influence the dominance of each strategy in a decision analysis model is determined by 1) the overall magnitude of the variable, 2) uncertainty associated with the baseline value of the variable, 3) the relative position of the variable in a decision arm, and 4) the number of decision arms in which the variable appears.

Consider the influence of the cost of oseltamivir on the overall cost of the Treat arm of the decision analysis model (see Figure 10.6). Oseltamivir is the third most costly input in the decision analysis model, and subsequently, we might expect it to have a big impact on the overall cost of the treatment arm. However, the cost of the medication remains relatively certain, so the cost of the medication need not be tested over a broad range of values. Because the cost of the medication does not fluctuate a good deal, it does not cause much fluctuation in the overall cost of the treatment arm. Moreover, the probability of actually incurring the cost is shaped by whether the patient becomes ill, whether the patient sees a physician, and whether the patient arrives in the doctor's office early enough for the medication to be efficacious, so the overall influence of oseltamivir is reduced by all of these other factors.

On the other hand, oseltamivir only appears in the treatment arm, so increasing the price of this medication does not increase the price of the vaccination or supportive care strategies. Therefore, a change in the cost of oseltamivir is more likely to cause changes in the dominance of the treatment strategy rather than a change in the cost of a medical visit, because the cost of a medical visit appears in all arms of the tree and subsequently causes changes in the overall cost of each strategy simultaneously. So, if the influence of a variable on the relative cost or effectiveness of a particular strategy is so complex, how do we know which variables are important to test and which are not?

FIGURE 10.6.   ONE-WAY SENSITIVITY ANALYSIS ON THE COST OF OSELTAMIVIR.

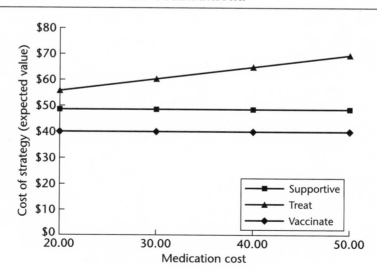

An **influence analysis** (also known under the more Wizard-of-Oz-like title, **tornado analysis**) is a handy way of determining how much influence each of the variables has on the overall model. Influence analyses are sometimes called tornado analyses because the graph that is produced assumes the appearance of a tornado. In this type of analysis, the decision analysis program will conduct a one-way sensitivity analysis on each of the variables and then produce a nice graph indicating which variable has the most influence, which has the second most influence, and so on.

In this type of analysis, each variable is tested independently. Students often assume that the program changes all the variables together over their plausible range of values in a mega-variable slugfest. This is not the case. An influence analysis does nothing more than save the researcher from having to test each variable in separate one-way analyses.

Determining the Plausible Range of Each Variable

Before we can conduct a tornado analysis, we must estimate the range of plausible values for each parameter we will use in our study. In Chapters Five and Six, we discussed some ways in which the highest and lowest values of a variable can be estimated. For example, in determining the efficacy of the influenza virus vaccine, we used the range of likely values published by the Centers for Disease Control and Prevention (CDC). In other instances, we used the highest and lowest values published in the medical literature. However, the high and low values published in the medical literature are sometimes implausibly high or low. For instance, Bridges and others (2000) estimated patient time costs using the wages of Ford employees, whose wages are twice that of the average citizen (U.S. Bureau of the Census, 1999). This, in turn, resulted in an implausibly high valuation for the cost of the influenza vaccine.

Guidelines for estimating plausible values. There are a few guiding principles one should follow in determining the range of plausible values for a given variable.

- If the parameter is based on an assumption or expert opinion, it should be tested over a very broad range of values in a one-way analysis. Expert opinion should be used to determine the high and low boundaries for the variable in other types of analyses if the variable influences the expected value of any strategy. For example, in the sample analysis we assumed that approximately 1 percent of all patients would experience side effects to vaccination. If we find that increasing this value to 10 percent results in a large increase in the cost of vaccination, relative to supportive care, we should attempt to obtain a better estimate of how high this value might be in the real world.

- If the parameter was derived from a representative sample, you may use 95 percent confidence intervals when no other source of error is likely. In some instances, a large portion of the error in the value of a parameter will be sampling error. For example, laboratory test values derived from the National Health and Nutrition Examination Survey (NHANES) are only subject to sampling error and error inherent to the tests. After adjusting the data for the false positive error rate and so on, it is acceptable to use the 95 percent confidence interval for the sampling error in these data.

- If multiple estimates of the value of a parameter are available, consider conducting a meta-analysis; then, use the 95 percent confidence interval of the combined data sources. This requires the assistance of a researcher skilled in the research methods of meta-analysis.

- If two sources of error are interdependent, conduct a two-way sensitivity analysis on each source of error.

- If the parameter was obtained from electronic sources, check the data documentation for error estimates. As noted in Chapter Four, most public use data are accompanied by very detailed descriptions of the types of error these data contain.

- If an input contains multiple subcomponents, disaggregate the subcomponents of the variable so that they can be tested separately in your decision analysis model. For example, when we derived the cost of transportation in Chapter Six, we included an estimate of the mileage driven and the cost per gallon of gasoline, among other subcomponents, in the overall cost of transportation, to make the decision analysis model easier to understand. This is not good practice in real-world models. Instead, it is best to include the overall cost of transportation as a formula in the model and to break the formula into separate variables that can be independently tested.

In addition to some of the principles highlighted here, Gold and others (1996) describe methods for conducting more sophisticated sensitivity analyses. Some of these methods will be described in the "Monte Carlo Simulation" section below.

Range of parameter values in the sample cost-effectiveness analysis. The derivation of some of the high and low values we used in our sample decision analysis was described in Chapters Five and Six. These values were described to highlight some of the ways in which the limits of an interval might be estimated. Because providing the methods for deriving high and low values would be overly space- and time-consuming, we will not include a full description of this process in this book.

Parameters excluded from model. In the sample analysis, we chose to exclude costs associated with secondary transmission, because the vaccination strategy was found to be cost-saving. This is a common practice in cost-benefit analyses (CBA) because the outcomes of the analysis are concrete. (If the intervention is associated with savings, it is preferred over the alternative.) Any future savings associated with an intervention can be safely omitted so long as the overall intervention is cost-saving. When savings are eliminated from an analysis, it is sometimes called a **biased design.** It is called a biased design because the researcher intentionally introduces bias that works against the outcome that is expected to be dominant.

It is only acceptable to use this design in a cost-effectiveness analysis in the rare instances in which an intervention is both cost-saving and more effective than the comparator program. In all other instances, an attempt should be made to estimate the cost or probability for all relevant events in a cost-effectiveness analysis. This may be achieved via expert opinion or, in the case of secondary transmission, mathematical modeling. If we had included the probability of secondary transmission, it would have been necessary to test the value using a broad one-way sensitivity analysis.

Generating an Influence Diagram

An influence diagram (also known as a tornado diagram) tells the researcher which variables exert the most influence over the dominance of the strategies being tested in the decision analysis model (see Figure 10.7). Each bar in the diagram represents the results of a single one-way sensitivity analysis. Those analyses that have the

FIGURE 10.7.   TORNADO DIAGRAM OF SELECTED VARIABLES IN THE DECISION ANALYSIS MODEL.

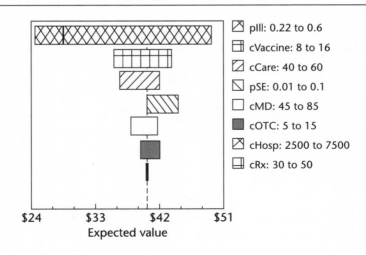

greatest effect on the expected value of the model are widest and appear at the top of the graph. Each variable is then ranked for its overall influence from top to bottom, giving it the appearance of a tornado.

In Figure 10.7, the expected value (x-axis) indicates the expected value of the entire tree over the range of values we assigned to each variable. The average expected value is represented by a dashed line spanning from the top of the graph to the bottom. (Some software packages do not produce this line.) We see that the variables with the most influence over outcomes are 1) the incidence rate of influenza-like illness (pIll), 2) the cost of the influenza vaccine (cVaccine), 3) the cost of the caregiving (cCare), 4) the probability of side effects, 5) the cost of a medical visit (cMD), and 6) the cost of over-the-counter medications (cOTC). The remainder of the variables had little influence on the overall model outcomes when tested over estimates of their plausible ranges.

It is also important to conduct a tornado analysis separately for each of the arms of the decision tree. Figure 10.7 provides information on the expected value of the entire model (all three branches together). If we generate a tornado diagram for each option separately, we will have a better idea of how variables individually influence each strategy under study. For example, if we were to generate an influence diagram for the vaccination strategy alone, we would see that the cost of the vaccine is more important in this branch than it is in the overall model.

Monte Carlo Simulation

When we tested our model over a range of plausible values using one-way and two-way sensitivity analyses, we were able to give readers of our study an idea of the robustness of the model. For example, we were able to demonstrate that vaccination would remain the dominant strategy if any variable were set to its highest or lowest plausible value. When using standard sensitivity analyses, though, there is no good way of testing what would happen if all of the variables were simultaneously tested.

In the real world, some of the variables are likely to be lower than the values we estimated, and some are likely to be higher. If the true average incidence rate of influenza-like illness, efficacy of the influenza vaccine, and the probability of hospitalization were each slightly lower than the values we estimated, it is possible that influenza vaccination would be more costly than providing supportive care alone. On the other hand, if the real cost of a hospitalization for influenza-like illness were higher, it might offset these lower probabilities. If we had information on how the expected value of each intervention might change when subtle changes occurred in many variables at the same time, we would get a better idea of how likely it is that vaccination would remain dominant in the real world.

Cost-effectiveness analyses may better simulate real-world conditions by using a **Monte Carlo simulation.** Named after the famous gambling enclave, this type of analysis tests the range of expected values of each intervention when the values of many variables are changed at the same time. Imagine that you had a giant decision analysis model, and you had 100 friends jog through it one at a time. Some of your friends would take a left turn right off the bat and end up at a terminal node in the supportive care arm. Others might run straight, then jog to the right, and end up in the Well branch of the treatment arm. Eventually, each of your friends would have made it to one of the terminal nodes in the model, where they would gather in small groups with others that happened to take the same route. If each one of your friends recorded the cost value and the effectiveness value at the terminal node they finished in, you would be able to obtain a mean value for each intervention, along with a standard deviation.

In a Monte Carlo simulation, a hypothetical cohort of subjects is entered into the decision analysis model. As subjects pass through the model, they encounter a number of different probabilities such as the chance of developing influenza-like illness, the chance of seeing a doctor, the chance of being hospitalized, and so on. Once a subject reaches the terminal node, he or she then incurs the cost associated with that node. This process is repeated hundreds or thousands of times, until the expected value of each arm of the decision analysis model is associated with a distribution of cost or effectiveness values.

A Monte Carlo simulation provides much more comprehensive information than standard one-way and two-way analyses. For example, a Monte Carlo simulation can also provide a range of high and low cost-effectiveness ratios for each strategy you evaluate in your model (Gold and others, 1996).

How Monte Carlo Simulations Work

In a Monte Carlo simulation, the chances of drawing a very high or a very low value for a given variable are smaller than the chance of observing a number closer to the baseline value. For example, in estimating the cost of hospitalization, our closest estimate of the actual cost was $5,728. We might estimate that the actual cost was as high as $7,454, or as low as $4,014, but neither the high nor the low cost would likely represent the actual cost of hospitalization.

We must therefore provide the model with some estimate of the chances of seeing these high and low values in the real world. Recall from Chapter Three that a probability distribution indicates the chances of observing any value within a range of numbers. For example, the chance of a hospital cost value of $5,000 should be assigned a fairly high probability, and the chance of a hospital cost of $4,000 or $7,000 should be assigned a lower probability. Using a probability distribution, we can influence the chances that the model will assign a particular value to any given subject (see Figure 10.8). Thus, in effect we are weighting the dice each time the Monte Carlo simulation selects a value from the range of values we have assigned to each variable.

Let us walk through an example of how the Monte Carlo simulation deals with the probabilities of different events (see Figure 10.9). After a subject (⚲) enters a particular arm of the study, that subject is exposed to a chance event at the first decision node the subject encounters. In the Support arm of the decision analysis tree, the subject is first exposed to a chance of developing an influenza-like illness. The chance that the subject will become ill is influenced by a triangular distribution of plausible incidence rate values.

FIGURE 10.8. IN A MONTE CARLO SIMULATION, THE VALUE EACH SUBJECT IS ASSIGNED IS DRAWN FROM A PROBABILITY DISTRIBUTION.

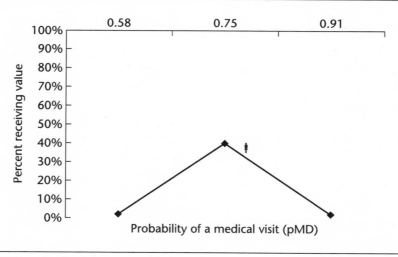

Note: In this example, the chance that a subject will visit a physician ranges from 0.58 to 0.91. While there is a 40 percent chance that the subject will be assigned a 0.75 probability of seeing a physician when ill with an influenza-like virus, the chance of being assigned a probability of either 0.6 or 0.9 is very small.

FIGURE 10.9.   PROGRESSION OF SUBJECTS THROUGH A MONTE CARLO SIMULATION.

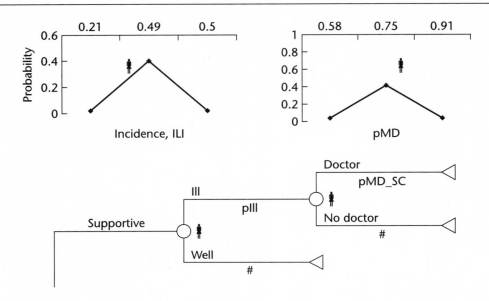

Defining Distributions

Estimates obtained from the medical literature are usually normally distributed, and the 95 percent confidence interval or the standard deviation is usually provided. If you are working with an electronic dataset, the distribution of a particular parameter can be obtained using a statistical software package. Once all of the variables have been assigned distributions using the high and low ranges previously defined, you will be ready to conduct a Monte Carlo analysis.

Oftentimes, though, you will not know the shape of the distribution or the range of error associated with an input. Assumed values, values obtained via expert opinion, and means obtained from data primarily subject to non-random error will not have a known distribution of error. In your published report, you must be careful to mention any assumptions that were made surrounding the distribution and the range of values assigned to any input. It is important to solicit expert opinion regarding the both the shape and the range of any unknown distribution you use in the model.

Tips and tricks. Always be certain to save a backup copy of your decision analysis tree under a different name before you assign distributions to the variables in your model. Once a distribution has been assigned to a variable, you will not be able to conduct further sensitivity analyses using fixed probabilities or costs.

Conducting a Monte Carlo Simulation

There are two major reasons to conduct a Monte Carlo simulation. The first is to estimate the mean and standard deviation of the expected value of each of the strategies in the decision analysis model. However, unless all of the high and low values you use in your model were derived from real statistical distributions, a Monte Carlo simulation does not produce a true standard deviation or 95 percent confidence interval for the error in your model.

The second goal is to determine the number of times each strategy would be expected to dominate the others, given the variability in the parameter estimates. This process is formally called a **strategy selection analysis.** For example, a Monte Carlo analysis will tell us the percentage of trials in which we would expect vaccination to produce the fewest costs or provide a superior cost-effectiveness ratio. This will provide more meaningful information on the robustness of the model as a whole than the mean and standard deviation of each strategy.

A Monte Carlo simulation should be conducted with a large number of hypothetical subjects, but not necessarily with the total number of subjects you are evaluating in your research question. In the influenza example, we are evaluating 175 million subjects between the ages of fifteen and sixty-five, which is far more than we need to get an idea of how the different interventions compare with one another. When a relatively basic model is used with five to ten terminal nodes, it is generally safe to enter 10,000 subjects in each Monte Carlo simulation, though this will vary depending on whether the Monte Carlo analysis is conducted to provide the reader with a general idea of the robustness of your model or is central to your analysis.

Figure 10.10 illustrates the outcomes of the strategy selection analysis. We see that the vaccinate option produced the fewest costs for over 85 percent of the subjects, and the treatment option produced the fewest costs for less than 5 percent of the subjects. In other words, we would expect vaccination to be the dominant strategy about 85 percent of the time when values are randomly selected from each of the variables in the model.

This is not bad. Subjects in the Vaccinate arm of the decision analysis model incur the cost of vaccination while subjects in the other arms of the decision analysis model can make it through influenza season without incurring any additional costs. Even so, the model predicts that vaccination will be less costly for the vast majority of subjects.

**FIGURE 10.10.   STRATEGY SELECTION FREQUENCY DIAGRAM
ON THE COST-EFFECTIVENESS RATIO OF EACH STRATEGY
IN THE SAMPLE ANALYSIS.**

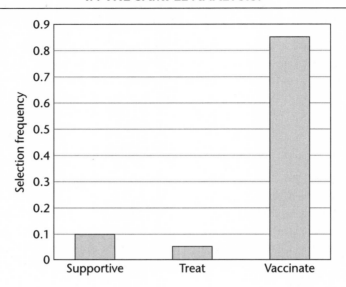

Each software package has a different set of features that are useful for conducting Monte Carlo analyses. It is worthwhile to read the user manual of the package you decide to use. The software packages commonly used in cost-effectiveness research are listed in Table 7.1.

Tips and tricks. When a tree containing distributions is rolled back, the average cost or effectiveness values assigned to each arm of the decision analysis model may differ from those generated from a tree that does not contain distributions. This occurs because the mean or midpoint value of the distributions you enter may not be equal to the baseline value you used for each variable.

CHAPTER ELEVEN

PREPARING YOUR STUDY FOR PUBLICATION

Overview

In this chapter, we will address the structure and format of journal articles on cost-effectiveness analysis. We will also provide advice on how to improve your chances of publication. You will learn how to format a cost-effectiveness analysis, which elements of your study should be described, what editors look for in an original research article, and which type of journal might be best for your analysis.

Project Map

1. Develop a research question.
2. Design your analysis.
3. Understand the sources of error in data.
4. Obtain data.
5. Organize data.
6. Construct a decision analysis model.
7. Calculate quality-adjusted life years.
8. Test and refine the decision analysis model.
9. Conduct a sensitivity analysis.
10. **Prepare the study results for publication or presentation.**

The publication format of cost-effectiveness analyses differs from that of other types of scientific investigations in subtle ways. In most prospective and retrospective studies, for example, the article begins with a brief introduction to the problem, including the impact of the disease under study, the need for the study, and a brief review of previous research on the disease or treatment under investigation. This is followed by a detailed description of the cohort, including the demographics of the cohort, the number of subjects who completed the study, inclusion and exclusion criteria, the laboratory methods used, and the statistical tests used. The methods section usually contains a table listing the characteristics of the subjects in the experimental and control groups, describes the study design, and describes the statistical tests used. The methods section is followed by a presentation of the results in tables and text. Usually, the primary outcomes are presented in the second table, and secondary outcomes are presented in the tables that follow. The article typically finishes with a discussion section in which the relevance of the findings is discussed, the limitations of the study are described, and concluding remarks are made.

In a cost-effectiveness analysis, the basic format is the same as that of other medical studies; however, the methodological details must be given greater attention, and the results are presented in a highly structured way. Unless the analysis is a piggyback study or a primary cost-effectiveness analysis, the description of the cohort is brief, and the first table is often used to describe either the assumptions made or the values assigned to each variable. The primary study results are presented using a cost-effectiveness table, which lists the incremental cost and effectiveness of each outcome in ascending order of effectiveness. These are listed at an undiscounted rate and at a standard discount rate of 3 percent (for studies outside the United States, the results should be listed at the prevailing discount rate). Secondary study results include the results of the various sensitivity analyses that were performed. As in prospective or retrospective studies, the discussion summarizes the findings, discusses the relevance of the findings, discusses the limitations of the study, and makes concluding remarks. Because cost-effectiveness analyses require a good deal of detailed work, it is sometimes necessary to prepare a technical appendix describing the details of your analysis.

Content and Structure of Cost-Effectiveness Articles

In presenting the results of a cost-effectiveness analysis, the researcher has to make a trade-off between the practical and the ideal. Ideally, a cost-effectiveness article will detail every assumption made, outline the event pathway, present every formula used, and convey all of the results of the analysis to the reader. In the real world, journal articles are limited to 3,000 to 5,000 words (about six to ten double-spaced pages excluding references). Therefore, it is important to be concise.

On the other hand, if critical information is omitted from the journal article, readers will not be able to verify that you have done the hard work necessary to produce a valid cost-effectiveness analysis. As with any other study, every cost-effectiveness article contains an introduction, methods, results, and discussion section. In the following sections, we will discuss the key aspects of each of these segments of a cost-effectiveness journal article.

Introduction

The introduction should begin by describing the impact of the disease under study and the need for a cost-effectiveness analysis that evaluates the interventions used to treat or prevent this disease. We will refer to the former as the "impact statement" and the latter as the "statement of need." The impact statement describes the epidemiological and economic impact of a disease on society. The statement of need outlines why there is uncertainty about the cost-effectiveness of medical interventions for the disease that warrant such an economic analysis. The introduction should also clearly state the research question and should include a description of the cohort, the setting, the interventions that were included and excluded, the perspective of the analysis, the geographic boundaries of the analysis, and the type of analysis conducted.

The impact of the disease on society usually includes facts pertaining to the incidence rate, the severity of the disease, and mortality rates of the disease. For example, the article might begin with the statement, "Influenza virus infections account for approximately 30,000 deaths, upwards of 200,000 hospitalizations, and over a million ambulatory care visits and days of lost work in the United States each year (Neuzil and others, 1999; Nichol and others, 1994)." If the economic impact of the disease has been published elsewhere, this data should be cited. When describing the need for a cost-effectiveness analysis, the researcher should indicate why it is unclear whether the costs, risks, and efficacy of one intervention might outweigh those of another. In our sample analysis, the cost-effectiveness of vaccination versus treatment hinges on the fact that, while treatment is only administered to those who become ill, vaccination must be administered to every healthy adult. The debate between vaccination and supportive care should focus on the fact that influenza virus infections tend to be less severe in healthy adults than in the elderly or chronically ill (in whom vaccination is already established as the intervention of choice).

If we were to prepare the sample analysis for publication, the reader should understand that the study examines the costs and benefits of vaccination in the workplace rather than the costs and benefits of vaccination in general, and that the analysis is targeted toward all adults residing in the United States for whom vaccination is not currently recommended (fifteen- to sixty-five-year-olds without heart disease, diabetes, or lung disease). Ideally, the study would briefly indicate why other anti-influenza virus medications were not included in the analysis and why a cost-effectiveness analysis was used instead of an alternate type of analysis. The impact of the disease, the need for a cost-effectiveness analysis, the research question, and the fundamental elements of the study must be tied together in three to six clear and concise paragraphs.

It is better to condense the information in the introduction into a few concise statements rather than painstakingly detail each point you are making. For instance, if you indicate, "While there is good evidence that the chronically ill and elderly will benefit from vaccination, healthy adults are at lower risk of hospitalization or death from influenza-virus infections. Therefore, there is uncertainty as to whether vaccination is cost-effective among healthy adults," you are telling the reader that 1) it is fairly certain that the elderly and ill would benefit from vaccination, 2) influenza-virus infections may lead to severe morbidity or death among the elderly and chronically ill persons, and 3) healthy adults are not as susceptible to severe complications of influenza as the elderly or persons with chronic illness.

A large part of the art of writing journal articles is in the prose. The use of jargon and painstaking detail should be avoided. The introduction and discussion sections are less formal and technical than the methods and results sections, so some leeway is provided for creative writing. For instance, rather than use technical descriptions such as, "We examined the cost-effectiveness of vaccination in institutional settings, such as the workplace, because such settings require only minimal marginal expenditures of social resources," it is better to state the problem in a simple and direct fashion. Instead, you might state, "When patients are vaccinated in the workplace or during a medical visit for an unrelated condition, they need not make an additional trip to their clinician for vaccination, so the institutional setting is intuitively more cost-effective than the noninstitutional setting." Because the introduction section must clearly set up the problem to the reader, it is more literary (and more fun to write) than the methods section, which must be highly concise and technical.

Methods

Unlike the introduction section, the methods section approaches a list of technical facts and sources. Though it should also be free of jargon, there is usually an extraordinarily large amount of information that must be conveyed to the reader.

Therefore, there is little room for detailed descriptions of statistical tests, rates, and so on. The methods section should mention:

- The demographic profile of the cohort or hypothetical cohort,
- The perspective of the study (if not mentioned in the introduction),
- The discount rate used,
- The year to which all costs were adjusted,
- All assumptions used in the analysis,
- Whether the model adhered to the reference case scenario recommended by the Panel on Cost-Effectiveness in Health and Medicine,
- The event pathway of your analysis,
- The sources used to obtain cost and effectiveness data, and
- The types of sensitivity analyses performed.

If you are using a hypothetical cohort, you should mention how the subjects from your data sources matched or deviated from your cohort. If differences existed, you should mention how the problem was addressed. In our analysis, it was not always possible to perfectly match data from electronic datasets to our cohort of healthy adults. For instance, we had to adjust the number of deaths we obtained from the CDC using information from Neuzil and others (1999) to reflect the number of deaths expected among healthy adults. We also had to adjust incidence rates and hospitalization rates for vaccination status.

Details such as the perspective of the analysis, the discount rate used, and the year to which all costs were adjusted can be fit into a single sentence. Likewise, the assumptions you used can be included in a table. Placing the assumptions in a table is convenient for a number of reasons. First, one of the nagging difficulties with writing a journal article is that the word count has to be kept within the journal's limits. By placing the assumptions in a table, they are not counted as words in the body text. Second, when the assumptions are listed in a table, the reader does not have to scan through the text to find them.

It is important to indicate whether your results include a reference case scenario (or whether the entire study is a reference case analysis). For example, some studies may assume an insurer's perspective, which is not compatible with the reference case scenario, but also present the results from a societal perspective. You should also indicate ways in which your results may have strayed from the reference case scenario. For instance, you may not have been able to capture an environmental cost that was likely to have been relevant.

The event pathway should be described and illustrated using a decision analysis model. Frequently, the decision analysis model will be too large to include in the analysis, and the event pathway will be too detailed to describe. If this is the case, be sure to highlight the key points of the pathway. If you generated the event pathway using clinical practice guidelines, you may wish to cite the guidelines you used.

The bulk of the methods section describes the sources of the cost and effectiveness data you used in your analysis. It should include descriptions of the ways in which you adjusted your data using secondary sources and formulas. It is convenient to structure the methods section into logical categories with subheadings such as "Event Pathway," "Cost Data," and so on.

Results

Like the methods section, the results section borders on being little more than a list of facts. The results section of a cost-effectiveness analysis should include the cost, effectiveness, and incremental cost-effectiveness (if the intervention is not cost-saving) of each intervention under study. It should also contain a presentation of the results of the sensitivity analysis.

Presenting the primary outcomes. There is a standard format for presenting the results of cost-effectiveness analyses in table form (see Table 11.1). Interventions are ranked in order from the least effective at the top of the table to the most effective at the bottom of the table. The incremental cost-effectiveness ratios are then sequentially calculated from top to bottom (Gold and others, 1996). Recall that this is the process we used to generate Table 9.8. Some decision analysis packages will generate a publication quality cost-effectiveness table for you.

TABLE 11.1.   COST-EFFECTIVENESS TABLE.

Row	Intervention	Total Cost A	Total Effectiveness B	Incremental Cost C	Incremental Effectiveness D	Cost- Effectiveness E
3 Percent discount						
1	Usual care	Cost of usual care	Total QALYs in usual care cohort	—	—	—
2	Intervention 2	(Cost of intervention) − (Savings from intervention)	Total QALYs in intervention cohort	A1 − A2	B1 − B2	C2/D2
3	Intervention 3	(Cost of intervention) − (Savings from intervention)	Total QALYs in intervention cohort	A2 − A3	B2 − B3	C3/D3
Undiscounted						
...						

In a cost-effectiveness table, interventions that are dominated (are both less effective and more costly than others) should not contain incremental cost-effectiveness ratios (Gold and others, 1996). Instead, the word "dominated" should appear where you would have placed the ratio. The table should be divided into two or three sections listing the results of the analysis at a 3 percent discount rate, undiscounted results, and (optionally) the results of the analysis at a 5 percent discount rate (Gold and others, 1996).

Presenting the results of the sensitivity analysis. The sensitivity analysis description should outline:

- The variables that exerted the most influence on the model,
- How these variables affected the dominance of each strategy,
- The results of bivariate analyses,
- How assumptions affected the model,
- The results of a sensitivity analysis on the discount rate,
- The results of statistical analyses, such as a Monte Carlo analysis, and
- Alternative questions of interest to policymakers. For instance, the vaccination study might include an analysis indicating different scenarios in which oseltamivir might be a reasonable option for unvaccinated persons.

Rather than use technical terms such as "tornado analysis," it is generally better to make descriptive statements. For example, in describing the influence of each variable, you might state, "The incidence of influenza-like illness, the cost of transportation, and the cost of caregiver support exerted the greatest influence over the relative cost and effectiveness of each intervention." This may be followed by a brief description of the one- and two-way sensitivity analyses that you performed on each of these variables. You should also describe how each assumption affected the relative dominance of each strategy in one-way sensitivity analyses.

Discussion

The discussion, as the name implies, provides an analysis of the overall study. Like the introduction section, the discussion section provides more leeway for descriptive prose and analysis. Generally, the researchers' thoughts on the interactions between variables and descriptions of the approaches used to collect or manipulate data should be described in the discussion section, rather than in the results section, because the discussion section is more geared toward analytical statements. This section is generally broken into a recap of the results, an analysis of the policy implications of the study, a discussion of the limitations of the study with an emphasis on the results of the sensitivity analyses you conducted, and a statement indicating the need for future research or for changes in current medical practice or public health policy.

After briefly highlighting the results, it is generally a good idea to discuss the policy implications of the study prior to mentioning the limitations of the study. Policy implications might include a review of the ethical dimensions of the dominant intervention and the ways in which the intervention might differentially affect low-income groups or racially defined groups. The limitations section should comment on the robustness of the model when tested for uncertainty and should discuss how different assumptions might affect the relative priority assigned to each strategy. The limitations of the data sources and the model design should also be discussed. The discussion section should end with a brief statement on the ways in which the research might be improved had more data been available or, if the results are felt to be conclusive, recommendations for implementing the results of your study.

The Technical Appendix

It is somewhat more difficult to effectively communicate the results of a cost-effectiveness analysis than it is to present the methods and results of a longitudinal study, so extra care must be taken to ensure that all of the relevant issues are addressed while the less important aspects of the analysis are left out. Still, most of the nuances of the cost-effectiveness cannot adequately be described within the word count limitations of most journals.

By including a technical appendix, the researcher will be able to present to the reviewer each and every assumption, each piece of data used, and all of the mundane details of the sensitivity analyses performed. The reference case recommends that the pathway of different events in the decision analysis model be described (including changes in the HRQL in each pathway). It is generally better to include this level of detail in the technical appendix, but some journals may not accept such supplementary materials. In this case, it is generally acceptable to provide the technical document on the Internet, so that all readers can have access to the details of the analysis if they so desire.

Publishing Your Research

In this section, we will briefly describe the process of publishing an article in a **peer-reviewed** journal and will provide tips for submitting an article to a journal. A peer-reviewed journal is a journal that verifies the quality and content of an original research article by sending the articles it publishes to experts in the field(s) the article addresses. When editors receive an article, they initially evaluate it for its importance, content, and quality. If the article is judged to be of sufficient interest to the journal's readership to merit further consideration, and it is judged to be scientifically sound, it is sent for peer review. Usually, two to four experts will then review the article and comment on its shortcomings, with the hope that the researcher will heed their recommendations and improve the analysis. They will also provide separate comments to the editor indicating their impressions of the article's relative importance in their field(s) of interest, as well as their impression of whether the study merits publication in that particular journal.

The editor will then reject the article based on the reviewers' comments, accept it with the provision that the authors address the reviewers' comments, or accept the article for publication. Usually, rejected manuscripts end up in the recycle bin in the editor's office, so be sure to request that professionally constructed graphs are duplicated prior to submission and always make a specific request in the cover letter of the article that the journal return such graphs.

What Editors Want

Cost-effectiveness analyses require the construction of complex decision analysis models, utilize multiple sources of data, and include a number of different assumptions. When publishing an article in the medical literature, all of this information must be clearly and concisely stated between the introduction to the problem and a discussion of the analysis. Editors are interested in ensuring that all of this information is clearly conveyed while meeting the word limits of the journal, that the article is relevant to the interests of their audience, and that the article will make a splash, or at least a small ripple, in the scientific pond of knowledge.

Editors are also impressed by well-packaged articles. Each journal has its own style and submissions requirements. By adhering to a journal's style, you are communicating that you have carefully considered the journal you are submitting to. You are also communicating that you are careful with details, which is an important personality trait for researchers to have. By attending to both the content and the form of your article, you will likely improve your chances of publication.

Content of the article. Editors will want the study to be presented in plain English, with little medical or economic jargon. The audience of medical journals is usually broad, and it includes clinicians, policymakers, journalists, public health professionals, and health managers. Many of these people will not be familiar with terms like "incremental cost-effectiveness." One of the many jobs of the editor, therefore, is to make certain that the study will be accessible to the journal's readership.

The first thing that any reader will see is the title, so it is important to ensure that the title conveys the nature of the analysis. The best place to turn for an adequate title is your research question. If the title concisely captures most or all of the elements of your research question, you will have captured the attention of both the editor and the ultimate readers at the outset. Recall from Chapter Two that the research question addresses what the analysis is, to whom it is targeted, and where it is applicable. Though U.S.-centric journals do not generally require that the country be mentioned in the title of the article, this is a must for international journals, because the results of a cost-effectiveness analysis are generally only applicable to one country.

Editors prefer to put their energy into articles that they believe will benefit their journal and their readership. If you can convey that the article is likely to be cited in the medical literature or the press, you may increase your odds of getting published. One of the best ways to sell an article to an editor is to open the paper with an impact statement. This is a well-argued and well-supported sentence or two describing the severity of the problem that the study addresses. The introduction should also include a sentence or two indicating the need for your analysis. The remainder of the introduction should be based upon these opening lines. A paper with a well-written, concise, and pointed introduction may determine whether your article is distributed to reviewers or tossed in the recycling bin.

It is also generally helpful to try to sell the article. For instance, in the cover letter that accompanies your article you might include an honest assessment of the implications of your study for the scientific community and perhaps an assessment of the potential interest the journal's readership might have in the study. At a minimum, this will show the editors that you chose their journal carefully. On the other hand, most editors are likely to be aware of the implications of an analysis on its face value and will not want to read through a lengthy cover letter, so be certain to summarize the implications of your analysis using no more than a few sentences.

It is equally important that you do not oversell your article. One team of researchers generated a good deal of negative press when they hyped up the impact and the results of their analysis (see Exhibit 11.1).

Form of the article. Editors are also concerned with the length, format, and general presentation of the document. One easy way to win points with an editor is to ensure that the paper conforms to that journal's style requirements. These requirements can be found at the journal's homepage on the Internet (see Table 11.2) or in the journal itself (usually, the style requirements are published in one issue of the journal each year). It is also important that the article fit within the journal's length requirements and contain a word count on the title page. Attention to these little details can make the difference between an article that is sent to reviewers and one that is rejected outright.

EXHIBIT 11.1.   WATCH THOSE RESULTS.

In their article appearing in the *New England Journal of Medicine,* Shulman and others (1999) examined the impact of gender and racial bias on a physician's recommendations for cardiac catheterization. In their study, they implied that women and African-Americans are much less likely to receive a costly diagnostic screening intervention than are men or whites. Though cardiac catheterization is a frequent event, they reported their results as odds ratios rather than as adjusted risk ratios (see Chapter Five), giving the impression that the problem was much more serious than it was. Though only African-American women had lower rates of referral for cardiac catheterization, the authors aggregated the data so that it seemed as if all women and all African-Americans were impacted by what appeared to be racial and gender discrimination on the part of physicians. The study was widely reported in the media, including ABC's *Nightline,* the nightly news, and the *New York Times.* The journal quickly published an editorial explaining where the authors went wrong in presenting the results of their study.

TABLE 11.2.   INTERNET ADDRESSES FOR SELECTED MEDICAL JOURNALS.

The New England Journal of Medicine. http://www.nejm.org.

The Journal of the American Medical Association. http://www.jama.com.

The Annals of Internal Medicine. http://www.acponline.org/journals/annals.

The American Journal of Public Health. http://www.apha.org/journal/AJPH2.htm.

Medical Care. http://www.medicalcare.org.

Medical Decision Making. http://www.hanleyandbelfus.com/journals/mdm.html.

American Journal of Preventive Medicine. http://www.elseiver.com.

Preventive Medicine. http://www.academicpress.com/pm.

With the exception of policy journals, most journals adhere to the Uniform Requirements for Manuscripts Submitted to Biomedical Journals available at: http://www.nejm.org/general/text/requirements/1.htm. These requirements dictate the format of bibliographic citations, text format, and other essentials of manuscript writing.

Finally, the overall presentation of your article is important. Editors prefer, and often require, a generic double-spaced manuscript over a manuscript with fancy fonts or formatting. Researchers should put all of their creative energy into producing high-quality graphs and tables rather than fancy text formatting.

Tips and tricks. Most decision analysis programs do not produce publication quality graphs; however, many programs allow the user to export the information used to build a chart into a spreadsheet program, such as Excel (Microsoft Inc.), a charting program, such as SPSS Graph (SPSS Inc.), or an illustration program, such as Adobe Illustrator (Adobe Systems Inc.).

When to call. There is little point in calling an editor that has rejected your manuscript outright. Editors tend to be busy people and will just become annoyed by persistent authors. Not only is the probability of success extremely low, but the editor may remember your name the next time you wish to submit to that journal.

On the other hand, an article that has been rejected after it has been peer-reviewed stands a much better chance of reconsideration. In this instance, the editor may feel more invested in the paper and may be willing to give it further consideration. Though most rejection letters kindly imply that the researcher should not call, researchers will occasionally have success in politely convincing an editor that the paper merits a second round of peer review. If you choose to ask an editor to reconsider an article, you should present the editor with very concrete reasons for why it should be reconsidered. For example, the reviewers may have misinterpreted the methods you used or did not understand the principles underlying cost-effectiveness analysis. In general, though, it is best to simply move onto the next best journal for your study.

Choosing the Appropriate Journal

Once the analysis is complete, the first step in deciding how to put the pieces together in prose is to decide which type of journal you are aiming for. The type of journal that you aim for will determine how much material you can fit into the article and will guide you in the way that it is written.

Journals that accept cost-effectiveness analyses generally fall into four classes: 1) public health journals, 2) policy journals, 3) clinical journals, and 4) methodological journals. The format, word limit, table limits, and content tend to be similar within these broader classifications, but there are no absolute rules.

The audience of your study should be the primary determinant of the type of journal you choose. You will want to communicate the results of your study to the parties that are most likely to have a stake in them. Moreover, the first thing an editor will consider is whether the research question is appropriate for the audience of his or her journal. Most papers that are rejected outright are rejected because the editor does not feel that the study fits the journal's theme or feels that the topic would not be of interest to the journal's readership. The following points should be considered when choosing a journal:

- If the study addresses a general policy question relevant to government agencies, academics, or institutions, a public health journal or policy journal may be most appropriate. Examples include analyses that recommend changes in the way health services are delivered, or evaluations of interventions that are delivered on a broad scale. Medical practitioners would not be very interested in whether folate should be added to cereal grains, but government agencies would. Because studies that are broad in scope tend to be technically complex, public health journals and policy journals tend to have higher word limits than other journals. However, policy journals tend to be less methodologically rigorous than general public health journals, and they may not always be appropriate for complex cost-effectiveness analyses. The format of policy journals often differs from that of other journals, so changing your target from a policy journal to a public health journal often requires reformatting the article.

- If the study evaluates a medical treatment or laboratory test, clinical journals may be most appropriate. Clinicians are predominantly interested in evaluations that will change the way they practice or will provide them with new clinical information. These journals tend to have lower word count limits than public health or policy journals. Because they must be short in length, cost-effectiveness analyses submitted to these journals should contain a technical appendix intended for reviewers only.
- If the study evaluates a preventive intervention, a public health journal or a clinical journal will be appropriate. Journals such as *Preventive Medicine* or *The American Journal of Preventive Medicine* are excellent venues for publishing cost-effectiveness analyses that examine clinical preventive strategies.
- If the study examines a problem specific to cost-effectiveness analysis or evaluates a novel way of conducting a study, a methods journal is probably most appropriate.

There are a number of Web sites that list the major journals by content area. For example, the online search engine PubMed (http://www.ncbi.nlm.nih.gov/entrez/query.fcgi) also allows search criteria by journal type.

CHAPTER TWELVE

ADVANCED CONCEPTS

Overview

Now you have completed a cost-effectiveness analysis! Most of the skills you have learned are applicable to any of the cost-effectiveness analyses you will later perform. However, there are a number of important issues in cost-effectiveness that were not illustrated by the influenza example. The primary difference between the influenza example and analyses that examine medical interventions geared toward preventing or treating illnesses of longer duration is that they require more complex decision analysis models.

In this chapter, we will cover:

- Advanced topics in risk measurement,
- Advanced topics in conditional probabilities,
- How to work with life tables, and
- How Markov models work.

Working with Measures of Risk

Cost-effectiveness analysis often requires researchers to calculate the amount of risk that is attributed to a particular risk factor. In Chapter Three, we learned that a risk ratio indicates the risk associated with an event in simple terms. For example, the risk ratio for lung cancer among smokers, 9.0, indicates that the risk of lung cancer among smokers is nine times higher than it is among non-smokers (Doll and Hill, 1956). In Chapter Five, we were also introduced to a measure for calculating the absolute differences in risk using the attributable risk, which takes the form:

$$\text{attributable risk} = \text{incidence}_{\text{risk factor}} - \text{incidence}_{\text{no risk factor}}$$
Equation 5.8

For example, if the incidence of influenza virus infections were 12 cases per 100 persons in smokers and 10 cases per 100 persons in non-smokers, then the attributable risk indicates that 12 cases per 100 persons − 10 cases per 100 persons = 2 cases of influenza in every 100 can be attributed to smoking.

Applications of risk ratios. Recall that the risk ratio indicates the risk of disease among people with a risk factor relative to people without that risk factor. For this reason, the risk ratio is often called the relative risk. In Chapter Three, we learned that the formula for relative risk takes the form:

$$\text{risk ratio} = \text{risk}_{\text{risk factor}} / \text{risk}_{\text{no risk factor}}$$
Equation 3.5

Because the incidence rate is generally equal to the risk of developing disease, the formula can also take the form:

$$\text{risk ratio} = \text{incidence}_{\text{risk factor}} / \text{incidence}_{\text{no risk factor}}$$
Equation 3.4

Risk ratios and attributable risk equations have many practical uses in cost-effectiveness analysis. For instance, when a risk ratio is expressed as a fraction, it can be used to calculate efficacy or to assign a probability to an event in a decision analysis model. For instance, the risk ratio for developing influenza-like illness if vaccinated can be expressed as:

$$\text{risk ratio} = \text{risk}_{\text{vaccinated}} / \text{risk}_{\text{unvaccinated}}$$
Equation 3.6

and the efficacy of the influenza vaccine is:

$$\text{efficacy} = 1 - \text{risk}_{\text{vaccinated}} / \text{risk}_{\text{unvaccinated}}$$
Equation 5.5

In Table 5.3, we calculated the efficacy of the influenza vaccine at preventing influenza-like illness (0.4). The relative risk of influenza-like illness among vaccinated people, $1 - 0.4 = 0.6$, was used in Chapter Nine to determine the proportionate change in HRQL among vaccinated persons relative to all persons. We also used the relative risk of hospitalization among people who are vaccinated against the influenza virus to calculate the probability of hospitalization in our decision analysis model in Chapter Seven (see Equation 7.8).

To determine the converse risk, the risk ratio is simply divided into 1.0. For example, the risk of influenza-like illness among unvaccinated persons is $1/0.6 = 1.67$.

Attributable risk proportion in the exposed. Let us explore some of the other measures of risk sometimes used in cost-effectiveness analysis. Imagine that you have constructed a decision analysis model that requires inputs specific to the risk of lung cancer attributable to smoking among smokers (see Figure 12.1). In this model, the probability of developing lung cancer (pDzSmoke) is a conditional probability; it must reflect the chance that people developed the disease because they smoked.

To determine the value of pDzSmoke, we would need to know the **attributable risk proportion in the exposed,** which takes the form:

$$\text{AR proportion}_{\text{exposed}} = \frac{\text{risk with risk factor} - \text{risk without factor}}{\text{risk with risk factor}} = \frac{(\text{RR} - 1)}{\text{RR}}$$

Equation 12.1

FIGURE 12.1.   DECISION ANALYSIS TREE EVALUATING A HYPOTHETICAL SMOKING CESSATION PROGRAM.

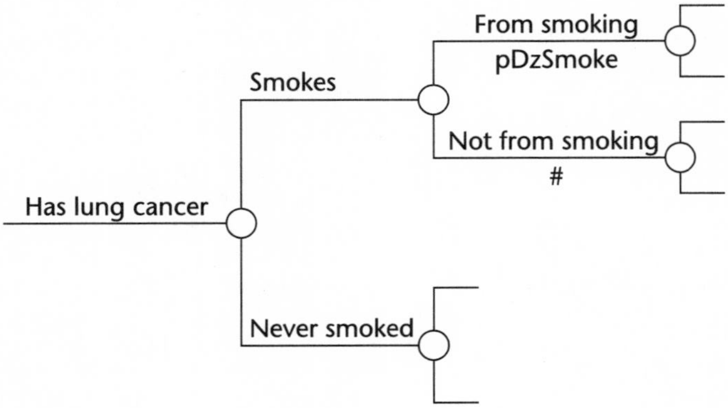

Here, we see that the risk ratio (RR) may be substituted for the direct measurement of the risk in the numerator of the equation. In the introduction to this section, we mentioned that the risk ratio for lung cancer is approximately 9.0, indicating that smokers are nine times as likely to develop lung cancer as nonsmokers. Applying Equation 12.1, we see that the attributable risk proportion in the exposed is $(9 - 1)/9 = 0.889$.

Population attributable risk proportion. Another measure that is sometimes used in large-scale public health interventions is the **population attributable risk proportion.** Imagine that you are a public health official in a developing country, and you must decide whether to spend your limited resources on a local water treatment facility or on providing all clinics in the country with oral rehydration solution and antibiotics. Although both of these interventions will reduce mortality from diarrhea, they are associated with a different efficacy and affect different populations.

On one hand, the water treatment plant will produce large benefits, but it can only be implemented within one geographic region in the country. On the other hand, the oral rehydration solution and antibiotics will reduce mortality from diarrhea nationwide, but they will be much less effective at reducing mortality on a case-by-case basis than the water treatment plant. In this instance, you will want to know whether the water treatment plant will result in a large enough improvement in the geographically limited region that the plant serves to justify depriving the remainder of the country of the benefits of oral diarrhea treatments.

The population attributable risk proportion will tell you the proportion of the total risk of death that is due to diarrhea *among the general population* that is attributable to a risk factor (lack of potable water or lack of access to oral rehydration solution).

The population attributable proportion is calculated as follows:

$$\text{population attributable risk proportion} = \frac{\text{total risk in population} - \text{risk without factor}}{\text{total risk in population}}$$

Equation 12.2

Bayes' Theorem

Bayes was an English clergyman who, like many clergymen before and after him, spent a good deal of time contemplating the meaning of life. Bayes was interested in conditional probabilities, or the chance that one event would occur (for example, hospitalization) given the occurrence of another event (for example, developing a secondary illness). As we saw in Chapter Five, decision analysis models usually require that probabilities placed further down on branches reflect changes in events closer to the decision node. For example, in each branch of the decision analysis tree we constructed in our sample cost-effectiveness analysis, we saw that the probability of a medical visit was modified by the chance that a patient would become ill.

Bayes' theorem is especially useful when conducting cost-effectiveness analyses that either evaluate laboratory tests as the intervention under study or include them when the presence of disease must be confirmed using tests.

Using Bayes' theorem to evaluate screening tests. Recall that the sensitivity of a test refers to the ability of a test to detect a disease *when it is present.* Therefore, the sensitivity of a test will only tell you how many times the test will correctly diagnose a case of disease when the test is administered to a group of people that actually have the disease. Likewise, the specificity of a screening test only tells us the probability that a test will correctly detect the absence of disease when it is administered a group of people without the disease.

But what happens when a test is applied to a group of people who may or may not have the disease we are interested in evaluating? In cost-effectiveness analysis, we will often need to know the proportion of subjects in a hypothetical cohort that a test will correctly identify with a disease (true positives) and without a disease (true negatives). We will also often need to know the proportion of subjects that will be misdiagnosed as having the disease (false positives) and the proportion of subjects with the disease who will test negative (false negatives). Unfortunately, we will usually only be able to obtain data on the sensitivity and the specificity of a screening test from the medical literature (or from the manufacturer of the test).

This is where Bayes saves the day. His formula allows us to predict the probability of disease among people who have a positive test result, so long as we know how many people in the population have the disease (the disease prevalence), the sensitivity of the screening test, and the specificity of the screening test.

The general formula for the positive predictive value of a screening test is:

$$\text{positive predictive value} = \frac{\text{true positive results}}{(\text{true positive results} + \text{false positive results})}$$

Equation 12.3

Using Bayes' theorem, we may derive the same values from the prevalence ratio, the sensitivity of a screening test, and the specificity of a screening test:

$$\text{positive predictive value} = \frac{\text{sensitivity} \cdot \text{prevalence}}{((\text{sensitivity} \cdot \text{prevalence}) + (1 - \text{specificity}) \cdot (1 - \text{prevalence}))}$$

Equation 12.4

Let us see how this information might be incorporated into a decision analysis model that incorporates conditional probabilities. If a woman is tested for breast cancer with a mammogram and is correctly diagnosed, she may be cured of the cancer. On the other hand, if she does not have breast cancer, but the test is positive, she may receive unnecessary surgery. Let us design a decision analysis model that will calculate the chances that a woman will have a true positive, false positive, true negative, or false negative mammogram (see Figure 12.2).

The chance that a woman will have a positive test result is represented by the variable pPositive. This variable is equal to:

$$\underset{\text{(number of true positives)}}{\text{sensitivity} \cdot \text{prevalence}} + \underset{\text{(number of false positives)}}{(1 - \text{specificity}) \cdot (1 - \text{prevalence})}$$

Equation 12.5

The variable pTP (or the probability that the positive test result is a true positive) is simply the proportion of all true positive test results over the proportion of all positive test results (the positive predictive value of the screening test). Of course, since we will not have this information, we shall have to enter Equation 2.4 into the decision analysis model instead. Thus, we see that Bayes' theorem allows us to assign a value to a conditional probability occurring anywhere in a decision analysis tree.

FIGURE 12.2. DECISION ANALYSIS TREE EVALUATING SCREENING MAMMOGRAPHY.

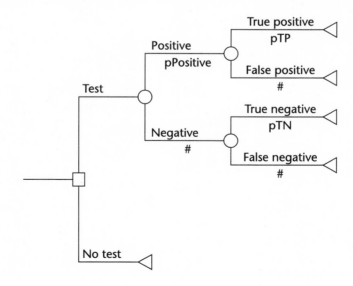

Other applications of Bayes' theorem. Bayes' theorem can also be used to assess the effectiveness of a screening program that is conducted on a periodic basis in a population. Suppose that we wanted to conduct cholesterol screening in a community with the hope of identifying people with hypercholesterolemia (high cholesterol). Not all of the people who have a high cholesterol test result will actually have chronically elevated cholesterol levels (in other words, some test results may be falsely elevated). Therefore, before conducting the test we should apply Bayes' theorem to determine the positive predictive value of the screening test. If the test is 85 percent sensitive and 95 percent specific, and the prevalence of disease is 10 percent, we obtain:

$$\text{postive predictive value} = \frac{0.85 \cdot 0.1}{(0.85 \cdot 0.1 + (1 - 0.95 \cdot 1 - 0.1))} = 0.65$$

We therefore now know that approximately 65 percent of people with positive test results will actually have hypercholesterolemia. Based on this information, we think the screening program will be worthwhile and decide to proceed. Suppose that thousands of people show up to receive the test in the first year that it is offered, and we are thanked by the people who were tested positive; most of these people are now receiving follow-up care with their physicians and have started rigorous diet and exercise programs. Because the first year of the program was a great success, we decide to reapply the screening test to the community a year later.

During the second year of our screening program, we make sure that none of the people who were already diagnosed with the condition are retested. Because we have removed many of the prevalent cases of hypercholesterolemia from the population, we will need to recalculate the positive predictive value of our screening test. (In other words, the prevalence of the condition in the remaining undiagnosed population will be lower the second time around, so there will be fewer cases to detect).

Of those who were not diagnosed with elevated cholesterol levels during the first year, some would have had a false negative test result (would actually have had elevated cholesterol levels). The proportion of false negatives during the first year would be equal to the disease prevalence $\cdot$ (1 − sensitivity) = 0.1 $\cdot$ 0.15 = 0.015 or 1.5 percent of all of those tested. The remainder of people in whom we might diagnose high blood cholesterol would have had to develop the condition over the last year.

If we knew the incidence rate of high blood cholesterol to be one case per 1,000 persons, then our prevalence is now 0.1 percent + 1.5 percent = 1.6 percent (0.016). The positive predictive value of the test has been reduced to 0.22 (22 percent), and the cost-effectiveness of the screening intervention has been dramatically reduced.

These types of calculations play an important role when a cost-effectiveness analysis analyzes the cost and benefits of repeated screening, such as annual mammography, in a population.

Generating Life Tables

In this section, we will learn how to calculate quality-adjusted life expectancy (QALE) using two methods. In the first method, you will learn how to calculate QALE using published sources of data by rebuilding the abridged life tables that are produced on an annual basis by the National Center for Health Statistics. These life tables will be quality adjusted using data from the National Health Interview Survey (NHIS), mortality data, and other published data tabulations (Adams and others, 1996; Anderson, 1999; Erickson and others, 1995). In the second exercise, you will learn how to generate a quality-adjusted life table using electronic mortality data or data from randomized controlled trials.

Though you will not need advanced mathematical or statistical skills to construct a life table using published mortality rates and existing life tables, constructing a life table using electronic data can be a laborious task. Therefore, we only recommend that students who are familiar with statistical software packages and electronic data attempt to construct a life table using this method.

Recall from Chapter Nine that the quality-adjusted life expectancy (QALE) is the product of the average HRQL of a cohort and the life expectancy of that cohort. The general formula for calculating the number of QALYs gained by an intervention is:

$$\text{QALYs gained} = \text{QALE}_{\text{intervention}} - \text{QALE}_{\text{no intervention}}$$
$$\text{Equation 9.1}$$

Suppose that we are interested in knowing the cost-effectiveness of a hypothetical new drug used to prevent stroke in people over the age of sixty-five, Stroke-ex, which has been shown to reduce mortality from stroke by preventing clots from forming in the arteries that feed the brain. Suppose that Stroke-ex is safe and inexpensive, and that this medication provides a 25 percent reduction in stroke (is associated with a risk ratio of 0.75 for stroke) among people over the age of sixty-five. Suppose further that this percentage represents a reduction in the lifetime risk of stroke, rather than the risk over some defined period. We might evaluate stroke-ex's use as a preventive therapy to reduce the incidence rate of stroke in the general population aged sixty-five and over.

As part of our analysis, we will need to calculate the total number of QALYs gained because of our intervention. Our first job, therefore, is to estimate the

QALE for all persons in 1997 ($QALE_{no\ intervention}$) and the QALE for the cohort that receives Stroke-ex every day ($QALE_{intervention}$). To do this, we must generate two abridged life tables, one representing the QALE of the general United States population and another representing a population that has been treated with Stroke-ex. If we subtract $QALE_{intervention}$ from $QALE_{no\ intervention}$, we will obtain the number of QALYs gained by that intervention. The first abridged life table will contain death rates and mean HRQL scores for all diseases. The second life table will also contain death rates and HRQL scores for all diseases, but it will reflect the reduced incidence rate of stroke due to Stroke-ex and the subsequent improvement in HRQL.

An abridged life table is constructed using a hypothetical population in which 100,000 persons are born each year. It is assumed that all persons in this cohort are at risk of dying or becoming ill, but that there is no migration into or out of the population. In other words, this is a "stationary population" because the hypothetical subjects are just sitting around, waiting to die.

Calculating QALE Using Published Data

To construct our life table using published tabular data, we must first obtain all-cause and cause-specific mortality data (http://www.cdc.gov/nchs/data/nvs47_19.pdf) and prevalence data for stroke (http://www.cdc.gov/nchs/data/10_200_1.pdf). Unfortunately, these printed tabulations of data use slightly different age intervals. Because the age intervals in our analysis must be the same across prevalence, mortality, and health-related quality of life (HRQL) data, we must find age intervals that are common to all three sources of data. When a life table is available in print, the process of generating a new life table is simple, because the total number of deaths in each age interval has already been calculated for us. As we proceed through these exercises, refer to the life tables in Appendix V.

Calculating $QALE_{no\ intervention}$. When using estimates of disease prevalence published by the National Center for Health Statistics (NCHS), we must use the four age intervals presented in Table 12.1, because these are the only age intervals common to both the mortality data and the prevalence data (Muennig and Gold, 2001). It is also necessary to adjust all rates to per capita parameters (the mortality rate, which is expressed as deaths per 100,000 persons, must be divided by 100,000, and the prevalence rate, which is expressed as the number of cases of disease per 1,000 persons, must be divided by 1,000).

Step 1. To begin, add the number of deaths due to all causes for persons aged zero to forty-five in the abridged life table and enter them in the first cell of Column 3 as in Table 12.1. (This is listed as "number dying during

TABLE 12.1. FIRST THREE COLUMNS OF A QUALITY-ADJUSTED LIFE TABLE.

	1		2		3
Age Interval	*Probability of Death in Interval*		*Number Alive at Beginning of Interval*		*Persons Dying During Interval*
	Step 5. ⇩ Enter rate	**Step 4.** Divide values	**Step 2.** ⇩ Enter the number 100,000 in 1st cell	**Step 3.** Subtract values in Column 3 from Column 2 and enter value in next Column 3 Row	**Step 1.** ⇨ Fill in number of deaths
				100,000 − 5,004 ⇩ = 94,996	
0–45	0.0500	⇦5,004/100,000	100,000		5,004
45–64	0.1420	⇦13,486/94,996	94,996⇦		13,486
65–74	0.2251		81,510		18,348
75+	1		63,162		63,162

age interval" in NCHS publications). Next, complete the remainder of the row values for Column 3 in the same way.

Step 2. An abridged life table cohort begins with 100,000 persons (Anderson, 1999). Enter this number as the value for the first row of Column 2.

Step 3. The number of persons alive in the subsequent age interval is simply the number of persons alive in the previous interval, less the number of persons who died. For the forty-five to sixty-four-year age group, this is $100,000 - 5,004 = 94,996$. This process is repeated until all the row values for Column 2 are completely filled out.

Step 4. Values in Column 1 are calculated by dividing values for Column 3 by values for Column 2.

Step 5. Enter the values from **Step 4** into Column 1. For example, the value in the first row of Column 1 is $5,004/100,000 = 0.05$.

Step 6. Now, let us fill in values for Column 4 (see Table 12.2). Column 4 is the number of **person-years** in the interval. One person-year represents one year of life lived per subject (Anderson, 1999). If the interval is twenty years in length, a person who survived to the next age interval would add twenty person-years, while a person who died at the midpoint of the interval would add ten person-years.

For the moment, let us forget about the <45 age group in the first row of Column 4 in Table 12.2, as well as the 75+ age group in the final row, and

TABLE 12.2.   CALCULATING THE TOTAL NUMBER OF PERSON-YEARS IN THE LIFE TABLE COHORT.

Age Interval	Interval Length (Years)	2 Number Alive at Beginning of Interval	3 Persons Dying During Interval	Step 6. Multiply the Length of The Interval by (Column 2 − 0.5 · Column 3)	4 Person-Years in Interval
<45	—	100,000	5,004		
45–64	20	94,996	13,486	$20 \cdot 94,996 - 13,486 \cdot 0.5 \Rightarrow$	1,765,060
65–74	10	81,510	18,348		723,360
75+	—	63,162	63,162		707,414

Note: Column 1 has been left out for brevity.

fill in all other values. Column 4 row values represent the total number of person-years in the interval and are calculated using the formula:

$$\text{interval length} \cdot (\text{number alive at beginning of interval} - 0.5 \cdot \text{number dying})$$

Equation 12.6

This formula assumes that all deaths occurred at the midpoint of the interval. Thus, because the second interval is 20 years long, those people who died in this age interval only added $0.5 \cdot 20 = 10$ years each. This assumption does not hold for the first year of life, because of infant mortality, or the final interval, because we do not know how long this interval is. Since birth is the riskiest time for a baby, the bulk of infant deaths tend to occur much closer to birth than to the midpoint of the age interval. This assumption is also not valid for the last age interval (75+ years of age), because the interval is of indeterminate length—some subjects will die right away, and a few subjects might make it all the way to 110 years of age.

Step 7. Now let us calculate the person-years in the first age interval, which is forty-five years in length. To obtain the total number of person-years in this age interval, calculate the person-years in the one- to forty-five-year interval (which is forty-four years in length and can be calculated using Equation 12.6). Next, add this number to the number of person-years in the zero to one age interval, which can be copied directly from an existing life table (see Table 12.3). The total number of person-years in the first interval is thus $99,371 + 4,366,048 = 4,465,419$.

TABLE 12.3.   CALCULATING THE TOTAL NUMBER OF PERSON-YEARS IN THE FIRST AGE INTERVAL.

Age Interval	2 *Number Alive at Beginning of Interval*	3 *Persons Dying During Interval*	*Step 7. Copy # of Person-Years for 0–1 Interval from a Life Table. Add this Value to the Person Years in the 1–45 Interval*	4 *Person-Years in Interval*
<45	100,000	5,004		
0 to 1	100,000	723	From life table ⇨	99,371
1 to 45	99,277	4,281	$44 \cdot 99,277 - 4281 \cdot 0.5$ ⇨	4,366,048

Step 8. Now let us calculate the number of person-years in the final age interval and complete Column 4 values (not shown). The total person-years in the final age interval (seventy-five or more years of age) is calculated as the product of the number living at the beginning of the interval and the life expectancy at the beginning of the age interval (each is readily obtained from the existing life table we are using). This can also be calculated from an existing life table by summing all of the person-year values from seventy-five on.

Step 9. To calculate Column 5 values, simply sum the person-years in Column 4 backwards (see Table 12.4). For example, the cumulative person-years for the 65–74 age interval is equal to the sum of the 65–75 row value of Column 4 and the 75+ row value of Column 4.

Step 10. Each row in Column 6 is calculated by dividing the row value of Column 5 by the corresponding row value for Column 2. If there are 7.66 million person-years from birth to death in a cohort of 100,000 people, the life expectancy is 7.66 million person-years/100,000 persons or simply, 76.6 years (see Table 12.5). Here, we see that the life expectancy at 75+ years of age is 707,414/63,162 = 11.2 years. The value of the first row in Column 6 is equal to the life expectancy at birth of the cohort, and it serves to validate the spreadsheet (this should be equal to the life expectancy obtained from the NCHS table).

Step 11. The values in Column 7 represent the health-related quality of life score for the average person in each corresponding age interval. These values can be obtained from a QALE table (see Appendix V). Be certain to use weighted mean values for HRQL scores. The values can be weighted using the number of person-years in each age interval and Equation 3.4.

TABLE 12.4.　CALCULATING CUMULATIVE PERSON-YEARS.

	2	3	4	Step 9. Sum the Person-Years from Column 4 Starting with the 75+ Age Interval	5
Age Interval	Number Alive at Beginning of Interval	Persons Dying During Interval	Person-Years in Interval		Cumulative Person-years
<45	100,000	5,004	4,465,419		7,661,253
45–64	94,996	13,486	1,765,060		3,195,834
65–74	81,510	18,348	723,360	Summed ⇨	1,430,774
75+	63,162	63,162	+707,414		707,414

TABLE 12.5. COMPLETE QUALITY-ADJUSTED LIFE TABLE.

	1	2	3	4	5	6	7	8	9	10
Age Interval	Prob. of Death in Interval	# At Beginning of Age Interval	# Dying During Interval	Person-Years in Interval	Total Person-Years	Life Expectancy	HRQL	QALYs	Total QALYs	QALE
<45	0.0500	100,000	5,004	4,465,419	7,661,253	76.6	0.91	4,074,604	6,504,173	65.04
45–64	0.1420	94,996	13,486	1,765,060	3,195,834	33.6	0.82	1,445,507	2,429,570	25.6
65–74	0.2251	81,510	18,348	723,360	1,430,774	17.6	0.75	543,005	984,063	12.1
75+	1	63,162	63,162	707,414	707,414	11.2	0.62	441,058	441,058	7.0

Step 12. Now let us finish the table. Column 8 values are equal to the product of corresponding Column 7 and Column 4 row values. (We performed these calculations in Chapter Nine.) Columns 9 and 10 are derived in the same way we calculated Columns 4 and 5 (see Step 9). For example, the Column 9 value for the <45 age group is equal to the sum of all Column 8 values. The corresponding Column 10 value is equal to the <45 row value in Column 9 divided by the <45 value for Column 2.

Calculating QALE$_{intervention}$. Now, we must calculate the QALE for the cohort receiving Stroke-ex. The life table for QALE in the intervention group is constructed in the same way as the QALE$_{no\ intervention}$ life table cohort; however, the probability of death and quality of life values must be adjusted to reflect the effects of Stroke-ex on the cohort.

In Column 1 of Table 12.5, the probability of death in the interval due to the disease under study (in this case, stroke) must be reduced using the risk ratio for stroke in people treated with the new drug (0.75). We must also adjust the mean HRQL score in Column 8 of Table 12.5 to reflect that of a cohort with a lower incidence rate of stroke; we do this by using the risk ratio for the disease and the prevalence of stroke in the general population. Because the construction of our QALE$_{no\ intervention}$ life table mostly involves copying values from other sources, we will not highlight the step-by-step process in the life table we generate. Instead, we will include a row mentioning the source of the data.

Step 1. To begin, we must obtain the predicted reduction in the total number of deaths due to stroke in the general population, as well as the subsequent gain in the total number of person-years in our cohort. (When a death due to a particular disease is prevented, the subject will go on to die of some other cause.)

Table 11 in the NCHS mortality report (*Deaths: Final Data for 1997*) indicates the number of deaths due to cerebrovascular disease (stroke) (ICD-9 code 430-438). To calculate the gain in person-years with the new therapy (see Table 12.6), we first enter the age-specific death rate due to stroke (Column 1). The table begins at age sixty-five because our intervention will only be applied to people over the age of sixty-five. Notice that the published age intervals for cause-specific death rates are different than the age intervals we used to generate our QALE$_{no\ intervention}$ table. We must therefore extend the age interval out another ten years, terminating in the eighty-five-and-over age interval.

Step 2. We then enter the total number of deaths due to all causes in each age interval (Column 2). These values are copied directly from a published life table.

TABLE 12.6. DEATHS, PREDICTED REDUCTION IN DEATHS, AND ADJUSTED LIFE EXPECTANCY FOR PERSONS TREATED WITH NEW DRUG.

	1	2	3	4	5	6	7	8	9	10	11
	Death Rate Due to Stroke	Number of Deaths	Person-Years in Interval	Life Expectancy in Interval	Treatment Efficacy	Number of Deaths Prevented	Person-Years Gained	Number at Beginning of Interval	Total Person-Years	Cumulative Person-Years	Adjusted Life Expectancy
Source	Mortality table	Life table	Life table	Life table	$1 - RR$	$C1 \cdot C3 \cdot C5$	$C4 \cdot C6$	See text	$C3 + C7$	C9 Summed backwards	$C10/C7$
65–74	0.000309	18,348	732,561	17.7	0.25	56.6	1,001.6	81,510	733,563	1,444,700	17.72
75–84	0.000721	28,940	495,484	11.2	0.25	89.3	1,000.3	63,219	496,484	711,138	11.25
85+	0.001249	34,221	214,232	6.3	0.25	66.9	421.4	34,368	214,653	214,653	6.25

Step 3. Next, enter the person-years in the interval (Column 3). These may also be copied directly from a published life table. Recall from Step 8 in the first life table we generated that the total number of person-years in the final interval may be calculated by multiplying the life expectancy at age eighty-five (6.3 years) by the number surviving at the beginning of the age interval. Alternatively, you may simply copy this number from the "85–90" row of Column 6 of the existing life table. (This is more accurate because the life expectancy figure is rounded.)

Step 4. Enter the life expectancy in each age interval (Column 4) from a published life table.

Step 5. Because the mortality rate is equal to the probability that one subject will die in a given year, the product of the total number of person-years in each age interval (Column 3) and the mortality rate from stroke (Column 1) yields the total number of deaths due to stroke. Therefore, the product of the age-specific mortality rate, the total person-years in the age interval, and the treatment efficacy yields the number of deaths prevented by Stroke-ex (Column 6).

Step 6. To calculate the number of person-years gained (C7), we multiply the life expectancy in the interval (Column 4) by the number of deaths prevented (Column 6).

Step 7. Now, we must recalculate the person-years at the beginning of each age interval, because this will change when Stroke-ex is administered. The value for the first row (sixty-five to seventy-five) is simply copied from the existing life table because people younger than sixty-five will not receive this treatment. To calculate the value for the seventy-five to eighty-five age interval, the number of survivors at the beginning of the sixty-five to seventy-five age interval (81,510) is reduced by the number of deaths in the sixty-five to seventy-five row (18,348) less the number of deaths prevented (56.6). Thus the value for the seventy-five to eighty-five age interval is $81,510 - (18,348 - 56.6) = 63,219$ (see Table 12.6).

Step 8. The adjusted number of person-years in the interval (Column 9) is equal to the original number of person-years in the interval (Column 3) plus the number of person-years gained (Column 7).

Step 9. The cumulative person-years and life expectancy in the interval are calculated as in steps 9 and 10 of the previous life table we calculated.

Step 10. Now, we must replicate Table 12.5, including the additional person-years gained by the medication. (On your spreadsheet, simply copy the original table to a new location.) Next, we will add the new values that reflect the total person-years in our treated cohort. To do this, add the number of person-years gained (Column 7) to the total person-years in each age interval (Column 3). In the final age interval (75+), we add the total number of person-years gained for persons seventy-five to eighty-five years of age and eighty-five years of age and over from Table 12.6. We then sum the total person-years backwards, as we did before, to obtain the total person-years in the interval and divide these values by the total person-years at the beginning of the age interval (see Table 12.7). Notice that the life expectancy of the cohort has increased to 76.8 years. Because stroke is a leading cause of death, we were able to noticeably increase the life expectancy of our cohort by reducing mortality from stroke by 25 percent.

To finish the life table, we will need to adjust the HRQL of the cohort to reflect the HRQL of persons with 25 percent fewer episodes of stroke (see Table 12.8). This is where the NHIS data becomes handy (Adams and others, 1996).

Step 11. Enter the risk ratio for stroke among treated persons (Column 2) and the age-specific prevalence rates for stroke you obtained from the NHIS (Column 3) into the table.

Step 12. To obtain the adjusted prevalence of stroke in the cohort (Column 4), we multiply Column 2 values by Column 3 values. We then enter the age-specific HRQL scores for stroke. In this case, we obtained the HRQL scores from the years of healthy life (YHL) measure (Gold and others, 1998).

Step 13. To adjust the mean HRQL for the reduced prevalence of stroke, the prevalence rates are multiplied by $(1 - \text{HRQL})$ for the disease under

TABLE 12.7. LIFE TABLE FOR THE COHORT RECEIVING STROKE-EX BEFORE QUALITY-ADJUSTMENT.

	1	2	3	4	5	6
Age Interval	Prob. of Death in Interval	# At Beginning of Age Interval	# Dying During Interval	Person-Years in Interval	Total Person-Years	Life Expectancy
<45	0.05	100,000	5,004	4,465,419	7,675,179	76.8
45–64	0.142	94,996	13,486	1,765,060	3,209,760	33.8
65–74	0.2251	63,219	18,348	733,563	1,444,700	22.9
75+	1	34,368	63,162	711,138	711,138	20.7

TABLE 12.8. DEATHS AND PREDICTED REDUCTION IN DEATHS FOR PERSONS TREATED WITH NEW DRUG.

	1	2	3	4	5	6	7	8	9
	Person-Years in Interval	Relative Risk of Stroke for Treated Persons	Prevalence of Stroke	Adjusted Prevalence of Stroke	HRQL for Stroke	Mean HRQL for Persons in the U.S.	QALYs	QALYs Remaining	QALE
	From table 12.7		From the NHIS	$C2 \cdot C3$	From YHL	$C4 \cdot (1 - C5) +$ YHL score	Column 1 · Column 6	Column 7 summed	
<45	4,465,419	—	—	—	—	0.912	4,072,462	6,541,874	65.42
45–64	1,765,060	—	—	—	—	0.818	1,443,819	2,469,412	25.99
65–74	733,563	0.75	0.0519	0.0389	0.43	0.767	562,643	1,025,593	16.22
75+	711,138	0.75	0.0988	0.0741	0.38	0.651	462,951	462,951	13.47

Note: Some columns have been removed.

study (in this case, the YHL score for stroke) in Column 5. These are then added to the mean HRQL for persons in each age interval, which we obtained from the YHL measure (see Appendix V, QALE table, Column 4). This is mathematically equivalent to averaging out the HRQL lost to stroke in the cohort.

Step 14. The remainder of the table values is calculated in the same way we calculated values for Table 12.5.

To obtain the QALE gained by the intervention, the QALE at birth in the reference cohort is subtracted from the QALE at birth in the treated cohort. Thus, the intervention results in a gain of 65.42 − 65.04 = 0.38 QALYs per person.

Generating QALE Using Electronic Data

To generate a life table from scratch, it is necessary to know how to use a statistical software package and how to format electronic data. This section is intended only for experienced researchers. To generate a life table, you will need a formatted death dataset, population data, and NHIS data. Because this section assumes greater than average mathematical expertise on the part of the reader, a more technical and more concise approach will be taken.

Most of the steps used in generating a life table using electronic data are identical to those used in generating a life table using published data. The only two points of difference are in calculating the probability of death values for the first column of a life table (see Table 12.5) and the total number of person-years in the final age interval of Column 4.

There are a number of ways to calculate the number of person-years in the first age interval (see Exhibit 12.1). The most accurate way to calculate the total number of person-years in this age interval is to use a **separation factor,** which is a weighting factor estimated by the NCHS and published annually along with life tables. Using NCHS nomenclature, the probability of death is q_x, where q is the probability of death and x is the year of life or row number. (Because the probability of death can be calculated for each year of life, there is no need to generate an abridged life table).

The first row value for Column 1 (q_0) is $D_0(1 - f)/B_x + D_0f/B_{x-1}$, where D_0 is the total number of infant deaths, f is the separation factor, and B_x is the total number of births in year x. The remainder of the values for Column 1 are generated using the formula $q_x = D_x/(P_x + 0.5D_x)$, where q_x is the probability of death during the interval, D_x is the total number of deaths observed at age x, and P_x is

EXHIBIT 12.1. CALCULATING PERSON-YEARS FOR THE FIRST INTERVAL.

Infant mortality is defined as a death to an infant in the first year of life, and the infant mortality rate is defined as the number of infant deaths divided by the number of live births. Some infants will die in the year under study but will have been born the previous calendar year. To correct for this, a separation factor is sometimes used, which accounts for the proportion of infants who died in the year of the analysis, but were born the previous year (Anderson, 1999). This is the most accurate way of measuring the number of person-years in the first age interval (zero years to one year of age) of a life table. However, this value is often not available in developing countries.

A slightly less accurate way of estimating the number of person-years in the first age interval is to simply use the infant mortality rate.

How much does each method affect the accuracy of the number of person-years in the interval? In 1996, the number of person-years predicted by a separation factor was 99,365. If we had used the infant mortality rate, the number would have been 99,280, which is not likely to introduce much error into the overall estimate of life expectancy.

the midyear population for persons aged x. The survivors at age x (s_x or Column 2 values in Table 8.5) may then be calculated as $s_{x-1}(1-q_{x-1})$. Column 3 values are simply the product of Column 1 and Column 2 values for the corresponding rows. All other values are calculated in an identical manner to those derived from a published life table, with the exception of total person years in the final age interval. This is equal to the number living at the beginning of the interval divided by the probability of death during the interval (s_x/q_x).

Using Markov Models

Recall from Chapter Seven that cost-effectiveness analyses that examine interventions intended to reduce chronic diseases are best evaluated using a Markov model. While it is sometimes possible to build a complex model using a basic decision analysis tree, Markov modeling greatly reduces the bulk and complexity of a tree. As a result, you will be less likely to make errors, will be able to complete the analysis in less time, and will likely be able to improve the precision of your analysis. This section is intended to introduce the basic concepts of Markov modeling. To actually build a Markov model, it will be necessary to sit down with the instruction manual for your decision analysis software, because each package handles Markov modeling differently. In this section, we will describe only the basic principles of Markov modeling.

Markov States

Simple decision analysis trees do not incorporate a measure of time. As far as the decision analysis program is concerned, all of the events in a simple decision analysis model occur at a single point in time. If the researcher wishes to include events that occur at some point in the future, all of these events have to be adjusted outside of the decision analysis program and then entered as adjusted events at terminal nodes. For example, in Chapter Nine, when we calculated QALYs using future life years lost we had to use a separate spreadsheet program to discount QALYs before entering the values at the terminal nodes.

A Markov model allows the researcher to model changes in the progression of disease over time by assigning subjects to different health states as they grow older. In a Markov model, subjects are followed from one time interval to the next (for instance, from one year to the next). As subjects age, the model records changes in their health status. Some subjects will die while others will develop medical conditions. When a subject develops a medical condition, he or she will incur the costs associated with that condition and experiences a change in HRQL. All of these events are captured in a Markov model using **Markov states.**

A Markov state is a particular health state. Each state is held constant over a fixed interval of time. This interval of time is sometimes called the **cycle length.** During each cycle, all information pertaining to a particular subject is held constant.

Consider the example of a woman recently diagnosed with early breast cancer. Throughout the year in which she is diagnosed, she will incur the cost of treatment and its associated risk of side effects. The year after she receives treatment, she will have health experiences similar to other women recovering from early stage breast cancer. As the years go by, she may remain well, may be diagnosed again with breast cancer, or may develop undiagnosed breast cancer. The logical unit of time for evaluating breast cancer is thus one year. If the Markov cycle is one year in duration, the cost and health information that the Markov model uses will not change until the end of each hypothetical year in the analysis.

At the end of the year, the model will then re-evaluate the subject based on the subject's probability of remaining healthy, experiencing a progression of breast cancer, developing other diseases, or dying from breast cancer or other causes of death during the next hypothetical year of the analysis. This process of re-evaluation is called **recursive** because once a subject reaches a terminal node, she is shuttled back to the beginning of the tree one year older. Figure 12.3 illustrates a recursive process. As the cohort naturally ages (1), some subjects may become ill (2), recover and re-enter the pool of healthy subjects (3), or die from their illness (4).

Because Markov models examine changes in health states over time, they are sometimes called state-transition models. Because they are recursive in nature, they are occasionally called recursive models.

FIGURE 12.3.   EXAMPLE OF A RECURSIVE PROCESS.

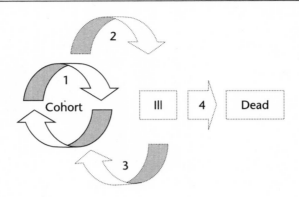

How Markov Models Work

Markov models are most useful and easiest to understand when they are conducted using a Monte Carlo simulation (see Chapter Ten). When a Monte Carlo simulation is employed, each subject in a hypothetical cohort is essentially treated as an individual. Each subject can be assigned very specific characteristics; for example, a subject can be assigned a particular age and can be assigned risk factors for a disease.

Let us see how a Markov model works when a Monte Carlo simulation is employed. Figure 12.4 shows a Markov model that is designed to evaluate screening mammography for breast cancer. The comparison node, No screening mammography, has been left off for simplicity. In this tree, subjects entering the mammography branch are assigned a probability of cancer, pCa, equal to 0 and a probability of being alive equal to 1.0. (The probability of being alive is typed below the Alive branch in this figure.)

Subjects are shuttled through the Alive branch, where they are exposed to a chance of cancer, pCa. Because the variable pCa was assigned a probability of 0, subjects automatically enter the "No cancer" branch. There, they will be screened, will return to the Alive branch at the beginning of the tree, or will die before they have a chance to receive screening during that Markov cycle (which, in this case, has been set to a period of one year). The name of each terminal branch indicates where the subject is moved to at the beginning of the next Markov state.

The chance that a particular subject will be assigned to have cancer is equal to the incidence rate of breast cancer for people in the subject's age group. If the subject is assigned to have cancer, that particular subject will be marked, so that the model knows to shuttle her to the Cancer arm of the model during the next Markov cycle. In other words, for that subject, pCa will be set to 1.0 until she is cured or dies.

If subjects are screened, they will either be assigned to have a true positive test, a false positive test, a true negative test, or a false negative test. All subjects

FIGURE 12.4. MARKOV MODEL EVALUATING SCREENING
MAMMOGRAPHY.

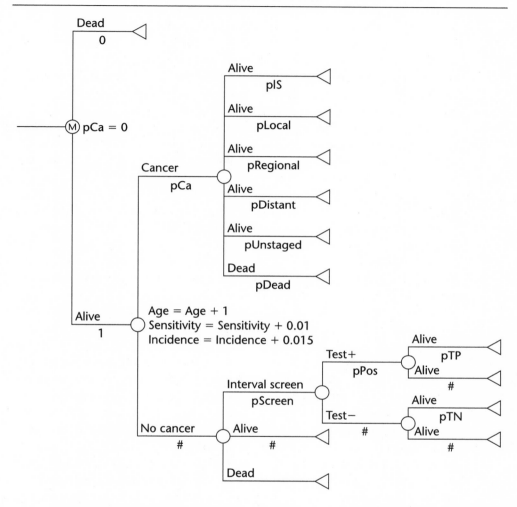

receiving a true positive or a false negative test will be assigned a probability of having cancer (pCa) equal to 1.0. All other patients are assigned a probability of cancer equal to 0. However, patients diagnosed as a false positive will incur the costs associated with further diagnostic tests, and patients receiving a false negative test result will be at a higher risk of death than patients with breast cancer who were screened until they are screened again and the cancer is detected.

After the screening exam, the subjects are then shuttled back to the first Alive branch emanating from the decision node. Women with breast cancer are staged (*in situ,* local, regional, distant, or unstaged), and women without cancer may or may not receive another mammogram. (Cancer staging is discussed in Chapter Five).

The model diligently keeps track of each subject and notes changes in the age of the subjects, health states, costs, tumor size, and the chance of death. Once all of the subjects are dead, subjects who have received a mammogram are compared with subjects who have not received a mammogram.

Tracking changes. Notice that the sensitivity of the mammography screening exam increases with the patient's age, as does the incidence rate of breast cancer. (These formulas are listed at the Alive probability node in Figure 12.4.) The sensitivity of the screening exam increases because breast tissue becomes less dense with age, and it becomes easier to detect cancer. The incidence of breast cancer naturally increases with age, so as the subjects grow older, the chance that they will develop breast cancer also increases.

Accounting for QALE. Because a Markov model is capable of predicting the changes in disease states over time, it can predict changes in life expectancy, quality-adjusted life expectancy and the total QALYs gained for persons who are exposed or not exposed to an intervention.

Let us consider a hypothetical example in which subjects who are diagnosed with advanced breast cancer will either be treated with surgery and chemotherapy or will receive surgery alone. Suppose that we turn to the SEER dataset (see Table 4.1) to calculate the expected survival of our cohort on a year-to-year basis. We find that surgically treated subjects will live an average of four years from the time of diagnosis, and that subjects receiving both surgery and chemotherapy will live an average of five years from the time of diagnosis. We also find that some subjects will live for eight years, and we decide to set the Markov model to complete eight Markov cycles, each one year in duration. The model will read mortality data and HRQL data specific to each stage of breast cancer from spreadsheet tables.

The results of our Markov analysis appear in Table 12.9. In the group that received surgery alone, the number surviving and the overall HRQL for the first two years is higher than in the group receiving both surgery and chemotherapy because the side effects of the chemotherapy have an initial adverse impact on quality of life and survivorship. Once the chemotherapy is completed, however, this group experiences a higher quality of life and greater survival rates than the untreated group.

The decision analysis model can calculate the product of the number surviving and the average HRQL of survivors to determine the total QALYs for each year. Summing over eight years, the model produces the QALYs lived in each group. When the sum total of the QALYs in the surgery alone group is subtracted from the surgery plus chemotherapy group, we obtain $158.5 - 142.2 = 16.3$ QALYs gained in the surgery plus chemotherapy group, relative to the surgery group alone. Because there are 100 patients, the average patient experiences a gain of 16.3 QALYs/100 subjects = 0.163 QALYs per subject.

TABLE 12.9. HYPOTHETICAL EXAMPLE OF THE HRQL OF 100 PERSONS RECEIVING SURGERY ALONE AND 100 PERSONS RECEIVING SURGERY PLUS CHEMOTHERAPY FOR ADVANCED BREAST CANCER.

Year	Surgery Alone			Surgery Plus Chemotherapy		
	Number Surviving	*HRQL*	*Product*	*Number Surviving*	*HRQL*	*Product*
1	95	0.54	51.3	92	0.39	45.1
2	87	0.39	33.9	81	0.32	25.9
3	75	0.35	26.3	75	0.38	28.5
4	52	0.32	16.6	65	0.39	25.4
5	35	0.29	10.2	48	0.35	16.8
6	12	0.27	3.2	35	0.29	10.2
7	3	0.24	0.7	22	0.27	5.9
8	0	0	0	3	0.24	0.7
Total			142.2			158.5

Note: In this example, the Markov state is set to one year.

Modeling mortality using formulas. In the last section, you learned that a Markov model can read information directly from a spreadsheet. It is also possible to model changes in life expectancy using formulas. Using a formula, such as the **declining exponential approximation of life expectancy (DEALE),** it is possible to quickly estimate the life expectancy of a hypothetical cohort. The formula for DEALE is:

$$(1 - e^{\text{rate} \cdot \text{time}})/\text{rate}$$

Equation 12.7

where the rate is the mortality rate over the time period, and e is the exponential function.

Benefits of Markov Modeling

As you can see, Markov modeling is a powerful and accurate way of modeling the changes in health states over time. Interventions to prevent or treat diseases of short duration are better evaluated with a simple decision analysis model because these models require much less effort to design, build, and test. However, interventions designed to prevent or treat chronic or complicated diseases are best evaluated using a Markov model.

Now that you have a basic understanding of how Markov models work, you should become acquainted with this function in your decision analysis software package. Not all software is capable of modeling Markov processes, so be certain to choose a package that does (see Table 7.1 for a list of software packages used in decision analysis modeling).

APPENDIX ONE

SOLUTIONS TO EXERCISES

Chapter One

1.1. The average cost-effectiveness of providing oseltamivir to persons with influenza is $100/0.5 QALYs = $200 per QALY gained. The average cost-effectiveness of providing supportive care only is $10/0.1 QALY gained = $100 per QALY gained. To calculate the incremental cost effectiveness ratio, the next most effective intervention is subtracted from the most effective intervention. The incremental cost-effectiveness of providing oseltamivir to persons with influenza is ($100 − $10)/(0.5 − 0.1) = ($90/0.4) = $225 per QALY gained.

1.2. The average cost-effectiveness of vaccination is $150/0.75 QALY gained = $200/QALY gained. To calculate the incremental cost-effectiveness ratio, the next most effective intervention is subtracted from the most effective intervention. The incremental cost-effectiveness of vaccination relative to treatment is thus ($150 − $100)/(0.75 − 0.5) = $200 per QALY gained.

Chapter Three

3.1. While people will have a difficult time remembering whether they had a common cold over the last year, they are much less likely to forget about the heart attack they had or whether they had a foot amputation. Because recall bias disproportionately affects acute diseases, survey data on chronic conditions are more reliable than data on acute conditions from which the patient may have recovered prior to answering the survey question.

3.2. Surveys that are administered using face-to-face interviews with patients are less likely to be affected by recall bias or misclassification bias, because the interviewer can prompt the patient to correctly remember or classify a disease. They way in which a question is asked can also affect the quality of the data provided.

3.3. If the estimate of a parameter is much more likely to produce an undercount than an overcount of the number of cases of disease, the sensitivity analysis should examine values that are larger than those produced by the data. For example, if the reported incidence of the common cold is twenty cases per 100 persons per year, the sensitivity analysis might examine study results when forty cases per 100 persons is used instead. Caution should be used with this approach, however. For example, influenza incidence rate data are subject to both **misclassification bias** and **recall bias.** While some subjects might not remember whether they had an influenza-like illness last influenza season, others might incorrectly classify the diarrhea they had after Thanksgiving as "influenza," because gastrointestinal illness is commonly referred to as the "flu."

3.4. In general, recall bias tends to exaggerate the impact of a risk factor. Consider the example of the study on birth defects presented in Chapter Three. Mothers of children without birth defects may not be as motivated to remember that they took a medication as mothers of children with birth defects. This would result in an undercount of the medications used by mothers with healthy children. Because more women in the experimental group would report having taken the medication, the medication may be incorrectly thought to be associated with the birth defect. Alternatively, if the medication did place infants at a small risk for birth defects, the magnitude of the effect may be exaggerated. For this reason, retrospective studies should not be used in cost-effectiveness analyses unless no other data sources are available. When they are used, the authors of the cost-effectiveness analysis should include a "no effect" value in the sensitivity analysis unless there are compelling reasons to believe that the study (or studies) contained little bias.

Chapter Four

4.1. To obtain total discharges, charges, and average length of stay for influenza with pneumonia (ICD code 487.0), go to http://www.ahrq.gov and follow the links to the "HCUP-3net" dataset (or go directly there: http://www.ahrq.gov/data/hcup/hcupnet.htm). Click on "Enter HCUPnet," then click the "Start HCUPnet" button on the following page. Click the "NIS" button (which stands for National

Inpatient Sample), then select "Choose Specific Diagnoses or Procedures." Select "ICD-9 CM Diagnosis Codes" from the pulldown menu on the following page. On the following screen, select "Principal Diagnosis." Next, type "Influenza" into the query box on the following screen. Finally, click on "Influenza and Pneumonia 487.0" on the next screen and proceed through the data query process until you have tables detailing the charges, discharges, and deaths by age group.

Save the page as an HTML file and then open the file from within your spreadsheet program. Data for the 1997 HCUP-3 year are listed in Table A1.1.

4.2. Recall that a rate is the number of cases over the population at risk. In this case, we are calculating the rate of discharges for influenza virus infections. The Census' population estimates are generated using data from the census of the United States population, which is conducted every ten years, and from the current population survey, which is conducted every month. Appendix III lists the United States population for the years 1994 through 1999. The 1997 hospitalization rate was $(433 + 721)/163,961,000 = 0.000007$. The rate you obtain may differ if you used more recent data.

4.3. Refer to Table A1.2. To calculate the weighted mean charge, multiply the number of discharges for each row in Column 1 of the table below by the charge for each row in Column 2, and then divide that number by the total

TABLE A1.1. HOSPITAL DISCHARGES AND CHARGES FOR INFLUENZA WITH PNEUMONIA, 1997.

Age Group	Discharges	Mean Charge	ALOS
18–44	433	13,984	5.4
45–64	721	14,534	5.9

TABLE A1.2. CALCULATION OF A WEIGHTED MEAN CHARGE FOR HOSPITALIZATION DUE TO INFLUENZA WITH PNEUMONIA.

Age Group	1 Discharges	2 Mean Charge	3 Weight (Column 1 · Column 2)
18–44	433	$13,984	6,055,072
45–64	721	$14,534	10,479,014
Total	1,154	—	16,534,086
Weighted mean (Total C3/Total C1)			$14,327.63

discharges for all rows. This yields the weighted mean charge for the two diagnoses for persons aged 18–64 (Column 3).

The weighted mean average length of stay (ALOS) is calculated in an identical fashion, substituting ALOS values for charge values listed in Table A1.2. In 1997, the weighted mean ALOS was 5.65 days.

4.4. To obtain total discharges by CCS code, follow the instructions outlined in Exercise 4.1, selecting "CCS Codes" rather than ICD-9 codes. In 1997, the use of CCS Code 123 produced a predicted 10,778 hospitalizations for influenza among persons eighteen to sixty-five years of age. The hospital discharge rate for this code is 10,778/163,961,000 or 0.0000657 (6.6 hospitalizations per 100,000 persons). This rate is larger because it contains discharges for a wider variety of influenza complications. The weighted mean hospitalization charge for influenza was $6,945.

4.5. While the ICD code we used included only hospitalizations for influenza with pneumonia, the CCS system encompasses all hospitalizations for illnesses arising from influenza virus infections. Because influenza with pneumonia is more severe than uncomplicated infections, we would expect the charges to be higher.

4.6. The data extraction tool allows us to select patients hospitalized with a primary diagnosis of influenza. It also allows us to break cases down by whether they were discharged to home, to another institution, or to a home health care program. If we only examine cases discharged to home, we will select out patients that are institutionalized and are thus severely ill. However, we will still include cases of other people with chronic conditions. If we were to examine the raw datafile for HCUP-3, we could exclude hospitalizations with other listed diagnoses that place people at risk for severe complications of influenza virus infection, such as persons with heart disease. Nevertheless, we should turn to the medical literature to determine whether extensive studies have been conducted on hospitalization rates for influenza infections among healthy adults.

4.7. Referring to Table 50 of the NHIS document, we may add up the incident cases of influenza, which will yield a rate of 15.9 + 5.8 + 4.9 + 14.6 = 41.2 cases per 100 persons.

Chapter Five

5.1. Treanor and others (2000) found that among untreated persons, influenza-like illness lasts 97 hours, and among untreated persons with confirmed influenza, the duration of illness was 103 hours. Among persons treated with oseltamivir, 75 mg per day for five days, the duration of influenza-like illness was 76.3 hours. In their study, influenza-like illness was defined as fever, respiratory symptoms, and constitutional symptoms.

5.2. The definition of influenza-like illness Treanor and others (2000) used is more stringent than the definition we decided upon—feverishness or a measured temperature of at least 37.7°C (100°F) plus cough or sore throat (Kendal and others, 1982). Had Treanor and others (2000) used our definition, the measured duration of illness would probably have been shorter. When a more stringent definition is used, subjects will have more severe illness because they will be more likely to actually be infected with the influenza virus.

5.3. Treanor and others (2000) found that persons treated with oseltamivir experienced 76.3 hours of influenza-like illness, and persons receiving placebo experienced 97 hours of influenza-like illness. The efficacy of oseltamivir in reducing the duration of illness is therefore $1 - (76.3/97) = 0.2134$ or approximately 21 percent.

5.4. Bridges and others (2000) examined the efficacy of the influenza vaccine over two influenza seasons, and Wilde and others (1999) examined the efficacy of the influenza vaccine over three seasons. Table A1.3 summarizes these data.

While Bridges and others (2000) tested 278 subjects for influenza virus infection, Wilde and others (1999) included 267 subjects. We may obtain a mean efficacy from the seasons in which the vaccine was effective (0.879), or we may average in the ineffective season (yielding an efficacy of 0.803). The vaccine will be ineffective in one in ten seasons. If we were to average in one ineffective season in ten, we would obtain a vaccine efficacy of 0.83 (work not shown). For our purposes, we will use the low value, 0.803.

We might examine high and low values of vaccine efficacy using data from the CDC. It estimates that the efficacy of the vaccine is between 0.7 and 0.9 during the average season, but it does not report a mean value and did not exclusively include studies of healthy adults ("Prevention," 1999).

TABLE A1.3. THE EFFICACY OF THE INFLUENZA VACCINE IN PREVENTING INFLUENZA VIRUS INFECTIONS FROM TWO RANDOMIZED CONTROLLED TRIALS.

Season	Vaccine Efficacy
Bridges and others (2000)	
1998 season	0.50
1999 season	0.86
Wilde and others (1999)	
1992–95 seasons	0.885

5.5. The influenza vaccine only prevents influenza virus infections. If influenza constitutes a large percentage of all influenza-like illnesses in any given study, the vaccine will appear to be more effective at preventing influenza-like illness. The higher efficacy of the influenza vaccine in preventing upper respiratory illness in the Nichol and others (1995) study likely reflects a higher proportion of influenza illnesses relative to other upper respiratory illnesses.

5.6. To calculate the probability that a person with influenza-like illness will receive antibiotics, divide the total number of antibiotics prescribed by the total illnesses in the placebo and vaccine groups listed in Table A2.1. The results of these calculations are listed in Table A1.4.

The rate of antibiotic prescription among ill vaccinated subjects is slightly *higher* than it is among unvaccinated subjects. This is occurs because influenza-like illness encompasses both viral illnesses, such as influenza, and bacterial illnesses, such as pneumonia. When subjects receive the influenza vaccine, they are much less likely to contract an influenza infection, which is viral and therefore does not require antibiotics. Thus, even though the vaccine may prevent some secondary bacterial infections, the influenza vaccine increases the overall proportion of ill subjects that have a bacterial infection that requires antibiotics. If you divide the number of subjects receiving antibiotics by the total number of subjects in each arm of this study, you will see that vaccination reduces antibiotic use overall.

5.7. The number of excess deaths estimated by the CDC includes deaths among persons with chronic lung disease, diabetes, and heart disease. In our analysis, we are only interested in death among "healthy" adults who do not have these conditions. If we know the percent of influenza deaths attributable to these three conditions, we can estimate the number of deaths that would occur when these conditions were not present. The attributable risk is discussed in the "Efficacy and Measures of Risk" section of Chapter Five.

TABLE A1.4. PROBABILITY OF RECEIVING ANTIBIOTICS AMONG PERSONS WITH INFLUENZA-LIKE ILLNESS IN THE VACCINE AND PLACEBO GROUPS OF BRIDGES AND OTHERS (2000).

	Placebo		Vaccine	
	# Receiving	Total	# Receiving	Total
Bridges and others	33	128	24	82
Proportion receiving antibiotics	0.258		0.293	

Chapter Six

6.1. The consumer price index and the annual change are listed in Table A1.5.

To inflate the cost of a medical visit reported by Nichol and others (1995) from 1994 dollars to 1997 dollars, simply divide the 1997 index by the 1994 index and multiply the result by the Nichol and others (1995) estimate, $69.71.

$$234.6/211 \cdot \$69.71 = 77.51$$

6.2. The Health Care Financing Administration (HCFA) maintains a list indicating the amount that Medicare recipients were charged for hospitalizations by DRG and what HCFA actually paid for each of these hospitalizations. Point your Internet browser to http://www.hcfa.gov/stats/medpar.htm. Click on the data that corresponds to the year of the HCUP-3 data you retrieved. A spreadsheet should open on your computer containing all of the data you requested. The cost-to-charge ratio is the ratio of HCFA reimbursements to HCFA charges. You should have generated a table that appears similar to Table A1.6.

TABLE A1.5. THE MEDICAL PORTION OF THE CONSUMER PRICE INDEX.

Index	Percent Change	Year
	1 − (Year X − 1/Year Y)	
162.8	—	1990
177	8.02	1991
190.1	6.89	1992
201.4	5.61	1993
211	**4.55**	**1994**
220.5	4.31	1995
228.2	3.37	1996
234.6	**2.73**	**1997**

TABLE A1.6. CHARGES AND REIMBURSEMENTS FROM THE MEDICARE MEDPAR SYSTEM AND THE WEIGHTED COST-TO-CHARGE RATIO.

DRG	Charge to HCFA	HCFA Reimbursement	Number of Discharges	Cost/ Charge	Weighted Ratio
079	$3,681,605,628	$1,836,679,551	248,773	0.49888	
080	$68,429,953	$32,042,390	8,337	0.468251	0.497887

6.3. Before comparing the charges, be sure to obtain the per patient charges on your Medpar spreadsheet by dividing the total cost by the total number of people that were hospitalized. (For example, in Table A1.6, the per patient charge would be $\frac{\$3,681,605,628}{248,773} = \$14,799$.) The charge obtained from HCUP-3 differs from the HCFA charge because the HCFA charge is based on the DRG system, rather than the ICD system, and is specific to elderly populations. The ICD system is much more specific than the DRG system. While the hospital charges obtained from the ICD system reflect only those for influenza virus infections, those obtained from the DRG system reflect all hospitalizations for inflammatory or infectious conditions of the respiratory system.

6.4. To convert the charges from HCUP-3 into costs, simply multiply the mean charge by the weighted cost-to-charges ratio. In 1997, the total *charge* obtained for influenza with pneumonia (ICD code 487) using the 1997 HCUP data was $14,328, resulting in a *cost* of $0.4979 \cdot \$14,328 = \$7,134$. The cost for the average hospitalization due to influenza using CCS code 123 was $0.497887 \cdot \$6,945 = \$3,458$.

6.5. Because we do not have data from the medical portion of the consumer price index for 2000, it will be necessary to use an average inflationary rate to deflate these costs to our reference year. In determining an average inflationary rate we could use the average rate between 1990 and 1997; however, medical inflation slowed significantly between 1994 and 1999. Therefore, it might be best to use the average inflationary rate between 1995 and 1997 to deflate these costs (see Table A1.7).

Assuming that the rate of inflation over the two-year period between 1995 and 1997 was similar to the rate of inflation during the two-year period 1997 to 1997, we can simply divide the 1995 index 220.5 by the 1997 index 234.6 to obtain the deflation factor, 0.94. Thus, all of the cost values obtained from Bridges and others (2000) should be multiplied by 0.94. The cost of an ambulatory visit becomes $34.39 \cdot 0.94 = 32.33$. When a co-payment is added, the cost of an ambulatory care visit becomes $32.33 + \$10 = \$42.33$.

TABLE A1.7.   USING THE MEDICAL PORTION OF THE CONSUMER PRICE INDEX.

Index	Percent Change	Year
	1 − (Year X − 1/Year Y)	
220.5	**4.31**	**1995**
228.2	3.37	1996
234.6	**2.73**	**1997**

6.6. Nichol and others (1995) conducted a complex analysis of the cost of an ambulatory care visit and included the cost of prescription medications (see Exercise 6.1). Though the cost estimate of Bridges and others (2000), $42.33, is much lower than the Nichol and others (1995) estimate, $77.51, when each is adjusted to 1997 dollars, Bridges and others (2000) did not include the cost of prescription drugs, $49.38 (see Appendix II).

If we deflate the cost of prescription drugs to 1997 dollars using the deflation factor (0.94) we calculated in Exercise 6.6, we obtain a cost of $49.38 · 0.94 = $46.42. Adding this to the cost of a medical visit, the total cost of an ambulatory care visit becomes $95.80. The difference between the two estimates is $95.80 − $77.51 = $18.29 more than the Nichol and others (1995) estimate.

6.7. To obtain the mean wage from the United States Census, visit the census homepage at http://www.census.qov. Click on "Income" in the center of the page (Alternatively, on the upper left hand corner of the page there is an alphabetical listing of topics. Click on "C" for current population report and follow the links through to "Money Income in the United States.")

Once the document "Money Income in the United States, 1997" has been downloaded in .pdf format, you can obtain the median individual income for persons fifteen to sixty-five years of age who worked full time year round ($25,978 for females and $35,126 for males in Table 7). To obtain an hourly wage, we must assume a thirty-five-hour workweek for fifty-two weeks per year.

Officially, the definition of a full-time year-round worker is someone who works thirty-five hours a week *or more* for at least fifty weeks a year (the hour lunch break is usually not included in a wage estimate). To estimate the opportunity cost of an hour of time lost, we must assume that the employee took the job knowing that he would be working overtime, that he would be paid for fifty-two weeks of work per year, and that two of these weeks would be vacation time.

Approximately 49 percent of United States citizens are male and approximately 51 percent are female, and influenza-like illness affects males and females in similar proportions. Because our hypothetical cohort is healthy adults in the United States, we do not need to adjust for the demographics of our cohort. The average hourly wage is:

(proportion female · median annual income female + proportion male · median annual income male)/weeks per year/hours per week

or

(0.51 · $25,978 + 0.49 · $35,126) year/52 weeks per year/35 hours per week = $16.74/hr.

6.8. If we add 1.5 hours of patient time costs to the cost of an ambulatory care medical visit, we obtain a cost of (1.5 · $16.74) + 42.33 = $67.44.

6.9. The average length of stay in 1997 was 5.65 days (see Exercise 4.1). Because every hour spent in the hospital is valued as a cost, we should multiply 5.65 days by twenty-four hours a day to obtain the total time cost of hospitalization. Because hospitalization for influenza virus infection is a rare event among healthy adults, we may use the person's wage to approximate this cost. The total cost of a hospitalization is calculated as follows:

$$\text{wage} \cdot \text{hours in hospital} + \text{cost of hospitalization}$$

or

$$\$16.74/\text{hr.} \cdot 5.65 \cdot 24 \text{ hours} + \$3,458 = \$5,727$$

6.10. There are a number of ways to approach this problem. Here, we present one example of how the cost of transportation may be estimated by combining micro- and gross-costing methods using data from the 1990 census (the latest available decennial census at the time of publication). To locate transportation costs, visit http://www.census.gov, click on "T" in the alphabetical listing that appears in the upper left hand corner, and scroll down to "Journey Time to Work." Cost estimates will differ if you are using data from the 2000 census. Table A1.8 itemizes costs based on the mode of transportation used, various assumptions, and the cost of a gallon of gas.

6.11. If the average cost of traveling to and from work is $0.97 and 2.8 days of work will be missed on average, then the cost-savings associated with reduced transportation are:

$$\$0.97/\text{day} \cdot 2.8 \text{ days} = \$2.71$$

The HRQL score should capture all components of costs associated with morbidity and mortality. When the person is sick, she will not be able to travel to work, and this is ideally taken into consideration when valuing the time spent ill in the HRQL score.

6.12. The cost of traveling to and from work will serve as an estimate of the cost of traveling to and from the doctor or the hospital because influenza-like illness is usually treated by a person's primary care provider (who, for most people, is probably not located much nearer or further than a person's place of work). We must add $0.97 to the cost of an ambulatory care visit ($67.44, see Exercise 6.8) and to the cost of hospitalization ($5,727, see Exercise 6.9), revising our cost estimates to $67.44 + $.97 = $68.41 for ambulatory care and $16,598 + $0.97 = $5,728 for hospitalization.

TABLE A1.8.   SAMPLE OF ITEMIZED MICRO- AND GROSS-COSTS THAT MIGHT BE USED TO CALCULATE THE COST OF TRANSPORTATION.

Input	Value	Source
Mean travel time		
Minutes	22.4	1990 Census of Population, STF3C
Hours	0.37	Minutes/60
Miles per gallon	25	Assumption
Distance traveled	11.2	1990 Census of Population, STF3C
Gallons consumed	0.45	Distance to work/miles per gallon
Cost per gallon	$1.25	Assumption
Percent driving	73%	1990 Census of Population, STF3C
Percent public transport	5%	1990 Census of Population, STF3C
Percent walking/carpooling	21%	1990 Census of Population, STF3C
Subtotals		
Driving	$1.12	Gallons consumed · cost per gallon · 2*
Public transportation	$3	Assumption (based on one way cost of $1.50)
Totals		
Driving	$0.82	Cost of driving · fraction driving
Public transportation	$0.15	Cost of taking public transport · fraction taking public transport
Total transportation	$0.97	

*Subtotals are multiplied by 2 because people must travel to and from work

6.13.   The wage of a registered nurse was $20.40 in 1997. We then determine the value of 5 minutes of the nurse's time: $20.40 per hour · 5 minutes/60 minutes per hour = $1.70. If you are standardizing to 1997 U.S. dollars, your data summary table should appear similar to Table A1.9.

6.14.   The estimated cost of vaccination by Nichol and others (1995) was $10. When this cost is inflated to 1997 dollars, it becomes $10.67. Bridges and others (2000) estimated that vaccination would cost $24.70 which, deflated to 1997 dollars, is $23.22. Nichol and others (1995) estimate is lower because they obtained costs from vaccination clinics at public health facilities, which conduct business on a shoestring budget. The estimate from Bridges and others (2000) is very high simply because they used the wages of Ford Motor employees, generous estimates of patient time, and a large amount of time required to administer the vaccine.

TABLE A1.9. COST OF THE INFLUENZA VACCINE USING THE MICRO-COSTING APPROACH.

Vaccine Cost	Cost	Notes
Patient time	$8.37	Wage · 0.5
Nurse time	$1.70	Wage nurse/60 · 5
Vaccine cost	$2.50	$2.66 deflated to 1997 dollars
Total	$12.57	

6.15. In Exercise 6.5, we calculated a deflationary ratio to lower costs from 1999 dollars to 1997 dollars, 0.94. The cost of antibiotics in 1997 dollars would be $49.38 · 0.94 = $46.42. The cost of oseltamivir is $53 · 0.94 = $49.82.

6.16. Oseltamivir, vaccination, antibiotics, and over-the-counter medications may all be associated with side effects. We do not have information on the mix of antibiotics or other prescription medications administered to patients who see physicians with an influenza-like illness. The easiest approach to this problem is to assume that the side effects to each of these medications will be similar and assign them a cost of $45.11 (see the "Side Effects" section of Chapter Six. If there was reason to believe that some of these side effects would be more severe or occur at a greater frequency than others and that these costs were likely to be relevant, we should solicit other sources of data or obtain expert opinion to identify, measure, and valuate these costs.

6.17. The cost of caregiver support is valued at the average wage of workers in the United States, $16.74. Keech and others found that the average worker with influenza-like illness will require 0.4 days of caregiver support. The cost is thus:

$$0.4 \text{ days} \cdot 8 \text{ hours/day} \cdot \$16.74/\text{hour} = \$53.56.$$

Chapter Nine

9.1. Treated subjects would be expected to live an additional year at an HRQL of 0.48. Thus, $1 \cdot 0.48 = 0.48$ QALYs are gained.

9.2. While subjects undergoing treatment will live an average of six years at an HRQL of 0.45, subjects not receiving treatment will live an average of five years at an HRQL of 0.48. Thus the number of QALYs in the treatment arm is $6 \cdot 0.45 = 2.7$ QALYs. The number of QALYs among subjects who do not receive treatment is $5 \cdot 0.48 = 2.4$. The total number of QALYs gained per person in the treatment arm is $2.7 - 2.4 = 0.3$.

9.3. In the "Distribution of Disease" section of Chapter Five, we calculated the percent change in an outcome, such as hospitalization or death, if no one in the United States were vaccinated (see Table 5.6). Doing so requires consideration of the vaccine efficacy and the percentage of people who were vaccinated. Table A1.10 provides one example of what your table might look like after adjusting for vaccine efficacy. Here, we inserted Column 2 containing the percent increase in deaths had no one been vaccinated. However, this column could have been inserted anywhere in the table.

9.4. In this exercise, we are interested in determining the chances that a person who dies from influenza virus infection will not have a chronic disease. Neuzil and others (1999) estimate that the risk of death from influenza among people with chronic illness is 1.1 deaths per 10,000 person-months, and the risk of death among people without chronic disease is 0.02 deaths per 10,000 person-months.

If we knew the number of excess deaths that occurred among persons with and without chronic disease, the chance that the decedent is free of chronic disease is equal to the number of excess deaths due to influenza virus infection among people without chronic disease divided by the total number of deaths due to the influenza virus ($deaths_{no\ disease}$/all deaths). However, we have been given rates, so the chance that a death will occur in a person that was otherwise healthy is equal to the incidence among persons without the disease over the overall incidence, or $0.02/1.12 = 0.0179$. Thus, if these authors are correct, less than two percent of all deaths due to influenza occur in healthy adults. The total number of QALYs lost to influenza-associated deaths thus becomes 472 (see Table A1.11).

9.5. The mean HRQL in the vaccination arm is 0.876 and subjects are expected to live $472 - 93 = 379$ QALYs longer in total. To obtain the QALYs in this arm, we need to sum these two numbers together. The HRQL score represents one year of life, but the 392 deaths are the total deaths that would be expected to occur in the 174,955,000 subjects in the cohort as a whole. The total gain in life per person is $392/174,955,000 = 0.0000022$ QALYs, and the total QALYs in the vaccination arm is $0.876 + 0.0000022 = 0.8760022$. Because the additional life gained is less than the rounding error, we can ignore the additional years of life gained altogether.

9.6. The number of QALYs in the supportive care arm is equal to the mean HRQL of the cohort, 0.872.

9.7. It is not possible to calculate the incremental cost-effectiveness ratio for vaccination relative to supportive care because this strategy was found to be cost-saving. Ratios containing negative numbers are deceptive (if vaccination were more effective, it would appear to result in smaller savings per QALY gained). Vaccination would result in an incremental cost-savings of $40.26 - $48.58 = -$8.32. The incremental gain in QALYs is $0.876 - 0.872 = 0.004$ QALYs.

TABLE A1.10. TOTAL NUMBER OF QALYs LOST TO INFLUENZA-ASSOCIATED CONDITIONS AFTER ADJUSTING FOR THE PROPORTION OF PERSONS VACCINATED IN THE GENERAL U.S. POPULATION.

Age Group	# Deaths 1	Percent Change 2 From Chapter 5	Projected Deaths 3 Column 1 · (1 + Column 2)	Years Lost 4 From Life Table	Total Years Lost 5 Column 3 · Column 4	Discounted Years Lost 6 Column 5/ (1.03)^{Column4}	HRQL 7 YHL Measure	QALYs Lost 8 Column 6 · Column 7
15 to 24	111	13.3	126	57.5	7,230	1,321	0.92	1,216
25 to 34	194	12.2	218	48.1	10,474	2,527	0.91	2,300
35 to 44	500	14.7	574	38.7	22,198	7,072	0.89	6,294
45 to 54	500	20.7	604	29.7	17,927	7,451	0.85	6,334
54 to 64	861	30.4	1123	21.4	24,027	12,764	0.79	10,083
Total					81,856	31,135		26,226

TABLE A1.11. TOTAL NUMBER OF QALYs LOST TO INFLUENZA-ASSOCIATED CONDITIONS AFTER ADJUSTING FOR THE HEALTH STATUS OF THE DECEDENT.

Age Group	# Deaths 1	Percent Change 2	Projected Deaths 3	Adjusted for Chronic Disease 4	Years Lost 5	Total Years Lost 6	Discounted Years Lost 7	HRQL 8	QALYs Lost 9
	From Chapter 5		Column 1 · (1 + Column 2)	Column 3 · 0.0179	From Table	Column 4 · Column 5	Column 6/ $1.03^{\text{Column 5}}$		Column 7 · Column 8
15 to 24	111	0.14	126.4	2.3	57.5	130	23.7	0.92	21.82
25 to 34	194	0.13	219.1	3.9	48.1	188	45.4	0.91	41.32
35 to 44	500	0.15	576.4	10.3	38.7	398	126.9	0.89	112.94
45 to 54	500	0.21	607.5	10.8	29.7	322	133.9	0.85	113.83
54 to 64	861	0.32	1,132.70	20.2	21.4	433	229.9	0.79	181.66
Total						1,471			472

9.8. The age-specific and mean HRQL is calculated using the formula:

$$\text{average HRQL} \cdot 1 - \text{efficacy oseltamivir} + \text{HRQL}_{\text{no ILI}} \cdot \text{efficacy oseltamivir}$$

for each age group. This method was illustrated when we calculated the HRQL after adjusting for vaccine efficacy in Table 9.6. The mean HRQL score in the treatment arm is 0.874.

9.9. The total QALYs lost to death from influenza virus infections is calculated in the same way that vaccine efficacy was calculated in Table 9.7. Under an assumed efficacy of 0.5, the total QALYs lost is 236. Alternatively, you may simply multiply the total QALYs lost to death from the influenza virus in the supportive care arm by 0.5.

Chapter Ten

10.1. At low incidence rates of influenza-like illness, few people will become ill and thus require treatment, which is a more expensive option than providing supportive care alone. As the incidence rate of influenza-like illness increases, more people will incur the cost of treatment, increasing the cost of the treatment arm relative to the supportive care arm of the analysis.

10.2. When the incidence rate of influenza-like illness is zero, vaccinated people will incur the cost of the vaccine and side effects, but unvaccinated people will not incur any costs. Therefore, the cost difference should be exactly equal to the cost of the vaccine and side effects.

10.3. The threshold of cost-savings for the treatment option relative to supportive care is approximately $5. (This value may differ for students who populated their model with more recent electronic data.) It would be necessary to reduce the cost of treatment dramatically for it to be the same price as supportive care.

10.4. The cost-effectiveness of treatment relative to supportive care is largely subjective; it is a more effective option but comes at a higher cost. For unvaccinated patients who develop influenza-like illness, the baseline incremental cost-effectiveness ratio for treatment relative to supportive care, $10,175, would likely be perceived as sufficiently "cost-effective" to merit administering to patients with an influenza-like illness.

JOURNAL SUMMARIES

Authors:	Bridges and others.
Title:	The Effectiveness of and Cost-Benefit of Vaccination of Influenza Vaccination of Healthy Working Adults.
Study design:	Double blinded randomized controlled trial.
Location:	Michigan.
# Subjects:	1,184 subjects for the 1997–1998 influenza season, 1,191 for the 1998–1999 influenza season.
Inclusion:	Subjects must have been eighteen to sixty-five years of age to enroll.
Exclusion:	Medical conditions that put subjects at risk for severe complications of influenza, an allergy to the vaccine, or an allergy to egg products.
Demography:	Subjects were recruited from a Ford Motor plant in Dearborn, Michigan. Approximately 78 percent of the subjects were male, and 76 percent had a median household income greater than $70,000—approximately twice the U.S. median income in 1999.

Tips and tricks. Males may be much less likely to seek medical care when needed, and the wealthy may be much less likely to require medical care than low-income persons.

Allocation: Subjects in the experimental and control groups were similar in demographic composition. Subjects in the experimental group in the 1997–1998 year were significantly more likely to have been exposed to secondhand smoke in the household. Over 90 percent of all enrolled subjects completed the study.

Notes: Influenza-like illness was defined as the presence of fever plus sore throat or cough. The authors also examined the incidence rate of upper respiratory illness so that the study outcomes could be compared with those of Nichol and others (1995). The authors examined all study outcomes over the 1997–1998 and 1998–1999 influenza seasons in Dearborn. All subjects were administered viral cultures, and a subsample of subjects was tested for influenza using serologic laboratory tests. The authors conducted a cost-benefit analysis from the societal perspective, but they used the wages of the employees under study rather than the wages of all workers in the United States and failed to include costs associated with severe events, such as hospitalization and death.

Twenty-three percent of the specimens collected from *ill* subjects during the 1997–1998 season tested positive for the influenza virus, and 4.4 percent of subjects in the placebo group had laboratory-confirmed influenza illness. During this season, the vaccine was poorly matched to the circulating viruses and was just 50 percent effective at preventing laboratory-confirmed influenza infection (3 of 138 vaccine recipients developed influenza, and 6 of 137 placebo recipients developed influenza). Twenty-three percent of the specimens obtained from ill subjects and 10 percent of the specimens collected in the placebo group tested positive for the influenza virus during the 1998–1999 season. The efficacy of the influenza vaccine was 86 percent during this season (2 of 141 vaccine recipients developed influenza and 14 of 137 placebo recipients developed influenza). The sample size for both of these years was too small to produce reliable estimates of vaccine efficacy of influenza virus infection. In the 1998–1999 season (the year in which the vaccine was matched to circulating viruses), vaccination resulted in 34 percent fewer influenza-like illnesses, 42 percent fewer physician visits, and 32 percent fewer lost workdays.

Vaccinated subjects queried during both seasons experienced a significantly higher incidence of arm soreness than subjects in the placebo group; however, no other side effects to the vaccine were noted, and no additional medical visits or lost workdays occurred because of vaccination.

The primary results of the study are summarized as in Table A2.1.

The cost of a physician visit and the cost of prescription drugs were obtained from the MEDSTAT MarketScan Databases (Medstat, 2001). The cost of over-the-counter drugs was obtained directly from patients. The cost values are summarized in Table A2.2.

TABLE A2.1. PRIMARY STUDY OUTCOMES OF BRIDGES AND OTHERS (2000).

	1997–1998 Season		1998–1999 Season	
	Vaccine Group n = 576	**Placebo** n = 554	**Vaccine Group** n = 582	**Placebo** n = 596
Influenza-like illness				
Illnesses	161	132	82	128
Physician visits	64	48	29	51
Medication use				
All prescriptions	47	45	26	40
Antibiotics	33	39	24	33
Over-the-counter	127	99	63	98
Upper respiratory illness				
Illnesses	259	232	137	156
Physician visits	84	62	41	50
Medication use				
All prescriptions	62	54	33	39
Antibiotics	46	48	30	34
Over-the-counter	200	170	103	118

TABLE A2.2.   COST VALUES FROM BRIDGES AND OTHERS (2000).

Costs	
Physician visits	$34.39
Physician co-payments	$10.00
Prescriptions	$49.38
Prescription co-payments	$12.40
Over-the-counter drugs[a]	$8.63

[a]Derived by dividing the average per person cost by the proportion of persons with influenza-like illness

These authors found that vaccination was associated with a cost of $65.59 per person during the 1997–1998 season and $11.17 during the 1998–1999 season. In their conclusion, they note that the Nichol and others (1995) study was conducted over an especially severe season, contradicting Nichol and others' concluding remark that the season was mild. Some of the differences between the two studies may be attributable to the demographics of the cohort, because this cohort was likely healthier and wealthier than the Nichol and others (1995) cohort.

Authors:	Campbell and Rumly.
Title:	Cost-Effectiveness of the Influenza Vaccine in a Healthy, Working-Age Population.
Study design:	Workers who volunteered to be vaccinated were compared with unvaccinated workers (non-randomized, non-case controlled study).
Location:	North Dakota.
# Subjects:	262 subjects.
Inclusion:	Subjects must have worked in one of the six textile plants under study over the study period.
Exclusion:	History of allergy to the vaccine or to egg products.
Demography:	Subjects were recruited from six textile plants. There were thirty-nine men and ninety-two women in both the experimental group and the control group. The median age was forty-five in the vaccinated group and forty-four in the unvaccinated group.

Tips and tricks. If the subjects in the vaccinated group were much older than subjects in the unvaccinated group, we would expect the vaccinated group to be less healthy than the unvaccinated group and to have poorer health outcomes.

Allocation: Subjects in the control group were matched by age, gender, and job duties to subjects in the experimental group.

Notes: The authors studied both influenza-like illness and upper respiratory illness. Influenza-like illness was defined as 1) respiratory illness of at least two days duration, 2) at least one of the following: fever, chills, or myalgias (muscle pain), and 3) coryza (runny nose), sore throat, cough, or hoarseness. An upper respiratory illness was defined using criterion 1 and criterion 3 above. Subjects were vaccinated through the month of November. The authors examined study outcomes over the 1992–1993 influenza season.

Tips and tricks. The definitions of both upper respiratory illness and influenza-like illness differ slightly from those used by Nichol and others (1995), Bridges and others (2000), and Treanor and others (2000).

A nurse at each of the six plants was assigned to follow subjects at his or her plant over the study period. The nurse administered a questionnaire to subjects once every two weeks. This questionnaire contained questions regarding the use of medical care, the number of workdays lost, and the number of influenza-like illnesses or upper respiratory illnesses each subject experienced during that time period.

The cost of the vaccine and supplies was $3.50. The incidence rate of influenza-like illness among subjects was 20 percent in the experimental group and 49 percent in the placebo group. Vaccination was associated with savings of $2.58 per person vaccinated relative to no intervention from the corporate perspective.

The vaccine was well matched to the circulating strains of influenza virus. Though patients were followed throughout March, influenza activity continued until May during the 1992–1993 season. The authors point out that the rate of influenza may have differed at each plant and that this may have contributed to the observed differences between the experimental and control groups (the mean distance between the plants was 120 miles). They also point out that the nurses were not blinded as to which subjects received the vaccine. Finally, they noted that the subjects receiving the vaccine were volunteers and may therefore have been subject to the healthy volunteer effect. However, care was taken to match the experimental subjects to the control subjects with respect to smoking, baseline medical care use, and the presence of chronic diseases.

Authors:	Keech and others.
Title:	The Impact of Influenza and Influenza-Like Illness on Productivity and Healthcare Resource Utilization in a Working Population.
Study design:	Survey.
Location:	England.
# Subjects:	411 subjects.
Inclusion:	Subjects were full-time employees of a pharmaceutical company.
Exclusion:	None.
Demography:	All subjects were workers, 85 percent were white and 55 percent were female. The mean age was 34.2.

Tips and tricks. Though the cohort is demographically similar (with respect to age, race, and gender) to the healthy adults in the United States, important differences in health status exist between countries. Most residents of developed countries have superior health outcomes compared to residents of the United States. Thus, the complications of influenza may be more severe in people from the United States than in English people.

Allocation:	411 out of 628 subjects completed the survey.
Notes:	Influenza-like illness was defined as fever plus two out of four of the following: cough, sore throat, myalgia (muscle pain), or headache. The primary purpose of this study was to examine the characteristics of unvaccinated subjects who become ill with influenza-like illness, including lost

work time, the amount of time a patient was confined to bed, and the number of days of caregiving required.

The major study outcomes were summarized in Table A2.3.

To limit recall bias, subjects were surveyed while ill at work or just after returning to work from convalescence.

Authors:	Lasky and others.
Title:	The Guillian-Barré Syndrome and the 1992–1993 and 1993–1994 Influenza Epidemics.
Study design:	Retrospective.
Location:	Multiple (hospitalization data from four states).
# Subjects:	180 subjects.
Inclusion:	N/A.
Exclusion:	N/A.
Allocation:	N/A.
Notes:	Subjects with Guillian-Barré syndrome were identified from electronic hospital data and were contacted to determine whether they had received an influenza vaccine within six weeks of developing their illness. Based on the odds of developing disease, these authors estimated that one in a million vaccinations will result in Guillian-Barré syndrome. The estimated range of cases ranged from 1 per 10 million vaccinated persons to 9 per million vaccinated persons. The authors were careful to note that the differences between persons who had received a vaccine within six weeks of developing the disease and those who developed the disease

TABLE A2.3. PRIMARY STUDY OUTCOMES OF KEECH AND OTHERS (1998).

Outcome	Mean Value	Standard Deviation
Lost work days	2.8	2
Days confined to bed	2.4	1.6
Effectiveness at work	4.6	1.9
Days of caregiver assistance	0.4	1
Visits to clinician (per 100 subjects)	0.32	N/R

Note: Effectiveness was measured on a scale of 1 to 10. 1 = "totally ineffective," 10 = "totally effective."

after six weeks from the time of vaccination were not significant. (It follows that the influenza vaccine may not be a cause of the Guillian-Barré syndrome).

Authors:	Nichol and others.
Title:	The Effectiveness of Vaccination Against Influenza in Healthy, Working Adults.
Study design:	Double blinded randomized controlled trial.
Location:	Minnesota.
# Subjects:	849 subjects.
Inclusion:	Subjects must be eighteen to sixty-five years of age and employed full time.
Exclusion:	Medical conditions that put subjects at risk for severe complications of influenza, a previous allergic reaction to the vaccine, or an allergy to egg products (the vaccine contains traces of the eggs that the vaccine was cultured in).
Demography:	Subjects were recruited from the community, but all were employed and the vast majority of subjects were middle class.
Allocation:	Subjects in the experimental and control groups were similar in demographic composition. Complete data were available for 99 percent of the subjects in the placebo group and 98 percent of the subjects in the experimental group.

Tips and tricks. Subjects who do not complete a study are often less healthy than subjects that complete a study. If a much lower percentage of subjects in the experimental group had completed the study (say, less than 80 percent), the benefits of vaccination might be understated.

Notes:	Subjects were enrolled beginning in October, but enrollment was not completed until November. The authors examined all outcomes over the 1994–1995 influenza season.

The authors examined upper respiratory illness (the presence of a sore throat plus fever or cough) as a primary outcome measure. Subjects were contacted by telephone once per month using a computerized phone response system. Subjects were required to report the number of illnesses, medical visits, and workdays lost over the previous month. The only difference in the number of reported side effects between the vaccine group and the placebo group was that significantly higher numbers of subjects in the vaccine group reported arm soreness with vaccination.

The primary study outcomes included cost values and event rates. They estimated the cost of a vaccine by surveying public health immunization clinics and estimated the cost of a medical visit using multiple electronic datasets. They estimated the cost of a vaccine to be $10 and the cost of a medical visit to be $69.51. The cost of a medical visit included the cost of medications prescribed by physicians. All costs were presented in constant 1994 dollars.

The vaccine was well matched to the circulating strains of influenza virus.

The major events were presented as a rate per 100 persons and were broken down in Table A2.4.

The overall incidence rate of upper respiratory illness was 0.69. Vaccination was found to be associated with *savings* of $46.85 per person vaccinated relative to providing no intervention.

The study minimized recall bias by requiring subjects to report illnesses each month throughout the study. The authors noted that influenza activity was reported as low to moderate in Minnesota during the study period.

TABLE A2.4. PRIMARY STUDY OUTCOMES OF NICHOL AND OTHERS (1995).

	Rate per 100 persons	
Outcome	Placebo	Vaccine
Episodes of upper respiratory illness	140	105
Visits to physicians' offices	55	31

Thus, the rate of influenza and upper respiratory illness may have been lower than the rate usually observed. They also pointed out that the study was not designed to detect differences in serious outcomes such as hospitalization or death. Overall, they felt that the outcomes represented a conservative estimate of differences in the rate of upper respiratory illness, physician visits, and monetary savings from the societal perspective.

Authors:	Treanor and others.
Title:	Efficacy and Safety of the Oral Neuraminidase Inhibitor Oseltamivir in Treating Acute Influenza.
Study design:	Double blinded randomized controlled trial.
Location:	Multi-center.
# Subjects:	629 subjects.
Inclusion:	To enroll, subjects must have been eighteen to sixty-five years of age who had a documented oral temperature of 38°C or higher at enrollment plus 1) cough, sore throat, or nasal symptoms, and 2) headache, malaise, myalgia (muscle pain), sweats and/or chills, or fatigue.

Tips and tricks. The definition of influenza-like illness used in this analysis is more stringent than the definition for influenza-like illness forwarded by the World Health Organization (Kendal and others, 1982) that we used in our study. Therefore, subjects will be more likely to be infected with the influenza virus in this study than in studies using a less stringent definition.

Exclusion:	Medical conditions that put subjects at risk for severe complications of influenza or vaccination against influenza within the past twelve months.
Demography:	The mean age was 32.6 years and 14 percent were smokers.
Allocation:	Subjects in the experimental and control groups were similar in demographic composition. There was a greater attrition rate in the treatment group than in the placebo group. Over 97 percent of the subjects completed the study.

Notes: See the "Inclusion" heading above for the definition of influenza-like illness used. The authors examined study outcomes over January through March of 1998. The authors tested subjects for the influenza virus using both cultures and serology. The primary outcome measure was the reduction in the duration of illness among persons with influenza virus infection and influenza-like illness. Subjects were treated twice daily for five days with either a placebo, oseltamivir 75mg, or oseltamivir 150mg. (The current recommended dosage is 75mg by mouth twice daily).

Approximately 60 percent of all the subjects were actually infected with influenza. Ninety-seven percent of the subjects in the placebo group and 98 percent of the subjects in the treatment group completed their medications. Subjects treated with oseltamivir had 50 percent fewer episodes of secondary complications, defined as sinusitis, otitis media, pneumonia, and bronchitis relative to the placebo group. Treated subjects had significantly higher rates of nausea and vomiting relative to subjects in the placebo group when both treatment groups were combined. No difference was noted between the placebo group and the 75mg treatment group. However, the total number of subjects experiencing side effects in this group was small.

The primary study outcomes are summarized in Table A2.5.

TABLE A2.5.   PRIMARY STUDY OUTCOMES OF TREANOR AND OTHERS (2000).

Outcomes Among Patients with an Influenza-Like Illness

	Placebo	Oseltamivir 75 mg
Duration of illness	97	76.3
Severity of illness	887	686
Return to normal health	178	134
Return to normal activity	230	173

The study was limited by too small of a sample size to firmly establish secondary illness rates and the rate of antibiotic use in the experimental and control groups. Nineteen out of 129 subjects in the placebo group, as well as a total of 17 out of the 245 subjects in both oseltamivir groups combined, experienced secondary complications to influenza-like illness (see Table A2.6). Fourteen out of the 129 subjects in the placebo group and 12 out of the 245 subjects in both treatment groups combined received antibiotics. The difference in the duration of illness was not significantly higher in the 75mg oseltamivir group than it was in the 150mg oseltamivir group.

Authors:	Wilde and others.
Title:	Effectiveness of Influenza Vaccine in Health Care Professionals.
Study design:	Double blinded randomized controlled trial.
Location:	Baltimore, Maryland.
# Subjects:	264 subjects.
Inclusion:	Subjects must be younger than fifty years, in good health, and willing to report illness.

Tips and tricks. This cohort is younger, and thus healthier, than the hypothetical cohort we chose to study. Because vaccine efficacy declines with age, Wilde and others' data may overstate the efficacy of the influenza vaccine in our cohort.

TABLE A2.6.   SECONDARY OUTCOMES FROM TREANOR AND OTHERS (2000). NUMBERS REPRESENT THE NUMBER OF SUBJECTS WITH COMPLICATIONS.

Complication	Placebo	Oseltamivir 75 mg	Oseltamivir 150 mg
Total subjects	129	124	121
Secondary complications	19	11	6
Antibiotic use	14	8	4

Exclusion: History of allergy to the vaccine, allergy to egg products, or the presence of chronic disease(s) that might put them at risk for severe complications of influenza infection.

Demography: Subjects were recruited from two large teaching hospitals. All subjects were physicians, nurses, or respiratory therapists, and the subjects were predominantly female.

Allocation: Subjects in the experimental and control groups were similar with respect to their demographic characteristics. Over 99 percent of the subjects completed the study.

Notes: Subjects were followed over three influenza seasons covering the years 1992 through 1995, or a total of 359-person-winters. (One subject over three winters is equal to three-person-winters). Serologic testing was used to determine the number of persons infected. Twenty-four of 179 control subjects and 3 of 180 vaccine recipients had laboratory evidence of influenza infection during the study period. The efficacy of the influenza vaccine was 88 percent for influenza A infections and 89 percent for influenza B infections.

APPENDIX THREE

CENSUS TABLES

THE UNITED STATES POPULATION 1995 THROUGH 1999.

Tips and tricks. Census data are often presented in abbreviated form as they are in this table. Be sure to multiply these numbers by 1,000 before using them.

July 1:	1999	1998	1997	1996	1995
Population, all ages (in thousands)					
	272,878	270,299	267,744	265,190	262,765
Summary indicators					
Median age	35.5	35.2	34.9	34.7	34.4
Mean age	36.4	36.2	36.1	35.9	35.8

(Continued)

THE UNITED STATES POPULATION 1995
THROUGH 1999. (*Continued*)

All Persons	1999	1998	1997	1996	1995
Five-year age groups					
Under 5	18,918	18,966	19,097	19,289	19,529
5 to 9	19,957	19,921	19,749	19,435	19,092
10 to 14	19,554	19,242	19,091	19,001	18,849
15 to 19	19,762	19,539	19,140	18,704	18,200
20 to 24	18,061	17,674	17,483	17,504	17,978
25 to 29	18,240	18,588	18,812	18,927	18,899
30 to 34	19,750	20,186	20,732	21,309	21,821
35 to 39	22,556	22,626	22,629	22,549	22,293
40 to 44	22,278	21,894	21,376	20,809	20,257
45 to 49	19,363	18,859	18,465	18,428	17,456
50 to 54	16,452	15,726	15,157	13,927	13,641
55 to 59	12,883	12,407	11,755	11,356	11,085
60 to 64	10,526	10,269	10,062	9,996	10,046
65 to 69	9,455	9,593	9,775	9,900	9,925
70 to 74	8,779	8,802	8,753	8,789	8,830
75 to 79	7,337	7,218	7,086	6,891	6,700
80 to 84	4,823	4,734	4,664	4,575	4,478
85 to 89	2,629	2,556	2,480	2,415	2,351
90 to 94	1,151	1,117	1,080	1,043	1,017
95 to 99	344	324	305	291	268
100 and over	60	57	54	51	48
Special age categories					
5 to 13	35,618	35,389	34,996	34,597	34,188
14 to 17	15,661	15,517	15,495	15,210	14,826
18 to 24	26,056	25,470	24,973	24,837	25,107
16 and over	210,627	208,277	205,919	203,666	201,492
18 and over	202,682	200,426	198,156	196,094	194,222
15 to 44	120,647	120,508	120,171	119,803	119,449
65 and over	34,578	34,401	34,198	33,955	33,618
85 and over	4,184	4,054	3,919	3,800	3,684

THE UNITED STATES POPULATION 1995
THROUGH 1999. (*Continued*)

Males	1999	1998	1997	1996	1995
Five-year age groups					
Under 5	9,668	9,696	9,768	9,867	9,991
5 to 9	10,213	10,195	10,105	9,946	9,773
10 to 14	10,015	9,855	9,778	9,733	9,656
15 to 19	10,159	10,046	9,841	9,617	9,357
20 to 24	9,197	8,996	8,894	8,902	9,138
25 to 29	9,067	9,247	9,370	9,439	9,441
30 to 34	9,780	10,007	10,288	10,589	10,853
35 to 39	11,221	11,256	11,259	11,219	11,087
40 to 44	11,045	10,845	10,577	10,287	10,011
45 to 49	9,505	9,252	9,058	9,044	8,565
50 to 54	8,001	7,648	7,372	6,765	6,629
55 to 59	6,186	5,956	5,639	5,447	5,315
60 to 64	4,973	4,849	4,745	4,707	4,723
65 to 69	4,339	4,393	4,466	4,510	4,505
70 to 74	3,866	3,857	3,818	3,824	3,839
75 to 79	3,060	2,997	2,927	2,828	2,729
80 to 84	1,816	1,764	1,721	1,671	1,616
85 to 89	848	814	780	749	723
90 to 94	308	294	280	267	258
95 to 99	76	70	65	61	55
100 and over	11	10	9	9	8
Special age categories					
5 to 13	18,231	18,114	17,911	17,710	17,502
14 to 17	8,059	7,985	7,974	7,829	7,631
18 to 24	13,294	12,993	12,734	12,659	12,790
16 and over	101,493	100,301	99,112	97,984	96,899
18 and over	97,395	96,251	95,107	94,076	93,147
15 to 44	60,468	60,396	60,229	60,052	59,886
65 and over	14,323	14,198	14,066	13,920	13,734
85 and over	1,242	1,187	1,134	1,086	1,045

(*Continued*)

THE UNITED STATES POPULATION 1995
THROUGH 1999. (*Continued*)

Females	1999	1998	1997	1996	1995
Five-year age groups					
Under 5	9,250	9,270	9,329	9,422	9,538
5 to 9	9,744	9,726	9,645	9,489	9,319
10 to 14	9,540	9,387	9,312	9,268	9,194
15 to 19	9,603	9,494	9,299	9,087	8,843
20 to 24	8,864	8,678	8,588	8,602	8,841
25 to 29	9,174	9,341	9,442	9,488	9,458
30 to 34	9,970	10,179	10,443	10,720	10,968
35 to 39	11,335	11,370	11,370	11,331	11,206
40 to 44	11,233	11,049	10,799	10,522	10,247
45 to 49	9,858	9,607	9,407	9,384	8,891
50 to 54	8,451	8,078	7,785	7,161	7,012
55 to 59	6,697	6,451	6,116	5,909	5,770
60 to 64	5,553	5,420	5,316	5,289	5,322
65 to 69	5,116	5,201	5,309	5,390	5,420
70 to 74	4,914	4,945	4,935	4,964	4,992
75 to 79	4,277	4,221	4,160	4,062	3,971
80 to 84	3,007	2,970	2,943	2,904	2,862
85 to 89	1,781	1,742	1,701	1,666	1,628
90 to 94	843	823	800	775	759
95 to 99	269	254	240	230	213
100 and over	49	47	45	42	40
Special age categories					
5 to 13	17,387	17,275	17,085	16,886	16,685
14 to 17	7,602	7,532	7,521	7,381	7,195
18 to 24	12,762	12,478	12,239	12,178	12,317
16 and over	109,134	107,976	106,807	105,682	104,593
18 and over	105,287	104,175	103,049	102,018	101,075
15 to 44	60,179	60,112	59,941	59,751	59,563
65 and over	20,255	20,203	20,132	20,035	19,884
85 and over	2,942	2,866	2,785	2,714	2,639

APPENDIX FOUR

HRQL SCORES DERIVED FROM THE YEARS OF HEALTHY LIFE MEASURE

Condition	Mean	Median	25 Percent	75 Percent
Cardiovascular				
Aneurysm, unspecified	0.45	0.47	0.25	0.67
Angina pectoris	0.56	0.55	0.34	0.84
Aortic valve disorder	0.64	0.67	0.52	0.84
Atherosclerosis, extremity	0.6	0.54	0.29	0.84
Atherosclerosis, unspecified	0.52	0.51	0.29	0.72
Athlosclerotic heart disease	0.47	0.43	0.25	0.68
Atrial fibrillation/flutter	0.67	0.65	0.55	0.84
Cardiac arrest	0.37	0.38	0.29	0.47
Cardiac dysrhythmia, other	0.62	0.6	0.38	0.84
Cardiac dysrhythmia, unspecified	0.67	0.72	0.48	0.87
Cardiomegaly	0.48	0.46	0.29	0.67
Carotid arterial occlusion	0.59	0.63	0.41	0.84
Cerebrovascular disease, unspecified	0.46	0.45	0.21	0.67
Chronic ischemic heart disease	0.6	0.63	0.38	0.84
Chronic ischemic heart disease, other	0.55	0.52	0.29	0.84
Conductive heart disturbance, unspecified	0.54	0.52	0.34	0.79

(Continued)

Condition	Mean	Median	25 Percent	75 Percent
Congestive heart failure	0.4	0.29	0.17	0.55
Coronary atherosclerosis	0.49	0.48	0.25	0.67
Endocarditis, unspecified	0.58	0.63	0.29	0.84
Endocardial fibroelastosis	0.75	0.84	0.52	0.96
Heart disease, unspecified	0.49	0.48	0.25	0.67
Heart failure, unspecified	0.49	0.49	0.21	0.63
Hypertension, unspecified	0.72	0.84	0.52	0.92
Hypertensive heart disease, unspecified	0.51	0.48	0.38	0.63
Hypertensive renal disease unspecified	0.49	0.29	0.17	0.84
Intracerebral hemorrhage	0.39	0.29	0.25	0.52
Mitral valve disorder	0.81	0.84	0.72	0.92
Myocardial degeneration	0.44	0.43	0.31	0.53
Nonruptured cerebral aneurysm	0.56	0.62	0.25	0.72
Premature beats	0.78	0.85	0.58	1
Pulmonary embolic infarction	0.47	0.41	0.25	0.84
Rheumatic endocarditis, unspecified	0.54	0.48	0.21	0.84
Rheumatic fever, no heart involvement	0.73	0.84	0.55	0.92
Rheumatic heart disease	0.57	0.55	0.38	0.82
Thrombophlebitis of leg, unspecified	0.61	0.63	0.36	0.84
Thrombophlebitis, unspecified	0.57	0.55	0.38	0.84
Transient ischemic attack	0.69	0.74	0.52	0.84
Varicose vein of leg, unspecified	0.76	0.84	0.63	0.92
Ventricular fibrillation/flutter	0.61	0.52	0.34	0.84

Cancer

Benign growth of ovary	0.69	0.84	0.52	0.92
Benign growth scalp/skin neck	0.76	0.92	0.63	0.96
Benign growth skin trunk	0.82	0.88	0.79	1
Benign growth skin upper limb	0.84	0.92	0.72	1
Benign growth skin, unspecified	0.89	0.92	0.84	1
Benign growth skin/face	0.77	0.84	0.72	0.92
Benign growth uterus, unspecified	0.83	0.92	0.84	0.92
Cancer breast, unspecified	0.64	0.67	0.45	0.92
Cancer bronchus	0.38	0.38	0.17	0.51

Condition	Mean	Median	25 Percent	75 Percent
Cancer colon, unspecified	0.54	0.52	0.36	0.84
Cancer ear	0.76	0.84	0.63	0.84
Cancer of stomach	0.39	0.38	0.17	0.63
Cancer prostate	0.65	0.63	0.38	0.84
Cancer scalp/skin neck	0.73	0.84	0.48	0.92
Cancer skin	0.68	0.79	0.38	0.92
Cancer skin low limb	0.49	0.47	0.29	0.72
Cancer skin trunk	0.85	0.92	0.84	1
Cancer skin upper limb	0.59	0.63	0.38	0.92
Cancer skin, other	0.73	0.84	0.55	0.92
Uterine leiomyoma	0.83	0.92	0.79	0.92
Endocrine/Metabolic				
Chronic lymphatic thyroiditis	0.88	0.92	0.84	0.92
Diabetes mellitus	0.62	0.63	0.38	0.84
Diabetes mellitus with retina complication	0.48	0.42	0.29	0.72
Goiter, unspecified	0.71	0.84	0.58	0.92
Gouty arthritis	0.66	0.7	0.47	0.92
Hypothyroidism, unspecified	0.77	0.84	0.63	0.92
Nontoxic nodular goiter	0.76	0.84	0.48	0.92
Thyrotoxicosis	0.74	0.84	0.55	0.92
Toxic diffuse goiter	0.7	0.72	0.48	0.92
Unspecified thyroid disorder	0.71	0.84	0.52	0.92
Nervous System				
Multiple sclerosis	0.49	0.45	0.36	0.63
Nonconvulsive epilepsy	0.73	0.84	0.63	0.92
Convulsive epilepsy	0.64	0.55	0.45	0.84
Epilepsy, unspecified	0.62	0.63	0.38	0.84
Migraine variant	0.83	0.84	0.74	0.92
Migraine, other	0.9	0.92	0.92	1
Migraine, unspecified	0.78	0.84	0.63	0.92
Retinal detachment, unspecified	0.63	0.67	0.46	0.84
Degenerative macula	0.68	0.72	0.45	0.92
Peripheral retina degeneration	0.56	0.52	0.29	0.84
Hereditary retinal dystrophy	0.61	0.6	0.46	0.83
Other retinal disorders	0.67	0.59	0.47	0.84
Retinal disorder, unspecified	0.66	0.72	0.38	0.92

(Continued)

Condition	Mean	Median	25 Percent	75 Percent
Glaucoma, open angel	0.66	0.72	0.45	0.92
Traumatic cataract	0.71	0.78	0.52	0.92
Cataract, unspecified	0.65	0.72	0.45	0.84
Color visual deficiency	0.89	0.92	0.84	1
Tinnitus	0.72	0.84	0.52	0.92
Respiratory				
Deviated nasal septum	0.81	0.87	0.72	0.96
Nasal sinus polyp other	0.82	0.84	0.67	1
Nasal polyp unspecified	0.75	0.84	0.63	0.92
Chronic sinusitis unspecified	0.82	0.92	0.79	1
Chronic tonsillitis	0.84	0.92	0.84	1
Tonsilar hypertrophy	0.86	0.92	0.81	1
Chronic tonsil and adenoid disease	0.68	0.84	0.25	0.92
Chronic laryngitis	0.75	0.84	0.63	0.92
Chronic laryngitis/tracheitis	0.73	0.74	0.48	0.92
Pollen rhinitis	0.88	0.92	0.84	1
Allergic rhinitis other	0.87	0.92	0.84	1
Allergic rhinitis, unspecified	0.86	0.92	0.84	1
Bronchitis, unspecified	0.75	0.84	0.63	0.92
Chronic bronchitis	0.72	0.74	0.55	0.84
Obstructive chronic bronchitis	0.72	0.84	0.55	0.92
Chronic bronchitis, unspecified	0.74	0.84	0.63	0.92
Emphysema	0.48	0.47	0.25	0.67
Extrinsic asthma	0.79	0.84	0.67	0.92
Asthma, unspecified	0.76	0.84	0.63	0.92
Coal worker's pneumoconiosis	0.46	0.38	0.25	0.68
Asbestosis	0.65	0.63	0.38	0.88
Silicosis	0.53	0.52	0.38	0.72
Pleurisy induced by tuberculosis	0.59	0.63	0.34	0.84
Post-inflammatory pulmonary fibrosis	0.6	0.7	0.34	0.92

LIFE TABLES AND QUALITY-ADJUSTED LIFE TABLES

1997 LIFE TABLES FOR THE UNITED STATES POPULATION.

Age Interval	Proportion Dying	Of 100,000 Born Alive		Stationary Population		Average Remaining Lifetime
Period of Life Between Two Exact Ages Stated in Years	Proportion of Persons Alive at Beginning of Age Interval Dying During Interval	Number Living at Beginning of Age Interval	Number Dying During Age Interval	In the Age Interval	In This and All Subsequent Age Intervals	Average Number of Years of Life Remaining at Beginning of Age Interval
(1)	(2)	(3)	(4)	(5)	(6)	(7)
x to $x \cdot n$	nq_x	l_x	nd_x	nL_x	T_x	e_x^c
0–1	0.00723	100,000	723	99,371	7,650,789	76.5
1–5	0.00144	99,277	143	396,774	7,551,418	76.1
5–10	0.00092	99,135	91	495,432	7,154,644	72.2
10–15	0.00116	99,043	115	494,997	6,659,212	67.2
15–20	0.00374	98,929	370	493,801	6,164,215	62.3
20–25	0.00492	98,558	485	491,596	5,670,414	57.5
25–30	0.00509	98,073	499	489,137	5,178,818	52.8
30–35	0.00630	97,574	615	486,397	4,689,680	48.1
35–40	0.00840	96,959	814	482,862	4,203,284	43.4
40–45	0.01196	96,145	1,149	478,017	3,720,422	38.7
45–50	0.01757	94,996	1,669	471,055	3,242,404	34.1
50–55	0.02618	93,327	2,443	460,915	2,771,349	29.7
55–60	0.04123	90,884	3,747	445,708	2,310,434	25.4
60–65	0.06457	87,136	6,627	422,450	1,864,727	21.4
65–70	0.09512	81,510	7,753	389,159	1,442,277	17.7
70–75	0.14365	73,757	10,595	343,402	1,053,118	14.3
75–80	0.20797	63,162	13,135	284,018	709,716	11.2
80–85	0.31593	50,026	15,805	211,466	425,698	8.5
85–90	0.46155	34,221	15,795	130,736	214,232	6.3
90–95	0.62682	18,427	11,550	60,800	83,496	4.5
95–100	0.77325	6,876	5,317	18,825	22,696	3.3
100 and over	1.00000	1,559	1,559	3,871	3,871	2.5

Source: National Vital Statistics Report, 47(19), Table 4.

LIFE EXPECTANCY AT SELECTED AGES, UNITED STATES, 1997 (BY RACE AND GENDER).

Exact Age in Years	All Races			White			All Other Total			Black		
	Both Sexes	Male	Female	Both Sexes	Male	Female	Both Sexes	Male	Female	Both Sexes	Male	Female
0	76.5	73.6	79.4	77.1	74.3	79.9	73.4	69.8	76.7	71.1	67.2	74.7
1	76.1	73.1	78.9	76.6	73.8	79.3	73.3	69.7	76.5	71.1	67.2	74.7
5	72.2	69.3	75.0	72.7	69.9	75.4	69.4	65.9	72.7	67.3	63.4	70.9
10	67.2	64.3	70.0	67.8	65.0	70.5	64.5	60.9	67.8	62.4	58.5	66.0
15	62.3	59.4	65.1	62.8	60.0	65.5	59.6	56.0	62.8	57.5	53.6	61.0
20	57.5	54.7	60.2	58.0	55.3	60.7	54.9	51.4	58.0	52.8	49.0	56.2
25	52.8	50.1	55.4	53.3	50.6	55.8	50.3	47.0	53.2	48.2	44.7	51.4
30	48.1	45.4	50.5	48.5	45.9	50.9	45.6	42.5	48.4	43.6	40.3	46.7
35	43.4	40.8	45.7	43.8	41.3	46.1	41.0	38.0	43.7	39.1	35.9	42.0
40	38.7	36.2	40.9	39.1	36.7	41.3	36.6	33.7	39.1	34.7	31.6	37.5
45	34.1	31.8	36.3	34.5	32.1	36.6	32.2	29.5	34.6	30.5	27.5	33.1
50	29.7	27.4	31.7	30.0	27.7	32.0	28.1	25.5	30.3	26.5	23.8	28.8
55	25.4	23.3	27.3	25.6	23.5	27.5	24.1	21.8	26.1	22.8	20.3	24.8
60	21.4	19.4	23.1	21.5	19.6	23.2	20.5	18.3	22.1	19.3	17.0	21.0
65	17.7	15.9	19.2	17.8	16.0	19.3	17.1	15.3	18.5	16.1	14.2	17.6
70	14.3	12.7	15.5	14.3	12.7	15.5	14.0	12.4	15.1	13.1	11.5	14.3
75	11.2	9.9	12.1	11.2	9.9	12.1	11.3	10.0	12.1	10.7	9.3	11.5
80	8.5	7.5	9.1	8.5	7.4	9.1	8.9	7.9	9.4	8.3	7.3	8.9
85	6.3	5.5	6.6	6.2	5.4	6.6	6.9	6.2	7.1	6.4	5.7	6.7
90	4.5	4.0	4.7	4.5	3.9	4.6	5.3	5.0	5.4	5.0	4.5	6.1
95	3.3	3.0	3.4	3.2	2.9	3.3	4.2	4.1	4.1	3.9	3.7	3.8
100	2.5	2.4	2.5	2.4	2.2	2.4	3.3	3.4	3.2	3.0	3.1	2.9

Source: National Vital Statistics Report, 47(19), Table 5.

QUALITY-ADJUSTED LIFE EXPECTANCY, 1990.

Age Interval Period of Life Between Two Exact Ages Stated in Years x to $x + n$ (1)	Number Living at Beginning of Age Interval of 100,000 Born Alive (l_x) (2)	Stationary Population in the Age Interval $({}_nL_x)$ (3)	Average Health-Related Quality of Life of Persons in the Age Interval (Q_x) (4)	Quality-Adjusted Stationary Population In the Age Interval $(Q_x \cdot {}_nL_x)$ (5)	Quality-Adjusted Stationary Population In This and All Subsequent Age Intervals (T'_x) (6)	Years of Healthy Life Remaining (7)	Life Years Remaining (8)
0–5	100,000	495,073	0.94	465,369	6,403,748	64.0	75.4
5–10	98,890	494,150	0.93	459,560	5,938,379	60.1	75.1
10–15	98,780	493,654	0.93	459,098	5,478,819	55.5	71.2
15–20	98,653	492,290	0.92	452,907	5,019,721	50.9	66.3
20–25	98,223	489,794	0.91	445,713	4,566,814	46.5	61.3
25–30	97,684	486,901	0.91	443,080	4,121,101	42.2	56.6
30–35	97,077	483,571	0.90	435,214	3,678,021	37.9	51.9
35–40	96,334	479,425	0.89	426,688	3,242,807	33.7	47.2
40–45	95,382	474,117	0.88	417,223	2,816,119	29.5	42.6
45–50	94,179	466,820	0.86	401,465	2,398,896	25.5	38.0
50–55	92,420	455,809	0.83	378,321	1,997,431	21.6	33.4
55–60	89,735	439,012	0.81	355,600	1,619,110	18.0	29.0
60–65	85,634	413,879	0.77	318,687	1,263,510	14.8	24.8
65–70	79,590	378,369	0.76	287,560	944,823	11.9	20.8
70–75	71,404	330,846	0.74	244,826	657,263	9.2	17.2
75–80	60,557	270,129	0.70	189,090	412,437	6.8	13.9
80–85	47,168	197,857	0.63	124,650	223,347	4.7	10.9
85 and over	31,892	193,523	0.51	98,697	98,697	3.1	8.3

Source: Erickson and others, Table 4.

THE EUROQOL INSTRUMENT

(English Version for the United Kingdom)

By placing a tick in one box in each group below, please indicate which statements best describe your own health state today.

Mobility

I have no problems in walking about ☐

I have some problems in walking about ☐

I am confined to bed ☐

Self-Care

I have no problems with self-care ☐

I have some problems washing or dressing myself ☐

I am unable to wash or dress myself ☐

Usual Activities (*e.g. work, study, housework, family or leisure activities*)

I have no problems with performing my usual activities ☐

I have some problems with performing my usual activities ☐

I am unable to perform my usual activities ☐

Pain/Discomfort

I have no pain or discomfort   ☐

I have moderate pain or discomfort   ☐

I have extreme pain or discomfort   ☐

Anxiety/Depression

I am not anxious or depressed   ☐

I am moderately anxious or depressed   ☐

I am extremely anxious or depressed   ☐

To help people say how good or bad a health state is, we have drawn a scale (rather like a thermometer) on which the best state you can imagine is marked 100 and the worst state you can imagine is marked 0.

We would like you to indicate on this scale how good or bad your own health is today, in your opinion. Please do this by drawing a line from the box below to whichever point on the scale indicates how good or bad your health state is today.

Your own health state today

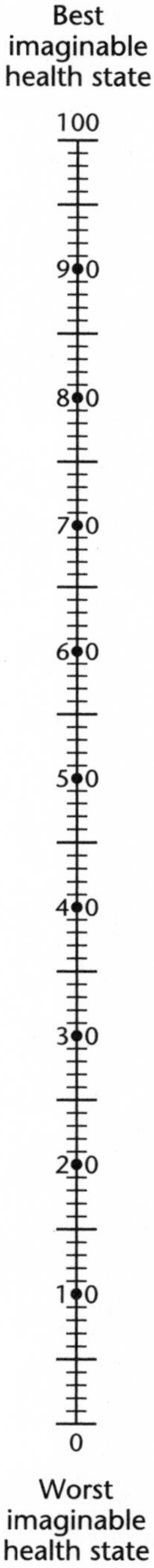

Best imaginable health state

100

9 0

8 0

7 0

6 0

5 0

4 0

3 0

2 0

1 0

0

Worst imaginable health state

Because all replies are anonymous, it will help us to understand your answers better it we have a little background data from everyone, as covered in the following questions.

1. Have you experienced serious illness?

	Yes	No
in you yourself	☐	☐
in your family	☐	☐
in caring for others	☐	☐

PLEASE TICK APPROPRIATE BOXES

2. What is your age in years?

3. Are you:

	Male	Female
	☐	☐

PLEASE TICK APPROPRIATE BOX

4. Are you:

a current smoker	☐
an ex-smoker	☐
a never smoker	☐

PLEASE TICK APPROPRIATE BOX

5. Do you now, or did you ever, work in health or social services?

	Yes	No
	☐	☐

PLEASE TICK APPROPRIATE BOX

If so, in what capacity? ....

6. Which of the following best describes your main activity?

in employment or self employment	☐
retired	☐
housework	☐
student	☐
seeking work	☐
other (please specify)	☐ ....

PLEASE TICK APPROPRIATE BOX

7. Did your education continue after the minimum school leaving age?

	Yes	No
	☐	☐

PLEASE TICK APPROPRIATE BOX

8. Do you have a Degree or equivalent professional qualification?

	Yes	No
	☐	☐

PLEASE TICK APPROPRIATE BOX

9. If you know your postcode, would you please write it here:

REFERENCES

Adams, P. F., Hendershot, G. E., and Marano, M. A. "Current Estimates from the National Health Interview Survey, 1996." *Vital Health Statistics*, 1999, 10, 1–212.

Adema, W., and others. *Net Public Social Expenditure. Labour Market and Social Policy*. Occasional Papers, No. 19. Paris: Organisation for Economic Co-operation and Development, 1996.

Anderson, R. N. "Method for Constructing Complete Annual U.S. Life Tables." *Vital Health Statistics 2*, 1999, 47, 1–20.

Arnesen, T., and Nord, E. "The Value of DALY Life: Problems with Ethics and Validity of the Disability-Adjusted Life Year. *British Medical Journal*, 1999, 319, 1423–1425.

Attaran, A., and Sachs, J. "Defining and Refining International Donor Support for Combating the AIDS Pandemic." *Lancet*, 2001, 357, 57–61.

Barendregt, J. J., Bonneux, L., and van der Mass, P. J. "The Health Care Costs of Smoking." *New England Journal of Medicine*, 1997, 337, 1052–1057.

Barker, W. H. "Excess Pneumonia and Influenza Associated Hospitalization During Influenza Epidemics in the United States, 1970–79." *American Journal of Public Health*, 1986, 76, 761–765.

Barker, W. H., and Mullooly, J. P. "Impact of Epidemic Type A Influenza in a Defined Adult Population." *American Journal of Epidemiology*, 1980, 112, 798–811.

Black, W. C. "The CE Plane: A Graphic Representation of Cost-Effectiveness." *Medical Decision-Making*, 1990, 10, 212–214.

Bridges, C. B., and others. "Effectiveness and Cost-Benefit of Influenza Vaccination of Healthy Working Adults." *Journal of the American Medical Association*, 2000, 284, 1655–1663.

Campbell, D. S., and Rumly, M. H. "Cost-Effectiveness of the Influenza Vaccine in a Healthy, Working-Age Population." *Journal of Occupational and Environmental Medicine*, 1995, 39, 406–414.

Centers for Disease Control and Prevention. "National Health and Nutrition Examination Survey." [http://www.cdc.gov/nchs/nhanes.htm]. Mar. 2001.

Chrischilles, E. A., and Scholz, D. A. "Dollars and Sense: A Practical Guide to Cost-Analysis for Hospital Epidemiology and Infection Control." *Clinical Performance and Quality Health Care,* 1999, 7(2), 107–111.

Dawber, T. R., Kannel, W. E., and Lyell, L. P. "Epidemiological Approaches to Heart Disease: The Framingham Study." *American Journal of Public Health,* 1951, 41, 279.

de Andrade, H. R. and others. "Chills, Cough and Fever: To Be or Not to Be Influenza." Program and Abstracts from Options for the Control of Influenza IV; September 23–28, 2000; Hersonissos, Crete, Greece. Abstract P2–79.

De Charro, F. "The EuroQol Group." [http://www.euroqol.org]. May 2001.

Doll, R., and Hill, A. B. "Lung Cancer and Other Causes of Death in Relation to Smoking: A Second Report on the Mortality of British Doctors." *British Medical Journal,* 1956, 2, 1071–1081.

Drug Topics Red Book. Medical Economics Co.: Montavaille, N. J., 2000.

Drummond, M. F., O'Brien, B. O., Stoddart, G. L., and Torrance, G. W. *Methods for the Economic Evaluation of Health Care Programmes,* 2nd ed., London: Oxford University Press, 1997.

Erickson, P., Wilson, R., and Shannon, I. "Years of Healthy Life." *Statistical Notes,* 1995, 7, 1–16.

EuroQol Group. "EuroQol: A New Facility for the Measurement of Health-Related Quality of Life." *Health Policy,* 1990, 16, 199–208.

Fahs, M. C., Mandelblatt, J., Schechter, C., and Muller, C. "Cost-Effectiveness of Cervical Cancer Screening for the Elderly." *Annuals of Internal Medicine,* 1992, 117, 520–527.

Fang, J., Madhaven, S., and Alerman, M. H. "Association Between Birthplace and Mortality from Cardiovascular Causes Among Black and White Residents of New York City." *New England Journal of Medicine,* 1996, 335, 1545–1551.

Feeney, D. H., Furlong, W., Burr, R. D., and Torrance, G. W. "Multiattribute Health States Classification Systems: Health Utilities Index." *Pharmacoeconomics,* 1995, 7, 490–502.

Fisher, M. J. "Better Living Through the Placebo Effect." [http://www.theatlantic.com/issues/2000/10/fisher.htm]. Oct. 2000.

Glezen, W. P., Decker, M., and Perrotta, D. M. "Survey of Underlying Conditions of Persons Hospitalized with Acute Respiratory Disease During Influenza Epidemics in Houston, 1978–1981." *American Review of Respiratory Disease,* 1987, 136, 150–155.

Gold, M. R., Franks, P., McCoy, K. I., and Fryback, D. G. "Toward Consistency in Cost-Utility Analyses: Using National Measures to Create Condition-Specific Values." *Medical Care,* 1998, 36, 778–792.

Gold, M. R., Siegel, J. E., Russell, L. B., and Weinstein, M. C. (eds.). *Cost-Effectiveness in Health and Medicine.* New York: Oxford University Press, 1996.

Gotzshe, P. C., and Olsen, O. "Is Screening for Breast Cancer with Mammography Justifiable?" *Lancet,* 2000, 355, 129–134.

Greenacre, M. J. *Correspondence Analysis in Practice.* London: Academic Press, 1993.

Haddix, A. C., Hillis, S. D., and Kassler, W. J. "The Cost Effectiveness of Azithromycin for Chlamydia Trachomatis Infections in Women." *Sexually Transmitted Diseases,* 1995, 22, 274–280.

Haddix, A. C., Teutsch, S. M., Shaffer, P. A., and Dunet, D. O. *Prevention Effectiveness: A Guide to Decision Analysis and Economic Evaluation.* New York: Oxford University Press, 1996.

Hayden, F. G., and others. "Use of the Selective Oral Neuraminidase Inhibitor Oseltamivir to Prevent Influenza." *New England Journal of Medicine,* 1999, 241, 1336–1343.

Healthcare Cost and Utilization Project. [http://www.ahrq.gov/HCUP]. May 2001.

Hendershot, G. E. "Health of the Foreign Born Population: United States 1985–86." *Advance Data Vital Health Statistics,* 1988, 156, 1–6.

Hoyart, D. L., Kochanek, K. D., and Murphy, S. L. "Deaths: Final Data for 1997." *National Vital Statistics Report,* 1999, 47, 1–146.

Jeckel, J. F., Elmore, J. G., and Katz, D. L. *Epidemiology, Biostatistics, and Preventive Medicine.* Philadelphia: W. B. Saunders Co., 1996.

Kaplan, R. M., and Anderson, J. P. "A General Health Policy Model: Update and Applications." *Health Services Research,* 1988, 23, 203–235.

Keech, M., Scott, A. H., and Ryan P. J. "The Impact of Influenza and Influenza-Like Illness on Productivity and Healthcare Resource Utilization in a Working Population." *Occupational Medicine,* 1998, 48, 85–90.

Kendal, A. P., Pereria, M. S., and Skehel, J. I. "Concepts and Procedures for Laboratory-Based Influenza Surveillance." Paper presented at the World Health Organization, Geneva, Switzerland, 1982.

Kolata, G. "Medical Fees are Often Higher for Patients Without Insurance." *New York Times,* Apr. 2, 2001, p. A1.

Kramarow, E., and others. *Health and Aging Chartbook. Health, United States, 1999.* Hyattsville, Md.: National Center for Health Statistics, 1999.

LaForce, F. M., Nichol, K. L., and Cox, N. J. "Influenza: Virology, Epidemiology, Disease, and Prevention." *American Journal of Preventive Medicine,* 1994, 10, 31–44.

Lantz, P. M., and others. "Socioeconomic Factors, Health Behaviors, and Mortality: Results from a Nationally Representative Prospective Study of U.S. Adults." *Journal of the American Medical Association,* 1998, 279, 1703–1708.

Lasky, T., and others. "The Guillain-Barre Syndrome and the 1992–1993 and 1993–1994 Influenza Epidemics." *New England Journal of Medicine,* 1998, 339, 1797–1802.

Laupacis, A. D., Feeny, D., Detsky, A. S., and Tugwell, P. S. "How Attractive Does a New Technology Have to be to Warrant Adoption and Utilization? Tentative Guidelines for Using Clinical and Economic Evaluations." *Canadian Medical Association Journal,* 1992, 146, 473–481.

Lui, K. J., and Kendal, A. P. "Impact of Influenza Epidemics on Mortality in the United States from October 1972 to May 1985." *American Journal of Public Health,* 1987, 77, 712–716.

Marseille, E., Kahn, J. G., and Saba, J. "Cost-Effectiveness of Antiviral Drug Therapy to Reduce Mother-to-Child HIV Transmission in Sub-Saharan Africa." *AIDS,* 1998, 12, 939–948.

Mauskopf, J. A., Cates, S. C., and Griffin, A. D. "A Pharmacoeconomic Model for the Treatment of Influenza." *Pharmacoeconomics,* 1999, 16, 73–84.

McNeil, D. G. "AIDS Stalking Africa's Struggling Economies." *New York Times.* Nov. 15, 1998, p. A1.

"Medstat Group." [http://www.medstat.com]. Apr. 2001.

Meltzer, M. I., Cox, N. J., and Fukuda, K. "The Economic Impact of Pandemic Influenza in the United States: Priorities for Intervention." *Emerging Infectious Disease,* 1999, 5, 659–671.

Monto, A. S., and others. "Zanamivir in the Prevention of Influenza Among Healthy Adults." *Journal of the American Medical Association,* 1999, 282, 31–35.

Monto, A. S., Ohmit, S. E., Margulies, J. R., and Talsma, A. "Medical Practice-Based Influenza Surveillance: Viral Prevalence and Assessment of Morbidity." *American Journal of Epidemiology*, 1995, 141, 502–506.

Muennig, P. "Influenza Vaccine for Healthy Working Adults." *Journal of the American Medical Association*, 2001, 285, 291–292.

Muennig, P., and Gold, M. R. "Using the Years of Healthy Life Measure to Calculate Quality Adjusted Life Years." *American Journal of Preventive Medicine*, 2001, 20, 12–17.

Muennig, P., Pallin, D., Sell, R., and Chan, M. S. "The Cost Effectiveness of Strategies for the Treatment of Intestinal Parasites in Immigrants." *New England Journal of Medicine*, 1999, 340, 773–779.

Murray, C. L. J., and Lopez, A. D. *The Global Burden of Disease: A Comprehensive Assessment of Mortality and Disability from Disease, Injury and Risk Factors in 1990 and Projected to 2020*. Vol. 1. Boston: Harvard University Press, 1996.

National Center for Health Statistics. *Healthy People 2000 Review, 1998–99*. Hyattsville, Md.: Public Health Service, 1999.

Neuzil, K. M., Reed, G. W., Mitchel, E. F., and Griffin, M. R. "Influenza-Associated Morbidity and Mortality in Young and Middle-Aged Women." *Journal of the American Medical Association*, 1999, 281, 901–907.

Nichol, K. L., and others. "The Effectiveness of Vaccination Against Influenza in Healthy, Working Adults." *New England Journal of Medicine*, 1995, 333, 889–893.

Nichol, K. L., Margolis, K. L., Wuorenma, J., and Von Sternberg, T. "The Efficacy and Cost-Effectiveness of Vaccination Against Influenza Among Elderly Persons Living in the Community." *New England Journal of Medicine*, 1994, 331, 778–784.

Olsen, M., and Bailey, M. J. "Positive Time Preference." *Journal of Political Economy*, 1981, 89, 1–24.

Oregon Office for Health Policy and Research. "Oregon Health Plan." [http://www.ohppr.state.or.us/]. May 2001.

Owings, M. F., and Lawrence, L. "Detailed Diagnoses and Procedures. National Hospital Discharge Survey, 1997. National Center for Health Statistics." *Vital Health Statistics*, 1999, 13, 1–163.

Petersen, M. "Lifting the Curtain on the Real Costs of Making AIDS Drugs." *New York Times*, Apr. 24, 2001, p. C1.

"Prevention and Control of Influenza: Recommendations of the Advisory Committee on Immunization Practices (ACIP)." *Morbidity and Mortality Weekly Report*, 1999, 48, 1–49.

"Prevention and Control of Influenza: Recommendations of the Advisory Committee on Immunization Practices (ACIP)." *Morbidity and Mortality Weekly Report*, 1998, 47, 1–25.

Schaller, D. R., and Olson, B. H. "A Food Industry Perspective on Folic Acid Fortification." *Journal of Nutrition*, 1996, 126, 761S–764S.

Schappert, S. M., and Nelson, C. "National Ambulatory Medical Care Survey, 1995–96. (1999). Summary. National Center for Health Statistics." *Vital Health Statistics*, 1999, 13(142), 1–123.

Schulman, K. A., and others. "The Effect of Race and Sex on Physicians' Recommendations for Cardiac Catheterization." *New England Journal of Medicine*, 1999, 340, 618–626.

Secker-Walker, R. H., and others. "Screening for Breast Cancer: Time in Travel and Out-of-Pocket Expenses." *Journal of the National Cancer Institute*, 1999, 91, 702–708.

Singh, G. K., and Siahpush, M. "All-Cause and Cause-Specific Mortality of Immigrants and Native-Born in the United States." *American Journal of Public Health*, 2001, 91, 392–399.

Sullivan, K. M., Monto, A. S., and Longini, I. M. "Estimates of the U.S. Health Impact of Influenza." *American Journal of Public Health*, 1983, 83, 1712–1716.

Tengs, T. O., and others. "Five Hundred Life-Saving Interventions and their Cost-Effectiveness." *Risk Analysis*, 1995, 15, 369–390.

The Real Price of Gas. International Center for Technology Assessment: Washington, D.C., 1998.

Thelle, D. S., Arnesen, E., and Forde, O. H. "The Tromso Heart Study. Does Coffee Raise Serum Cholesterol?" *New England Journal of Medicine*, 1983, 308, 1454–1457.

Treanor, J. J., and others. "Efficacy and Safety of the Oral Neuraminidase Inhibitor Oseltamivir in Treating Acute Influenza." *Journal of the American Medical Association*, 2000, 283, 1016–1024.

U.S. Bureau of the Census. *Current Population Reports. Money Income in the United States: 1998*. Washington, D.C.: Government Printing Office, 1999.

Urgert, R., and others. "Comparison of Effect of Cafetiere and Filtered Coffee on Serum Concentrations of Liver Aminotransferases and Lipids: Six Month Randomised Controlled Trial." *British Medical Journal*, 1996, 313, 1362–1366.

Wennberg, J., and Gittelsohn A. "Variations in Medical Care Among Small Areas." *Scientific American*, 1982, 246, 120–134.

Wilde, J. A., and others. "Effectiveness of Influenza Vaccine in Health Care Professionals." *Journal of the American Medical Association*, 1999, 281, 908–913.

World Health Organization. World Health Report 2000. [http://www.who.int/whr/]. May 2001.

Wynn, M., and Wynn, A. "Fortification of Grain Products with Folate: Should Britain Follow the American Example?" *Nutrition and Health*, 1998, 12, 147–161.

THE AUTHOR

Peter Muennig is the director of the Program in Cost-Effectiveness and Outcomes at the Robert J. Milano Graduate School of Management and Urban Policy at New School University, where he teaches courses in cost-effectiveness, decision analysis, and epidemiology. He attended medical school at the University of California San Diego and completed a public health residency at the New York City Department of Health/Columbia University residency program. While still a resident, he published a seminal study on the cost-effectiveness of strategies to prevent parasitic infections in immigrants.

Dr. Muennig has worked as a cost-effectiveness consultant for the Centers for Disease Control and Prevention (CDC), Health Canada, and for various medical schools. He has published numerous studies in the medical literature and has contributed to textbooks and governmental reports. In addition to cost-effectiveness research, Dr. Muennig is interested in immigrant health and socioeconomic disparities.

INDEX